ATLAS OF

Clinical Urology

ATLAS OF
Clinical Urology

VOLUME III

The Kidneys and Adrenals

VOLUME EDITORS

CANCEROUS DISEASE SECTION

Andrew C. Novick, MD
Chairman, Urological Institute
The Cleveland Clinic Foundation
Cleveland, Ohio

NONCANCEROUS DISEASE SECTION

Michael Marberger, MD
Professor and Chairman
Department of Urology
University of Vienna
Vienna, Austria

SERIES EDITORS

E. Darracott Vaughan, Jr., MD
James J. Colt Professor of Urology
Chairman, Department of Urology
Weill Medical College of Cornell University
New York, New York

Aaron P. Perlmutter, MD, PhD
Director, Brady Prostate Center
Weill Medical College of Cornell University
New York, New York

With 28 Contributors

Developed by Current Medicine, Inc., Philadelphia

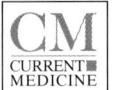

Current Medicine, Inc.

CM
CURRENT
MEDICINE
400 Market Street
Suite 700
Philadelphia, PA 19106

Managing Editor	Charles Field
Books Supervisor	Fran Klass
Commissioning Supervisor	Nicole Garron
Senior Developmental Editor	Marian A. Bellus
Editorial Assistant	Annmarie D'Ortona
Art Director	Wendy Vetter
Design and Layout	Christine Keller-Quirk
Illustration Director	Ann Saydlowski
Illustrators	Larry Ward, Ann Saydlowski
Cover Design	Jerilyn Bockorick
Cover Illustration	Debra Wertz, Wiesia Langenfeld
Production Director	Lori Holland
Assistant Production Manager	Simon Dickey
Indexing	Alexandra Nickerson

Library of Congress Cataloging-in-Publication Data

Atlas of clinical urology / series editors, E. Darracott Vaughan, Jr.,
Aaron J. Perlmutter.
        v. <1-2   >: ill. (some col.) ; 32 cm.
    Includes bibliographical references and index.
    Contents: v. 1. Impotence and infertility -- v. 2. The prostate.
    ISBN 1-57340-119-6 (v. 1)
    ISBN 1-57340-123-4 (v. 2)
    ISBN 1-57340-122-6 (v. 3)
    1. Urology--Atlases.
    [DNLM: 1. Urologic Diseases--atlases. WJ17 A8615 1999] I. Vaughan,
E. Darracott, 1939- II. Perlmutter, Aaron J., 1955-
    RC872 .A87 1999
    616.6--dc21

                         98-043304

For more information please call 1-800-427-1796 or email us at inquiry@phl.cursci.com
www.current-science-group.com

ISBN 1-57340-122-6

Printed in Singapore by Imago
10 9 8 7 6 5 4 3 2 1

SERIES PREFACE

As urology enters the 21st century, it is appropriate that the *Atlas of Clinical Urology* series captures and explains the major areas of modern urologic practice using a unique combination of images, schematics, tables, and algorithms. It does so in a compelling fashion, by combining a multilevel approach that includes the individual volumes and the internet. Urology is a specialty of great breadth, and visual images provide much of the backbone of urologic diagnosis and endoscopy and are key to surgical technique. The increasingly complex diagnostic and treatment paths are best depicted and understood as visual algorithms.

The editors of this five-volume series have not only contributed their world-renowned expertise to the chapters but have also assembled an outstanding group of individual chapter authors. Together, they provide each volume with completeness, depth, and—most important in this age of rapidly expanding science and technology—*current* urologic thinking.

In Volume I, Tom Lue and his contributors cover the expanding area of impotence from anatomic considerations through many of the new treatment modalities. As our population ages, urologists are evaluating and treating an expanding number of impotent patients. This section provides an excellent understanding and practical approach. In the second half of Volume I, Marc Goldstein and his expert colleagues provide a beautiful series of images that depict the important aspects of reproductive anatomy and endocrinology, as well as detailed surgical schematics demonstrating their ever-evolving "standard" surgery for infertility in addition to new assisted-reproduction techniques.

It would be fair to say that the 1990s are the decade of the prostate, and Volume II captures the paradigm changes that occurred in the management of both prostate cancer and benign disease. Management of prostate cancer is challenging, and the section by Peter Scardino provides a clear, concise, factual background for understanding the new treatment modalities available for benign prostatic hyperplasia (BPH). The choices of pharmacologic management and device therapies continue to challenge even the most seasoned urologist, and the diagnostic and treatment schematics provided in the section have been constructed by leaders in the field.

Renal carcinoma is covered in Volume III by section editor Andrew Novick. Radiologic images play an increasing role in our diagnosis and management of renal cancer, and the visual image format of the Atlas is ideal. The challenges of nephron sparing and vena caval surgery are clearly illustrated and are combined with an understanding of the appropriate patient populations for these procedures. This section also includes the management of benign and malignant adrenal disorders. Michael Marberger has assembled an extremely diverse and important set of noncancerous diseases of the kidney. Nephrolithiasis management is covered from medical therapy to endoscopy to incisional surgery. The important role that laparoscopy has established in both excisional and reconstructive renal surgery is visually depicted and explained. The evolution of the techniques illustrated in this section will likely provide the basis for renal intervention in the 21st century.

Volume IV covers the diversity of pediatric urology under the editorship of Dix Poppas and Alan Retik. This volume provides images illustrating the most important diseases that confront the pediatric urologist. In addition, the changes in management and thinking in classic conditions such as vesicoureteral reflux and neurogenic vesical dysfunction are illustrated. This volume will not only be of great value to the practicing pediatric urologist but also to general urologists as well as pediatricians and pediatric nephrologists.

Bladder diseases cause many patients to seek urologic care. In Volume V, Donald Skinner and John Stein have assembled state-of-the-art contributions in the management of bladder and urethra cancer. The combination of a better understanding of bladder cancer and new options in surgical urinary diversions is changing the management of bladder cancer. The role of surgery and surgical approaches to bladder cancer are illustrated in this volume by the innovative surgeons who contributed chapters to the section. Voiding dysfunction and incontinence as well as inflammatory and infectious conditions of the bladder are covered by Alan Wein's section. The excellent contributions to this section provide an illustrated understanding of the neuromuscular function of the lower urinary tract, and the images reproduced in this volume allow an easy understanding of the diagnosis and management of incontinence, inflammatory conditions, and fistulae.

These section editors and authors deserve tremendous credit for this *Atlas of Clinical Urology*, which was initiated by Abe Kreiger, President of Current Medicine. We thank Abe, the developmental editors, and the excellent illustrators of Current Medicine for their outstanding efforts.

E. Darracott Vaughan, Jr.
Aaron P. Perlmutter

CONTRIBUTORS

Demetrius H. Bagley, MD
Professor
Department of Urology and Radiology
Jefferson Medical College;
Jefferson Urology Associates
Philadelphia, Pennsylvania

Ronald M. Bukowski, MD
Director
Experimental Therapeutics Program
Cleveland Clinic Cancer Center
Cleveland, Ohio

Steven C. Campbell, MD, PhD
Assistant Professor
Department of Urology
Northwestern University Medical School
Chicago, Illinois

John W. Dushinski, BSC, MD, FRCSC
Clinical Assistant Professor
Department of Surgery
University of Calgary
Calgary, Alberta, Canada

Hamdy El-Kappany, MD
Professor
Department of Urology
Mansoura Medical College;
Urology and Nephrology Center
Mansoura, Egypt

Ibrahiem Eraky, MD
Associate Professor
Department of Urology
Mansoura Medical College;
Urology and Nephrology Center
Mansoura, Egypt

Robert C. Flanigan, MD
Albert J., Jr., and Claire R. Speh Professor and Chairman
Department of Urology
Loyola University
Maywood, Illinois;
Chief Urologist
Hines VA Hospital
Hines, Illinois

Mohamed A. Ghoneim, MB, BCH, MCH, MD
Professor and Chairman
Department of Urology
University of Mansoura
Mansoura, Egypt

Clemens Hammer, MD
Department of Urology
Rudolfstiftung
Vienna, Austria

Frederick L. Hoff, MD
Assistant Professor
Department of Radiology
Northwestern University School of Medicine;
Medical Director, Computed Tomography
Northwestern Memorial Hospital
Chicago, Illinois

Günter Janetschek, MD
Professor
Department of Urology
University of Vienna School of Medicine
Vienna, Austria

Francis X. Keeley, Jr., MD, FRCS
Consultant Urologist
Bristol Urological Institute
Southmead Hospital
Bristol, UK

Fernando J. Kim, MD
Chief Resident
Department of Urology
Loyola University Medical School;
Loyola University Medical Center
Maywood, Illinois

W. Marston Linehan, MD
Chief
Urocologic Oncology Branch
National Cancer Institute
Bethesda, Maryland

James E. Lingeman, MD
Clinical Professor
Department of Urology
Indiana University School of Medicine;
Director of Research
Methodist Hospital Institute for Kidney Stone Disease
Indianapolis, Indiana

Michael Marberger, MD
Professor and Chairman
Department of Urology
University of Vienna
Vienna, Austria

Fray F. Marshall, MD
Department of Urology
Emory University
Atlanta, Georgia

Villis R. Marshall, MB, BS, MD, FRACS
Professor and Chairman
Department of Surgery
The Flinders Institute;
Chairman
Surgical and Specialty Services Division, Flinders Medical Centre, Bedford Park
Adelaide, South Australia

James E. Montie, MD
Professor
Departments of Surgery and Urology
Head
Section of Urology
The University of Michigan
Ann Arbor, Michigan

Andrew C. Novick, MD
Chairman
Urological Institute
Cleveland Clinic Foundation
Cleveland, Ohio

Thomas J. Polascik, MD
Assistant Professor
Division of Urologic Surgery
Duke University Medical Center
Durham, North Carolina

Massimo Perachino, MD
Department of Urology
Santi Antonio E. Biagio Hospital
Alessandria, Italy

Paolo Puppo, MD
Professor
Department of Urology
Trieste Medical School;
Chief of Urology Unit
Galliera Hospital
Genoa, Italy

Silas Pettersson, MD, PhD
Emeritus Professor
Department of Urology
University of Göteborg;
Sahlgrenska University Hospital
Göteborg, Sweden

Norm D. Smith, MD
Chief Resident
Department of Urology
Northwestern University School of Medicine
Chicago, Illinois

Walter Stackl, MD
Professor
Department of Urology
Vienna Medical School;
Chairman
Ludwig Boltzmann Institute/Rudolfstiftung
Vienna, Austria

David A. Tolley, MD, FRCS, FRCSE
Honorary Senior Lecturer
Department of Surgery
Edinburgh Medical School;
Director
The Scottish Lithotriptor Center
Western General Hospital
Edinburgh, Scotland

Paul J. Van Cangh, MD
Professor
Department of Surgery
Universite Catholique de Louvain;
Chairman
Department of Urology
St. Luc University Hospital
Brussels, Belgium

J. Stuart Wolf, Jr., MD
Associate Professor of Surgery
Department of Surgery/Urology;
Director
Michigan Center for Minimally Invasive Urology
The University of Michigan
Ann Arbor, Michigan

CONTENTS

Section I — Cancerous Disease

Andrew C. Novick

Approximately 30,000 new cases of renal cell carcinoma (RCC) are detected annually in the United States, and this disease accounts for approximately 12,000 deaths per year. The number of cases of incidentally detected RCC is increasing as a result of the widespread use of noninvasive abdominal imaging modalities. A variety of renal imaging modalities are now available for diagnosis and clinical staging of patients with RCC. More efficient protocols for the evaluation of solid renal masses, complex renal cysts, and venous thrombi have evolved, and the indications for percutaneous renal biopsy have been refined.

In recent years there have been several important advances in our understanding of the biology and genetics of RCC that have had an impact on our evaluation and management of this disease. The von Hippel-Lindau tumor suppressor gene has been isolated and sequenced, and its role in both sporadic and familial forms of RCC has been defined. New pathology subtypes have been identified and characterized, and the histologic classification of RCC has been expanded to reflect these changes.

Significant progress has also occurred in the management of RCC. The indications for nephron-sparing surgery have expanded considerably, although not without some controversy. Expectant management of small, solid renal masses in select patients has been evaluated and placed into proper perspective. Modern cardiovascular surgical techniques have enhanced the safety and efficacy of operative therapy for patients with RCC involving the inferior vena cava. The promise and limitations of immunotherapy for the management of patients with metastatic disease have come into clearer focus. The combination of surgery and immunotherapy can extend survival for selected patients with RCC. The final chapter in this section reviews the contemporary evaluation and management of adrenal tumors, which is also relevant to the practicing urologic clinician.

This section of the *Atlas of Clinical Urology* relies heavily on radiographs, operative photographs, pathologic images, and tables to illustrate the most important aspects of kidney and adrenal tumors. These are further highlighted in the relatively brief accompanying text to provide a coherent view of each topic. Distinguished authors from several institutions have contributed generously of their knowledge and experience toward this volume. I am grateful for their efforts that blend together so well to enhance our understanding of this field.

The Radiologic Evaluation of Renal Masses

1

CANCEROUS DISEASE SECTION

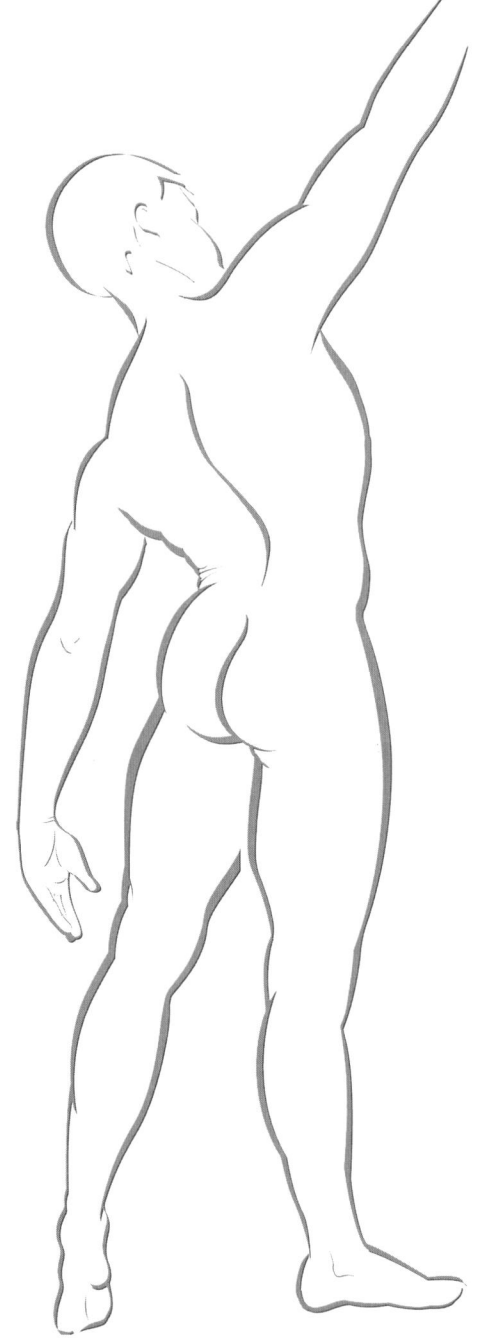

Norm D. Smith,
Frederick L. Hoff
Steven C. Campbell

The detection and evaluation of renal masses have changed significantly with improved radiographic techniques such as ultrasonography, CT, and magnetic resonance imaging (MRI). Historically, due to their retroperitoneal location, renal masses often remained clinically silent until large enough to cause local signs and symptoms, a frequent harbinger of advanced disease [1]. Currently, in an era of ubiquitous imaging with ultrasonography or CT for various complaints, incidental discovery by cross-sectional imaging with ultrasonography or CT has become the most common presentation of a renal mass [2–4]. Significantly, increased detection has led to diagnosis of renal cell carcinomas (RCCs) that are smaller and of a lower stage, with fewer patients presenting with metastatic disease [2,5–7]. Ultimately, serendipitous discovery of smaller lesions should correspond to improved cure rates and increased patient survival.

Each imaging modality commonly used to evaluate renal masses or their symptom complexes renders distinct advantages or disadvantages. Intelligent use of the various studies is necessary to maximize diagnostic yield, particularly in this cost-conscious era. This is clearly still a field in evolution, because many traditional techniques such as intravenous urography (IVU), angiography, and percutaneous renal biopsy have been replaced by more sensitive and discriminating noninvasive studies.

Intravenous urography with nephrotomography has traditionally been the cornerstone of urinary tract imaging. IVU provides physiologic information regarding uptake and excretion of contrast by the kidneys, as well as anatomic detail of the renal parenchyma, pelvocalyceal system, ureters, and bladder. Indications for IVU have lessened with the advent of more sophisticated technologies such as ultrasonography, CT, and MRI. However, IVU reserves a prominent role in uroradiology and remains the gold standard for initial assessment of suspected structural abnormalities, infection, urolithiasis, and hematuria [8]. Because hematuria is the presenting sign in many patients with RCC [1], IVU will continue to play a significant role in evaluation of renal masses.

If a renal mass is suspected on IVU, ultrasonography is frequently used next for imaging because it is noninvasive and readily available in most hospitals. The main value of renal ultrasonography is the characterization of cystic lesions and their differentiation from solid masses. Ultrasonography can detect cystic lesions less than 1.0 cm and solid renal masses greater than 1.0 to 2.0 cm in diameter [9,10]. The majority of renal masses identified on IVU are simple cysts, for which ultrasonography is quite accurate in diagnosis. A complex cyst or solid mass on ultrasonography mandates further evaluation with CT.

CT remains the gold standard for the diagnosis and staging of RCC, the characterization of complex cystic lesions, and the diagnosis of benign masses such as AML and inflammatory renal lesions. Fat density on CT is virtually diagnostic of AML, and in the absence of calcification excludes RCC from consideration [11,12]. In contrast, CT findings for oncocytoma are nonspecific; this lesion cannot be reliably differentiated from RCC preoperatively. The diagnosis of inflammatory masses such as acute diffuse or focal pyelonephritis, abscess, or xanthogranulomatous pyelonephritis is commonly made by clinical presentation and characteristic CT findings. Precontrast and postcontrast scans are crucial for an optimal examination. Noncontrast CT delineates high-density cysts or cystic carcinomas often misconstrued as simple cysts with postcontrast films only [13]. Intravenous contrast enhances characterization of renal masses, allows differentiation of lymphadenopathy from vascular structures, and optimizes assessment of renal vein or caval involvement by RCC.

Spiral CT virtually eliminates respiratory misregistration and minimizes partial volume averaging by continuous acquisition of contiguous images [3,14]. Spiral CT therefore has distinct advantages in the appraisal of renal masses smaller than 3.0 cm [14–17]. Further refinements of spiral CT with multiphasic scanning are even more sensitive for detecting small renal lesions, but routine use of this technology remains controversial [17,18]. Newer applications of helical CT, such as three-dimensional reconstruction of renal tumors, hold considerable promise as an adjunct to partial nephrectomy [19].

At present, the role of MRI in the evaluation of renal masses is relegated to diagnosis or staging that remains equivocal despite imaging with ultrasonography or CT [3,20,21]. Still, the capacity of MRI to appraise renal lesions is expanding with advances in technique, such as fat saturation sequences, fast spin echo, gradient-echo acquisition, and enhancement with gadolinium [21]. MRI is superior to CT and ultrasonography in staging venous involvement by RCC [3,22] and is at least as accurate as venacavography [23]. Moreover, MRI is often chosen over venacavography in staging IVC tumor thrombus because it is noninvasive, does not require intravenous contrast, and provides information about both the caudad and the cephalad extent of thrombus [21]. The development of paramagnetic contrast was a major advance in the MRI examination of renal masses, because gadolinium enhancement could then be used to discriminate cystic from solid masses, similar to a contrast-enhanced CT [3]. In addition, gadolinium-DTPA (diethylenctriaminepenta-acetic acid) has markedly fewer hypersensitivity reactions and no nephrotoxic side effects, thus making gadolinium-enhanced MRI the diagnostic test of choice for indeterminate renal lesions in patients with previous allergy to iodinated contrast [20] or with renal insufficiency [24,25]. Besides gadolinium enhancement, improved technology such as fat-suppressed spin echo and FLASH (fast low-angled shot) sequences yield similar results to those of CT for characterizing renal masses [26,27]. Despite the tremendous potential of MRI, CT remains the gold standard in characterizing renal lesions because of greater resolution, more widespread availability, and decreased cost. MRI may be advantageous for the diagnosis of cystic RCC with hemorrhage [28] and for identification of bone metastases or direct organ invasion seen with large, advanced carcinomas [20,29,30].

With highly sensitive noninvasive imaging such as ultrasonography, CT, and MRI, angiography and percutaneous renal biopsy are seldom used in evaluating renal masses. Angiography is still valuable in selected cases, including patients with RCC and severe hypertension, vascular disease, or other findings suggestive of concomitant renal artery disease [31–33]. Arteriography is also useful in ruling out a purely vascular lesion such as an arteriovenous malformation, which can mimic RCC [34]. Similarly, angiography remains important for vascular mapping for planned nephron-sparing surgery. Current indications for percutaneous renal biopsy are also limited, reserved primarily for patients suspected of having metastatic disease, abscess, or renal lymphoma.

The role of nuclear scanning in the assessment of renal lesions has also diminished. Infrequently, a contour abnormality detected on IVU is not confirmed with ultrasonography, raising suspicion for an isoechoic renal mass or pseudotumor such as persistent fetal lobulations, dromedary hump, or hypertrophied column of Bertin. Historically, ^{99m}Tc-DMSA (dimercaptosuccinic acid) renal scans were performed in this setting because the normal parenchyma of a pseudotumor concentrates radionuclide, whereas a renal cyst or tumor remains a photopenic defect [35,36]. Contrast-enhanced CT also distinguishes pseudotumor from RCC or cystic lesions and is currently the test of choice to rule out pseudotumor [37]. Nuclear studies are perhaps most useful for evaluating differential function in planning radical versus partial nephrectomy in patients with renal insufficiency.

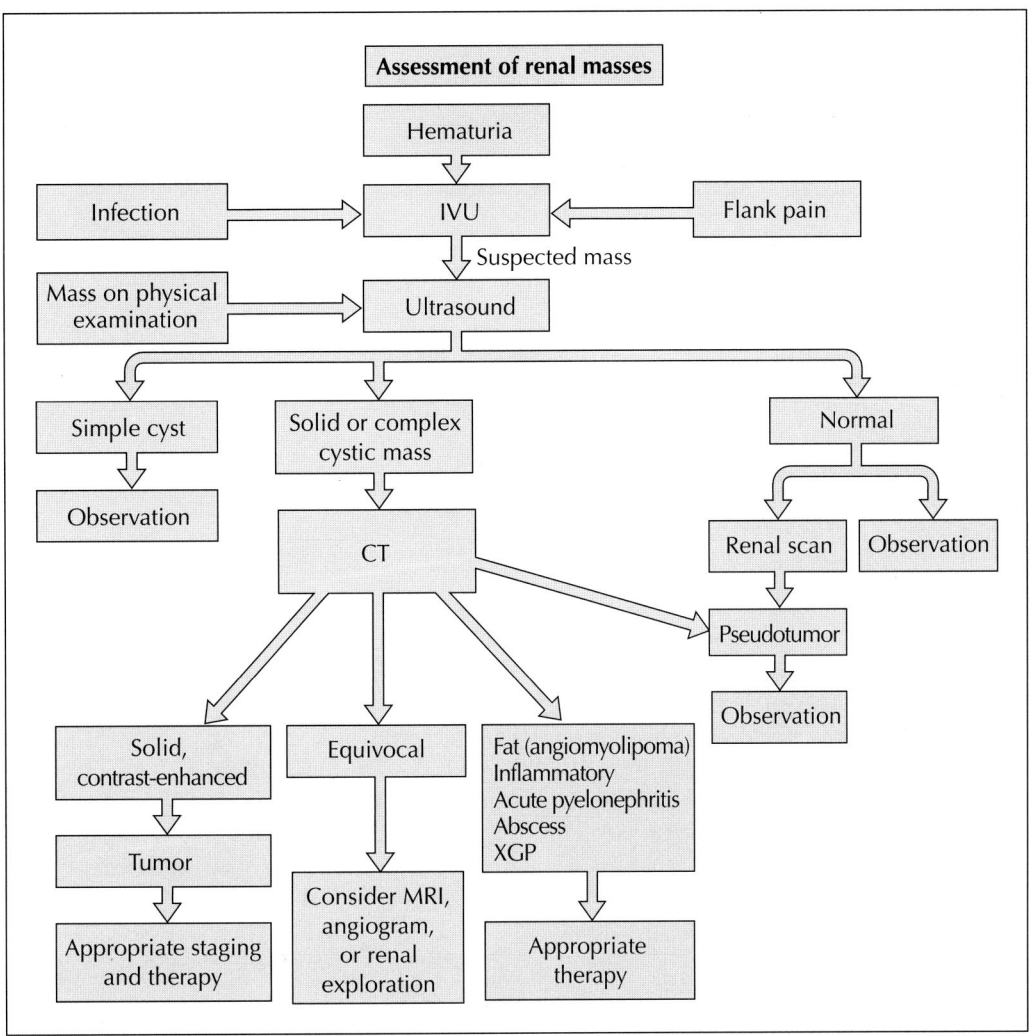

Assessment of renal masses

Hematuria → IVU

Infection → IVU ← Flank pain

IVU → Suspected mass → Ultrasound

Mass on physical examination → Ultrasound

Ultrasound → Simple cyst → Observation

Ultrasound → Solid or complex cystic mass → CT

Ultrasound → Normal → Renal scan, Observation

Renal scan → Pseudotumor → Observation

CT → Pseudotumor

CT → Solid, contrast-enhanced → Tumor → Appropriate staging and therapy

CT → Equivocal → Consider MRI, angiogram, or renal exploration

CT → Fat (angiomyolipoma) / Inflammatory / Acute pyelonephritis / Abscess / XGP → Appropriate therapy

▶ **FIGURE 1-1.** Algorithm for the assessment of renal masses. Renal cell carcinoma (RCC) may present in myriad ways. The classic triad of flank pain, abdominal or flank mass, and hematuria was considered pathonomic for RCC, but only a minority of patients now present with these findings, mostly those with advanced disease. Hematuria was previously the most common presentation, occurring in approximately 60% of patients [1]. The initial radiographic study for evaluation of hematuria remains intravenous urography (IVU) with nephrotomography because it provides functional information as well as visualization of the renal parenchyma, collecting system, and bladder. Still, the IVU is inferior to other modalities (ultrasonography, CT, and magnetic resonance imaging [MRI]) for identification of parenchymal lesions [3,5,6]; a reasonable alternative in high-risk patients with gross hematuria is to combine ultrasonography with cystoscopy and retrograde pyelography. If a renal mass is suspected on either physical examination or IVU, ultrasonography is then considered to determine whether the mass is solid or cystic. The majority of masses on IVU are benign cysts [1]; only lesions failing to meet ultrasonographic criteria for simple cysts require further evaluation. Solid, complex cystic, or indeterminate masses on ultrasonography need further evaluation with CT for characterization, diagnosis, and staging. MRI is valuable when explicit diagnosis or accurate staging remains in question. Angiography, renal scan, and percutaneous renal biopsy are also useful in selected circumstances. When the lesion remains indeterminate after fastidious evaluation, surgical exploration may be required to provide definitive diagnosis [36,37]. XGP—xanthogranulomatous pyelonephritis.

Differential Diagnosis of Renal Masses

Benign renal tumors
Angiomyolipoma
Oncocytoma
Adenoma
Fibroma
Leiomyoma
Hemangioma
Lipoma
Juxtaglomerular tumors
Primary malignant tumors
Renal cell carcinoma
Transitional cell carcinoma of the
  renal pelvis or calyces
Sarcoma
Primary renal lymphoma

Secondary malignant tumors
Hematogenous
  Lung cancer
  Breast cancer
  Gastrointestinal malignancy
  Malignant melanoma
Direct invasion
  Retroperitoneal sarcoma
  Pancreatic cancer
  Colon cancer
Other
  Lymphoma
  Leukemia

Cystic disease
Simple cyst
Complex cyst
Hyperdense cyst
Multilocular cystic nephroma
Inflammatory renal masses
Acute diffuse or focal pyelonephritis
Renal abscess
Xanthogranulomatous pyelonephritis
Vascular mass
Arteriovenous malformation
Normal variants
Pseudotumor

▶ **FIGURE 1-2.** The differential diagnosis of renal masses is complex and includes benign and malignant neoplasms, cystic lesions, inflammatory masses, vascular lesions, and normal variants of parenchymal architecture. Angiomyolipoma is a benign tumor usually distinguished from renal cell carcinoma (RCC) by imaging, whereas a plethora of other benign neoplasms have mostly pathologic diagnoses [1,3,36,37]. Primary malignant renal tumors include RCC and transitional cell carcinoma (TCC) of the renal pelvis and calyces, as well as rare malignancies like sarcoma or primary renal lymphoma [1]. Lung cancer is the most common metastatic neoplasm of the kidney, with other hematogenous metastatic deposits (breast, gastrointestinal), direct extension from adjacent organs (colon, pancreas), leukemia, lymphoma, and retroperitoneal sarcoma accounting for most other secondary neoplasms [3,38]. Cystic lesions are assigned malignant risk based on specific CT criteria (Bosniak classification) [39]. Nevertheless, enough overlap is present between complex cystic lesions and RCC to raise questions in diagnosis often requiring surgical intervention. Inflammatory masses include acute focal or diffuse pyelonephritis, abscess, and xanthogranulomatous pyelonephritis; diagnoses are often based on characteristic clinical presentation and radiographic findings [3]. Arteriovenous malformations are reported to mimic RCC but can be differentiated by angiography [34]. Pseudotumors are normal variants of renal parenchymal structure that may present with abnormal renal contour suspicious for mass on IVU or US but are readily recognized as normal parenchyma on either contrast-enhanced CT scan or radionuclide imaging [3,35–37].

RENAL CELL CARCINOMA

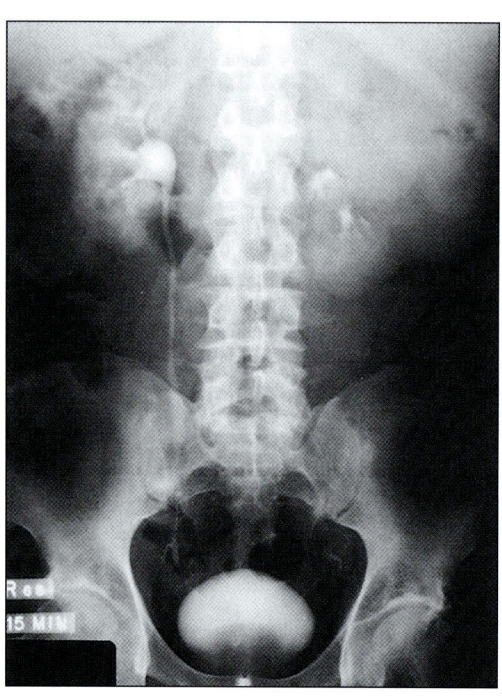

▶ **FIGURE 1-3.** Intravenous urography (IVU) study. Renal cell carcinoma (RCC) accounts for approximately 90% of all primary malignant renal neoplasms and in 1998 is estimated to be responsible for roughly 28,000 new cancer diagnoses and 11,000 cancer-related deaths in the United States alone [40]. IVU is often the initial diagnostic study because many patients present with hematuria [1]. This IVU study illustrates findings suspicious for RCC, including a large left renal mass with obliteration of calyceal architecture and grossly abnormal renal contour.

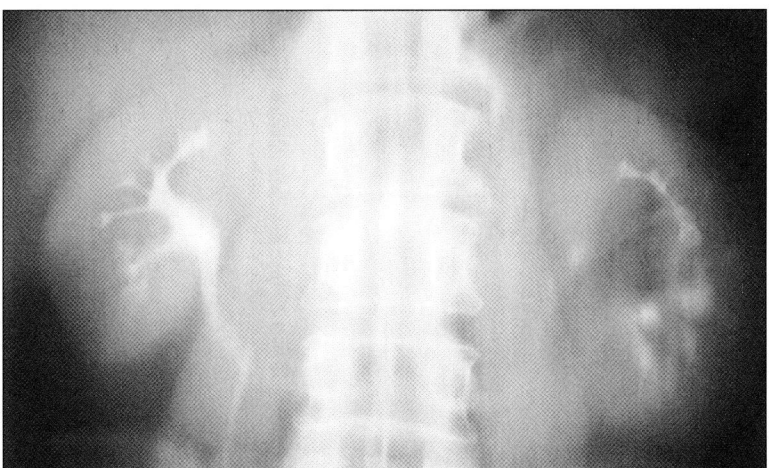

▶ **FIGURE 1-4.** Nephrotomogram of kidneys. Nephrotomography improves visualization of the collecting system and renal parenchyma by excluding structures not in the desired imaging plane [8]. This tomogram demonstrates displacement of the collecting system and subtle abnormality in the outline of the left kidney, which indicates a mass. Despite refinements such as tomography, intravenous urography (IVU) remains inferior to other modalities in assessing renal lesions [3,6,36]. IVU is especially poor in detecting small anterior or posterior masses that do not distort the renal contour or collecting system [5,6,36]. The suggestion of mass on IVU or nephrotomography demands further characterization with ultrasonography or CT.

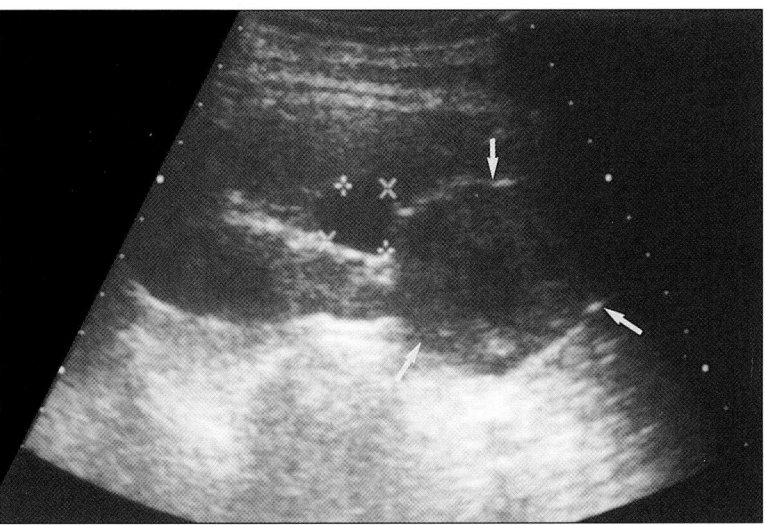

▶ **FIGURE 1-5.** Ultrasound image of kidneys. The diagnosis of renal cell carcinoma (RCC) is complicated due to the high prevalence of renal lesions, the vast majority of which are benign cysts. Autopsy series reveal that up to 50% of individuals over 50 years of age have renal cysts [3]. It is essential to distinguish benign cystic disease from RCC by radiologic rather than pathologic examination, but this can be difficult because of the heterogeneous appearance of both benign and malignant lesions. This ultrasonographic image demonstrates a simple cyst and solid mass (*arrows*) in the same kidney.

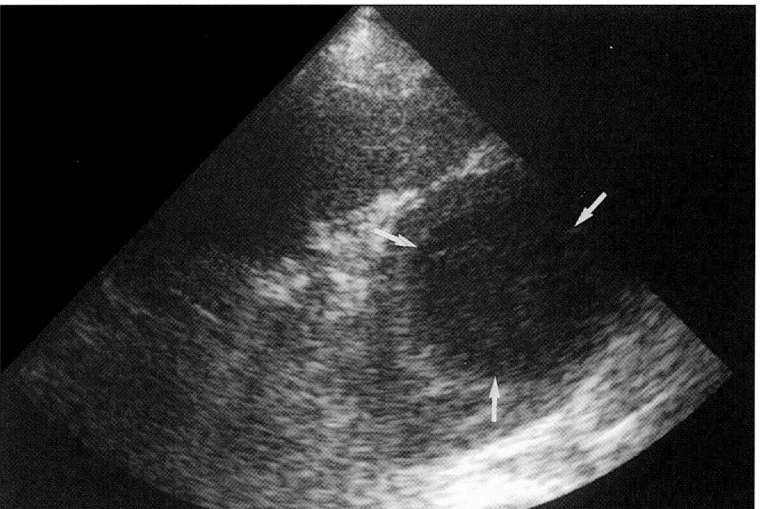

▶ **FIGURE 1-6.** Renal ultrasonogram. The ultrasonographic characteristics of a solid renal mass include acoustic impedance, heterogeneous shape with indiscriminate borders and the presence of internal echoes [9,10]. This renal ultrasonograph image illustrates a large solid mass (*arrows*) with a thickened wall, ill-defined borders, and multiple internal echoes. Ultrasonography often cannot distinguish benign solid lesions from renal cell carcinoma; a solid mass on ultrasonography requires further characterization and staging with CT.

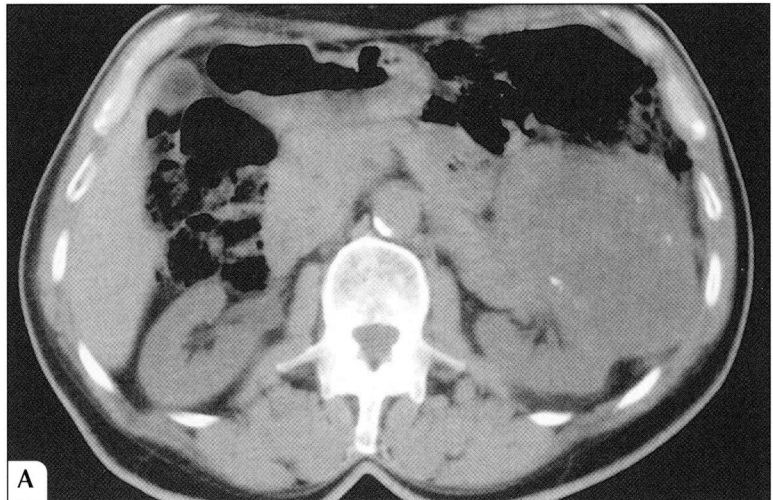

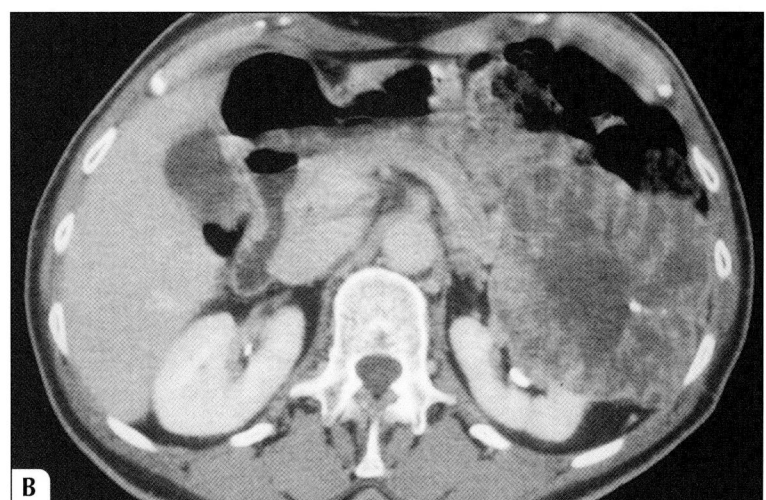

▶ **FIGURE 1-7.** Computed tomographic images of renal cell carcinoma (RCC). CT characteristics of RCC are diverse, including solid mass with contrast enhancement, speckled or irregular calcifications, asymmetric margins with a thick or nodular wall, hypervascularity, hemorrhage, and necrosis [3,36]. **A,** Nonenhanced CT scan of the abdomen with a heterogeneous left renal mass with irregular shape and non–border-forming calcifications. **B,** Postcontrast film of the same tumor showing obvious contrast enhancement and central necrosis, consistent with RCC.

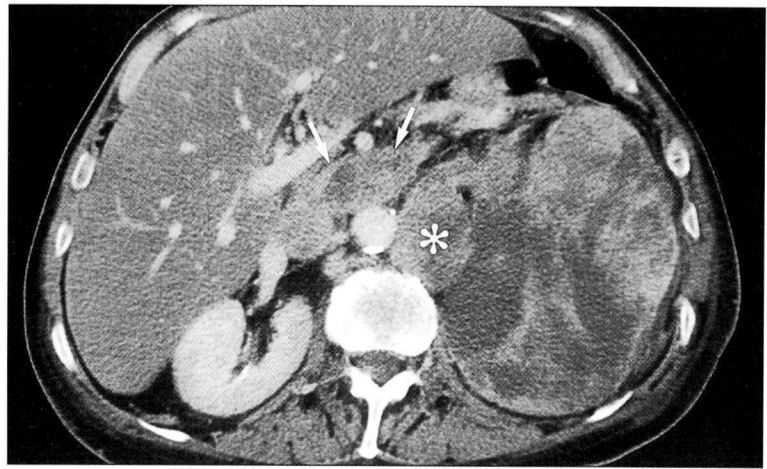 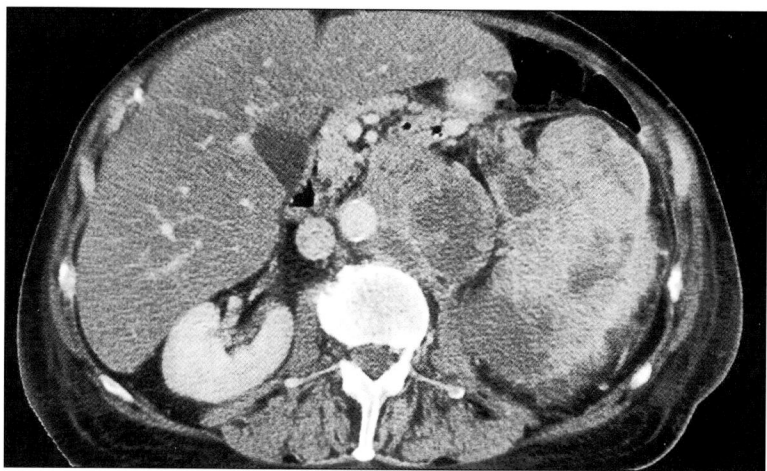

▶ **FIGURE 1-8.** Computed tomographic image of renal cell carcinoma (RCC). Not only is CT imaging important in the diagnosis of renal cell carcinoma (RCC), it is critical for staging as well. Overall, the accuracy of CT staging varies from 60% to 90% [41,42]. CT has particular difficulty with determination of perinephric tumor invasion, but this level of differentiation is often not clinically important because management is similar for stage T2 and T3a tumors. CT findings of venous involvement include filling defects or areas of decreased density, changes in intraluminal vein caliber, and venous enlargement [42]. This scan shows a large, variegated left renal tumor with para-aortic lymphadenopathy (*asterisk*), an enlarged left renal vein (*arrows*) displacing the superior mesenteric artery anteriorly, and apparent tumor involvement of the inferior vena cava. The accuracy of CT detection of renal vein and IVC tumor thrombus is 78% and 96%, respectively [42].

▶ **FIGURE 1-9.** Computed tomographic image of regional lymph node metastasis. Regional lymph node metastasis by renal cell carcinoma portends a dismal prognosis, with only approximately 10% survival at 5 years [1]. Lymph node involvement by tumor is suggested by enlarged nodes or by the clustering of several normal-sized nodes [41,42]. Lymph nodes greater than 2.0 cm in diameter usually contain metastatic disease [41]. Size criteria for lymph node involvement are uncertain, however, because enlargement to 1.0 to 2.0 cm may also be caused by reactive hyperplasia; surgical assessment is often required to discriminate. Further, micrometastatic deposits are not detected by any current imaging modality [41,42]. This CT scan reveals a huge, contrast-enhancing left renal tumor with massive retroperitoneal lymphadenopathy distinct from the primary tumor mass that displaces the aorta across the midline. Overall, staging of retroperitoneal lymph node metastases by CT has sensitivity and specificity exceeding 80% [41,42].

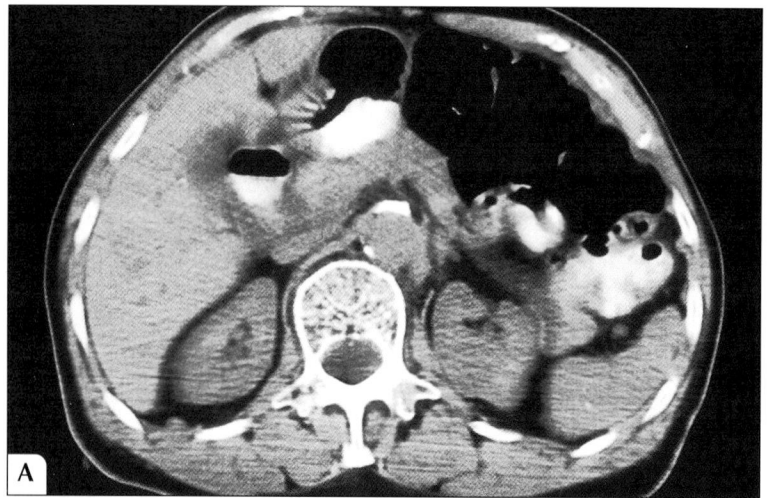 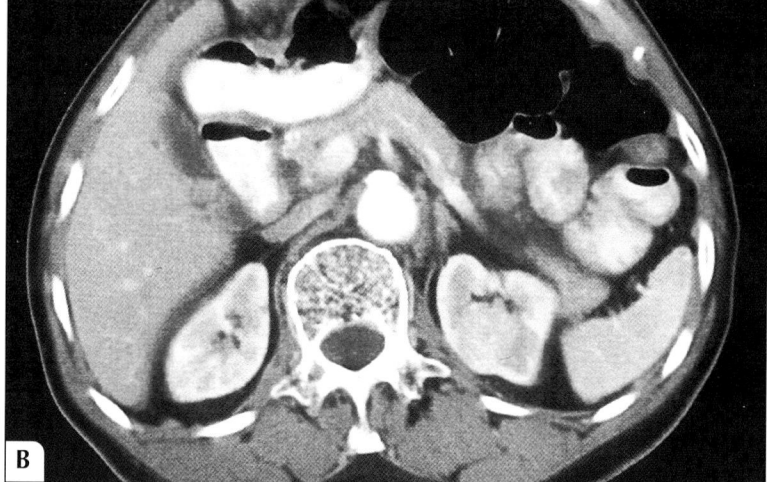

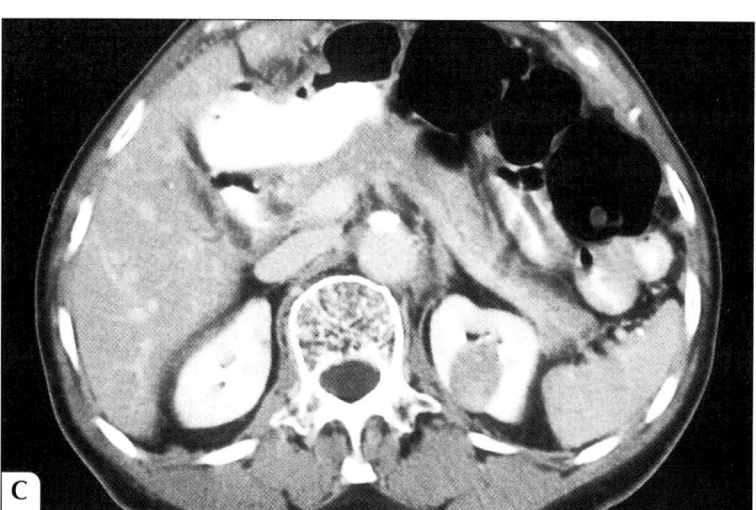

▶ **FIGURE 1-10.** Proper technique with 5- to 10-mm sections before and after administration of intravenous contrast is essential for optimal assessment of renal lesions, especially those smaller than 3.0 cm [3,17,18,42,43]. Technologic advances such as multiphasic helical CT improve imaging of small renal masses, with the nephrographic phase superior to the corticomedullary phase in detection of masses less than 3.0 cm [17,18]. **A,** Noncontrast CT scan reveals a subtle contour abnormality in the left kidney suspicious for mass; this could easily be overlooked. **B,** The same image during the corticomedullary phase, which is more suggestive of a solid renal mass. **C,** The nephrographic phase, which demonstrates an obvious solid tumor of the left kidney, with contrast enhancement and distortion of the collecting system. The corticomedullary phase has a higher incidence of both false-positive and false-negative results compared with the nephrographic phase due to lack of enhancement of the medulla [17]. Monophasic scanning with the nephrographic phase only or multiphasic helical imaging remain controversial because each technique has prominent strengths and weaknesses [18].

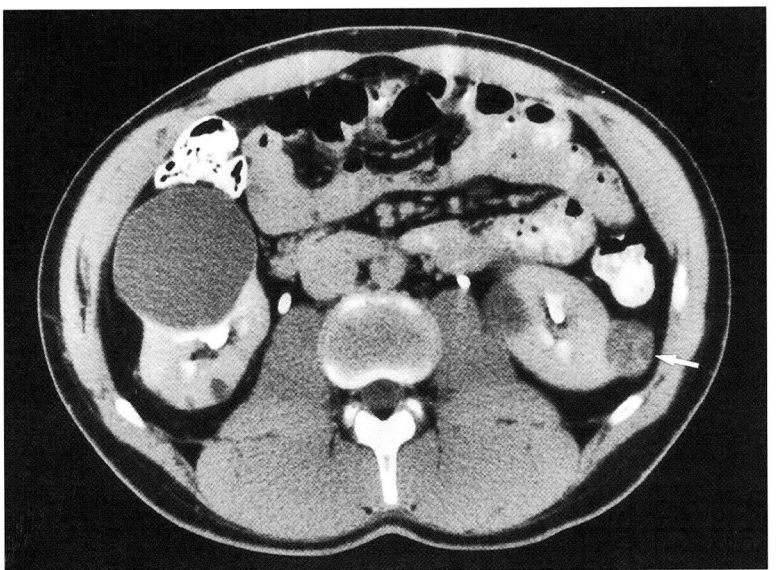

▶ **FIGURE 1-11.** Image of renal cyst. A familial form of renal cell carcinoma (RCC) characterized by genetic alterations on chromosome 3 is seen in patients with von Hippel-Lindau (VHL) syndrome. In addition to RCC, the spectrum of VHL syndrome includes a proclivity for renal cysts, pancreatic cysts and tumors, retinal hemangiomas, central nervous system hemangioblastomas, and pheochromocytoma [1]. RCC associated with VHL syndrome tends to be multifocal and bilateral, with presentation at an earlier age than sporadic RCC, all in accord with Knudson's hypothesis regarding cancer associated with mutation of a tumor suppressor gene. RCC occurs in roughly one half of patients with VHL syndrome [41]. CT is important in patients with VHL syndrome for assessment of renal cysts and of malignant risk, as well as for examination of potential pancreatic pathology. This scan reveals multiple bilateral renal cysts, the largest of which on the right is merely a simple cyst. However, the lateral aspect of the left kidney contains a solid, enhancing mass (*arrows*) highly suspicious for RCC. RCC with VHL syndrome is best treated with nephron-sparing surgery due to the propensity for multifocal and bilateral disease. Further, patients with VHL syndrome require lifelong interval screening with CT due to persistent risk of RCC [36].

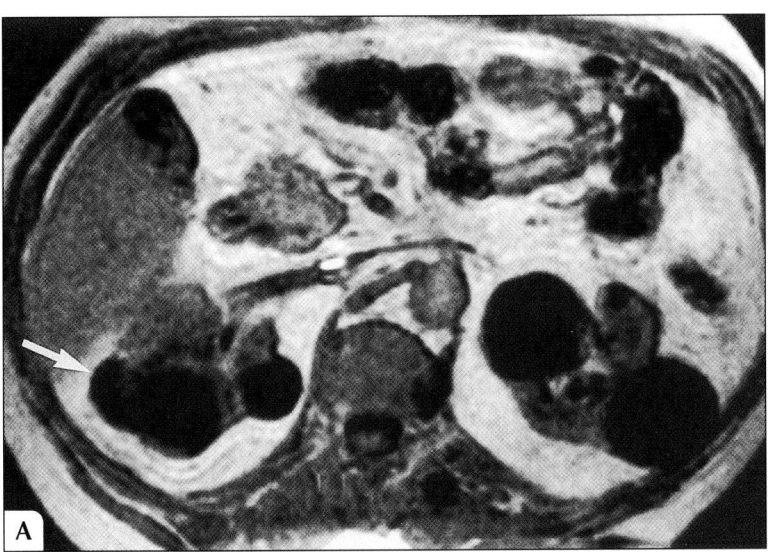

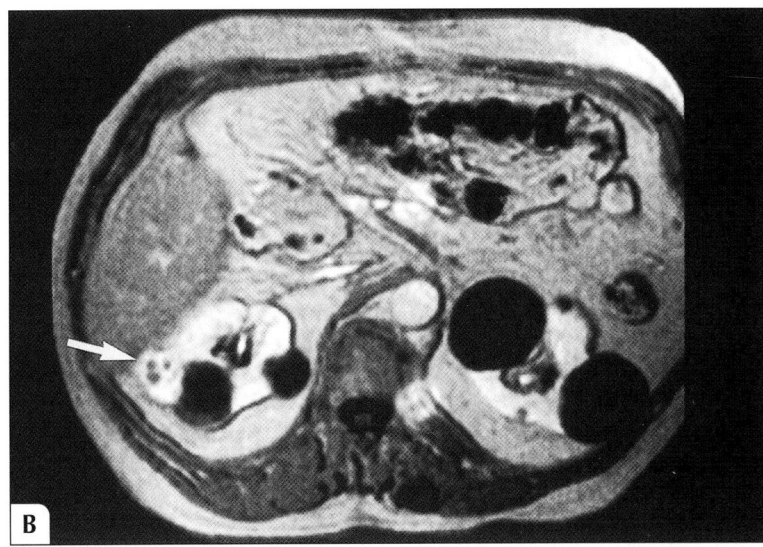

▶ **FIGURE 1-12.** Magnetic resonance images of renal lesions. Improvements in magnetic resonance imaging (MRI), including intravenous gadolinium and specialized pulse sequences such as fat suppression and breath-hold techniques, make MRI increasingly valuable in the appraisal of renal lesions, particularly those smaller than 3.0 cm [3,21,26,27,41–43]. Gadolinium was a major improvement in MRI; paramagnetic contrast enhancement is now used to differentiate cystic from solid masses, akin to contrast-enhanced CT [3,21]. In addition, gadolinium is not nephrotoxic and thus extremely beneficial in patients with renal insufficiency [24,25]. **A,** Axial T_1-weighted image without paramagnetic contrast in a diabetic patient with renal insufficiency who was found on ultrasonography to have a cystic mass in the right kidney. MRI shows that multiple cysts are present bilaterally, with debris or potentially solid components associated with the complex cyst on the right (*arrow*). **B,** The same image with gadolinium showing a complex cystic lesion on the lateral aspect of the right kidney with septae and unequivocal gadolinium enhancement, consistent with RCC (*arrow*).

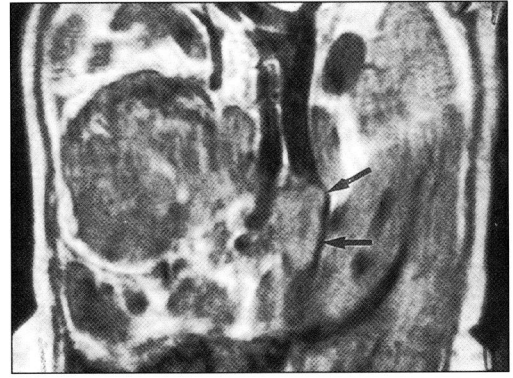

▶ **FIGURE 1-13.** Magnetic resonance image of renal masses. In the evaluation of renal masses, magnetic resonance imaging (MRI) serves most appropriately as an adjunct to CT when accurate diagnosis or staging remains in doubt [3,21,41,42]. Compared with CT, the staging advantages of MRI include superior definition of tissue planes and improved ability to detect local tumor extension and venous involvement [42]. MRI is especially useful for assessing tumor extension to the renal vein or inferior vena cava (IVC); it is superior to ultrasonography and CT and at least as sensitive as venacavography in detecting venous tumor thrombi [3,21,23]. MRI is also valuable in depicting the cephalad extent of caval thrombus in relation to the diaphragm, hepatic veins, and right atrium [41]. This T_1-weighted coronal image reveals a massive renal cell carcinoma of the left kidney with venous extension into the infrahepatic IVC (*arrows*). Invasion into the wall of the IVC is apparent, detected by MRI with an accuracy of roughly 60%. The overall staging accuracy of MRI ranges from 80% to 90%, with particularly high specificity (97%) for IVC involvement [42].

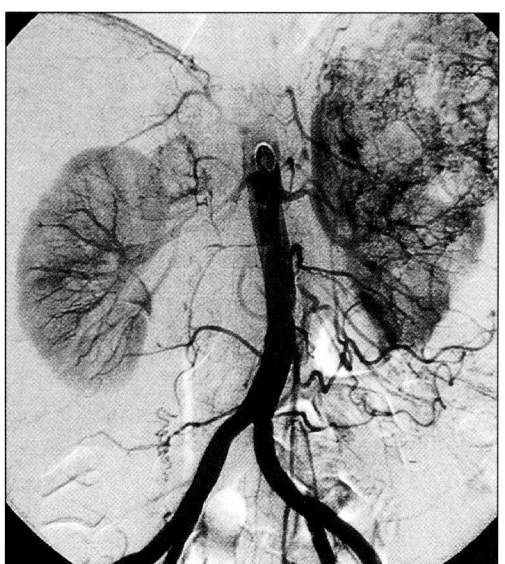

▶ **FIGURE 1-14.** Abdominal aortic arteriogram. Arteriography has only limited utility in the evaluation of renal cell carcinoma [3,13,37,41,42]; it is the most expensive and invasive of all modalities used in assessing renal masses and has been virtually replaced with accurate, noninvasive studies such as ultrasonography, CT, and magnetic resonance imaging [41,42]. This abdominal aortic arteriogram demonstrates classic tumor neovascularity of the left kidney with prominent venous pooling of contrast and arteriovenous shunting [13,41], as well as a contralateral adrenal metastasis.

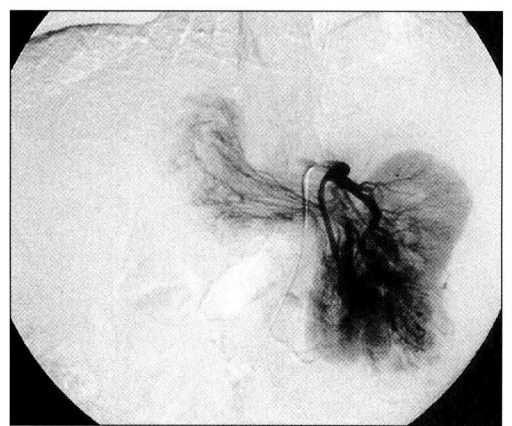

▶ **FIGURE 1-15.** Angiography in staging of renal cell carcinoma (RCC). Angiography is occasionally useful for staging RCC [13,41,42]. Arteriographic evidence of venous extension includes vascularization of the tumor thrombus itself or failure of the renal vein to opacify after injection of a sufficient amount of contrast into the renal artery [41,42]. This selective left renal arteriogram shows tumor hypervascularity, extreme venous blush, and prominent arteriovenous communications. Impressive neovascularity of the tumor thrombus in the left renal vein and inferior vena cava is indicative of venous involvement by RCC. The angiographic staging of RCC is poor, with overall accuracy ranging from 36% to 44% [42].

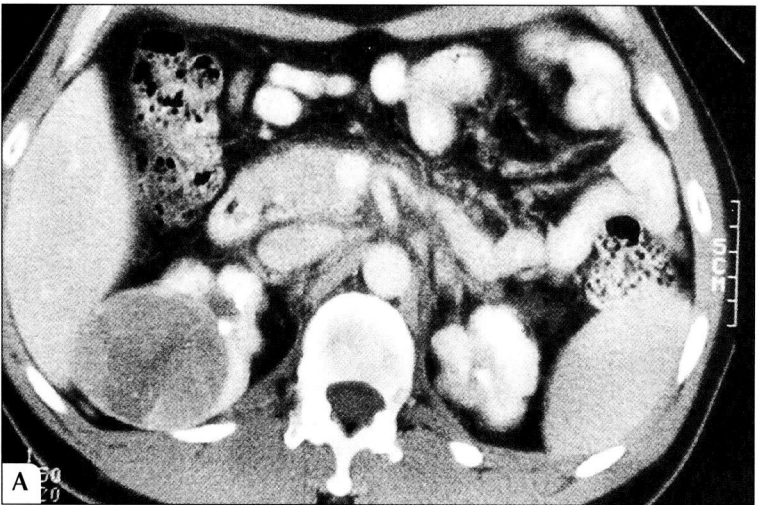

▶ **FIGURE 1-16.** Diagnostic angiography. Currently, the primary role of diagnostic angiography in patients with renal cell carcinoma (RCC) is that of vascular mapping prior to nephron-sparing surgery. Specific indications include bilateral RCC, tumors in patients with von Hippel-Lindau syndrome, RCC in a solitary or horseshoe kidney, and tumor embolization [41,42]. **A,** A well-circumscribed, enhancing right renal mass on CT, increased density in the retroperitoneum surrounding the aorta, inferior vena cava, and superior mesenteric artery, and scarring with parenchymal loss in the left kidney. Due to these findings and a history of lymphoma, the patient had angiography prior to planned open renal biopsy and possible partial nephrectomy. During the study, two renal arteries were discovered. **B,** Selective catheterization of the right upper pole renal artery outlining a relatively hypovascular tumor. **C,** Selective arteriography of the lower pole artery with normal vascular distribution and parenchyma. Open biopsy revealed RCC; partial nephrectomy was performed, with selective clamping of the upper pole renal artery.

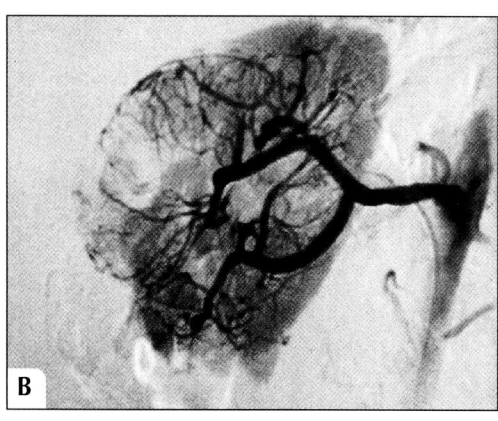

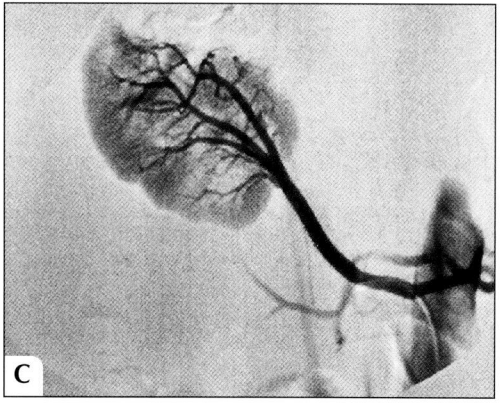

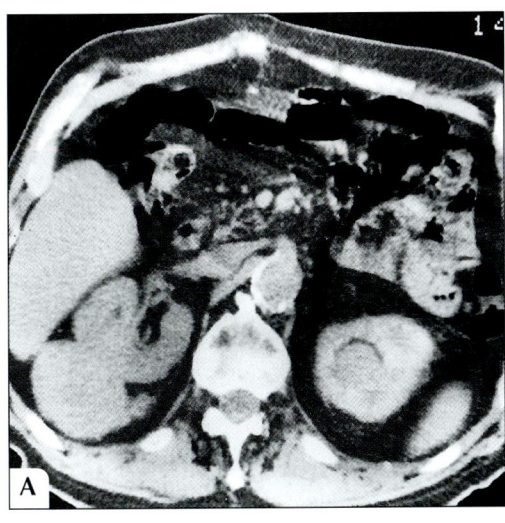

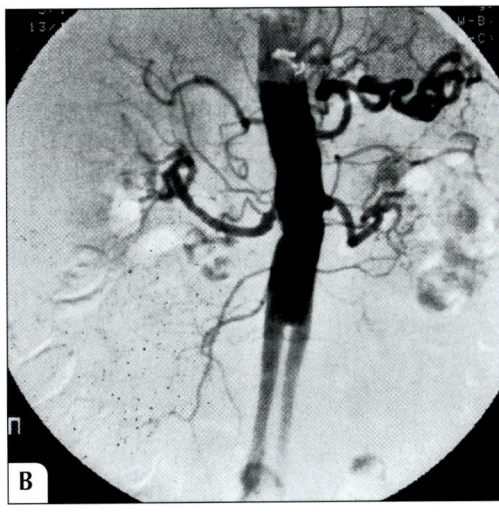

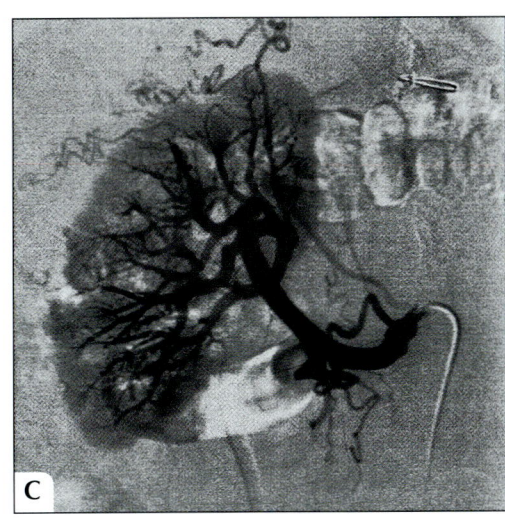

▶ **FIGURE 1-17.** Angiography in the evaluation of coexistent renal artery disease. Angiography is also beneficial for evaluating renal masses in patients with severe hypertension, vascular disease, or other history suggestive of coexistent renal artery disease [31–33]. **A,** Postcontrast CT scan in a patient with a history of hypertension, coronary artery disease, and previous abdominal aortic aneurysm repair who presented with left flank pain. Left hydronephrosis was diagnosed; the right kidney was incidentally found to have delayed enhancement and excretion of contrast, as well as an exophytic mass. Renal cell carcinoma (RCC) with concomitant renal artery stenosis was suspected. Further work-up of the left hydronephrosis revealed a distal ureteral stricture, presumably a sequelae of the patients prior abdominal surgery. **B,** Abdominal aortogram demonstrating renal artery stenosis at the origin of the right renal artery. **C,** Selective arteriography past the area of stenosis illustrating tumor neovascularity consistent with RCC. The preoperative serum creatinine level was 1.3 mg/dL. Renal scan demonstrated 63% function on the affected side; partial nephrectomy was subsequently performed. The postoperative creatinine level stabilized at 1.2 mg/dL.

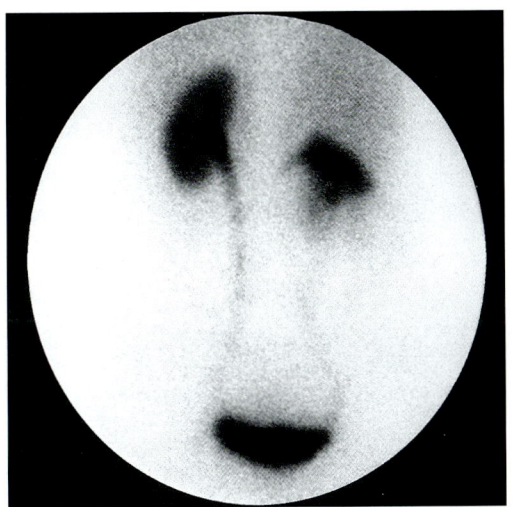

▶ **FIGURE 1-18.** Nuclear imaging for assessment of renal cell carcinoma (RCC). Nuclear imaging has a limited role for assessment of RCC and best serves to provide an estimate of differential function in patients with borderline renal reserve, which can be important for deciding partial versus radical nephrectomy. This renal scan shows a large right upper pole photopenic defect in a patient with RCC. However, this is a nonspecific finding because radionuclide imaging is unable to distinguish benign masses from cystic disease or RCC [35,36].

CYSTIC RENAL MASSES

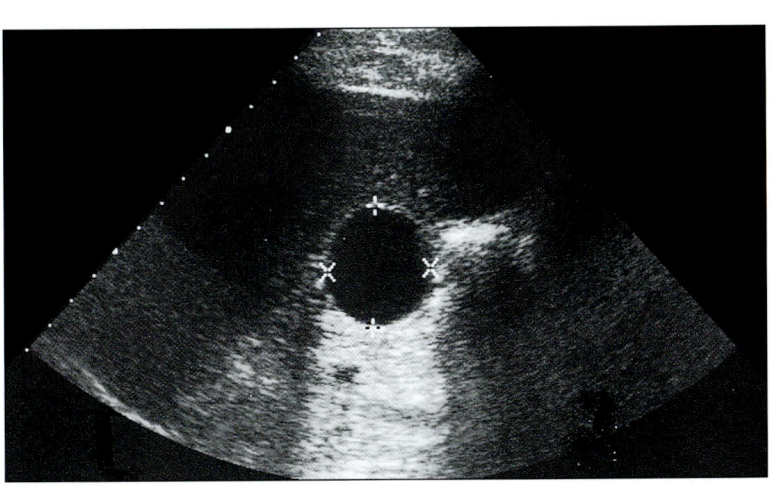

▶ **FIGURE 1-19.** Radiography of suspicious masses. The vast majority of renal cysts are incidentally discovered on abdominal imaging for unrelated reasons [39]. Simple cysts are the most common renal masses and must be differentiated from complex cystic lesions and solid masses by radiographic means to avoid unnecessary procedures. Lesions with a lack of internal echoes, good through transmission, and sharply marginated borders meet ultrasonographic criteria for simple cysts and require no further assessment [9,10].

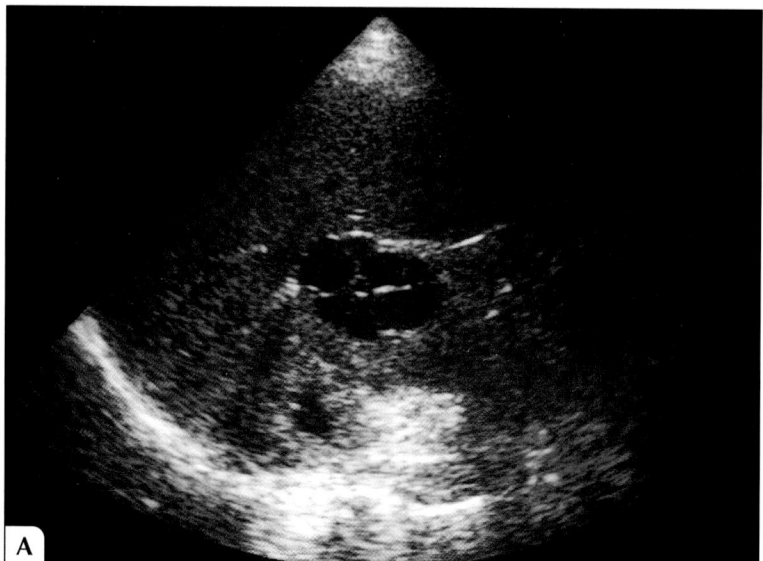

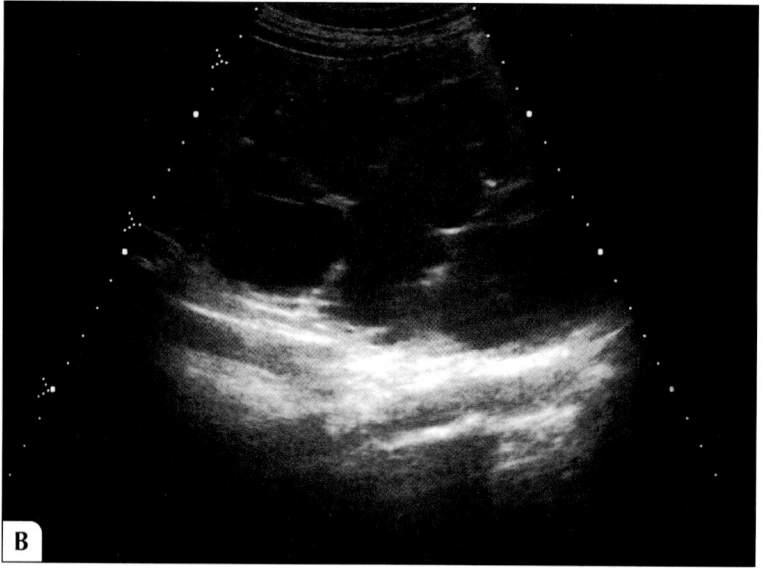

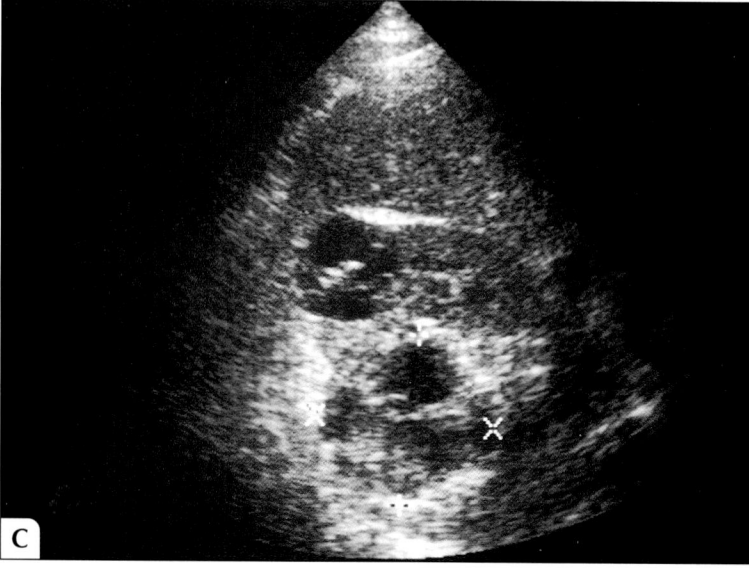

▶ FIGURE 1-20. Complex cystic lesions. On ultrasonography, complex cystic lesions are characterized by variability in shape, indistinct borders, the presence of septae or calcifications, and varying degrees of internal echoes [9,10]. **A,** A minimally complicated cyst with ovoid shape and thin, branching septae. **B,** A complex cystic lesion with irregular shape and multiple thick septae. **C,** A complex cystic lesion with a thickened wall and solid, nodular components. RT LONG—right longitudinal.

Bosniak Classification of Cystic Renal Masses

Bosniak Category	CT Characteristics	Malignant Risk	Management
1) Simple benign cysts	Uniform water density Low attenuation (0–20 Hounsfield units) Sharply marginated borders Smooth walls Absence of contrast-enhancement	None	Observation
2) Minimally complicated lesions	Thin septae Minimal or curvilinear calcification very low Hyperdense cysts	Very low	Observation
2F) Minimally complicated lesions: require follow-up	Unusual hyperdense cysts More calcium in cyst wall Slightly more complex lesions	Most likely benign	Interval follow-up imaging
3) Equivocal lesions: moderately complicated	Thick or irregular calcifications Dense or irregular calcifications Small, nonenhancing nodules	~50% Benign, 50% malignant	Exploration or biopsy, partial or radical nephrectomy as indicated
4) Cystic malignancy	Solid components Irregular margins Heterogeneous Presence of contrast-enhancement	Malignant	Partial or radical nephrectomy as indicated

Data from Bosniak [37,39,45]; Aronson, et al. [44].

▶ **FIGURE 1-21.** Bosniak classification of cystic renal masses. In an effort to accurately delineate malignant risk, the Bosniak classification of cystic renal masses categorizes cystic lesions based on CT findings [37,39,43–45]. Bosniak category 1 includes simple cysts with CT characteristics such as uniform water density (0–20 Hounsfield units [HU]), sharply defined borders with indiscernible walls, and absence of contrast enhancement. The presence of these strict criteria virtually excludes malignancy from consideration. Bosniak category 2 lesions contain thin, nonenhancing septae or linear, border-forming calcifications. Category 2 also includes the hyperdense cyst, which is homogeneously hyperdense (40–90 HU) on CT and almost always benign [45]. In fact, the vast majority of all category 2 lesions are benign, although there are certainly exceptions [3]. These exceptions have led to the development of Bosniak category 2F, or minimally complex cysts that require follow-up imaging due to more equivocal radiographic findings. Unfortunately, criteria for differentiation between category 2 and 2F lesions are not well defined. Bosniak category 3 includes suspicious lesions with thickened or complex septae and dense, irregular calcifications. The malignant risk of these lesions is indeterminate and they vary from complicated, multilocular cysts to multilocular cystic nephroma to cystic renal cell carcinoma (RCC). Category 3 lesions warrant surgical excision by either radical or partial nephrectomy because approximately 50% ultimately prove malignant [3]. Bosniak category 4 includes cystic masses with solid or nodular components; irregular, thick margins; or the presence of unequivocal contrast enhancement. These lesions are considered RCC until proven otherwise and are managed as such. Although the Bosniak classification is clinically useful in the radiologic evaluation of renal masses, more data about pathologic correlates of these lesions and improved techniques to better discriminate category 2 and 3 lesions are necessary. (*Data from* Bosniak [37,39], Aronson *et al.* [44], and Bosniak [45].)

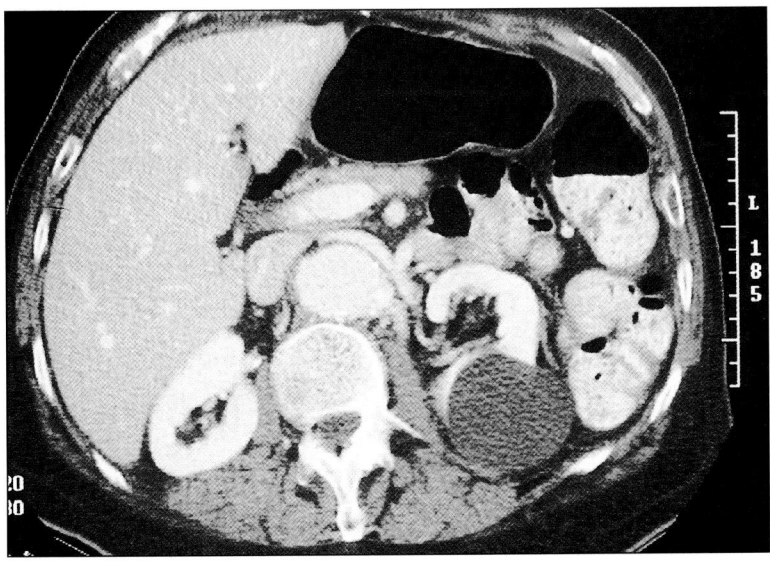

▶ **FIGURE 1-22.** Bosniak category 1 lesion. Criteria for this simple cyst include a round or oval shape, uniform water density, sharply defined borders with indiscernible walls, and absence of contrast enhancement.

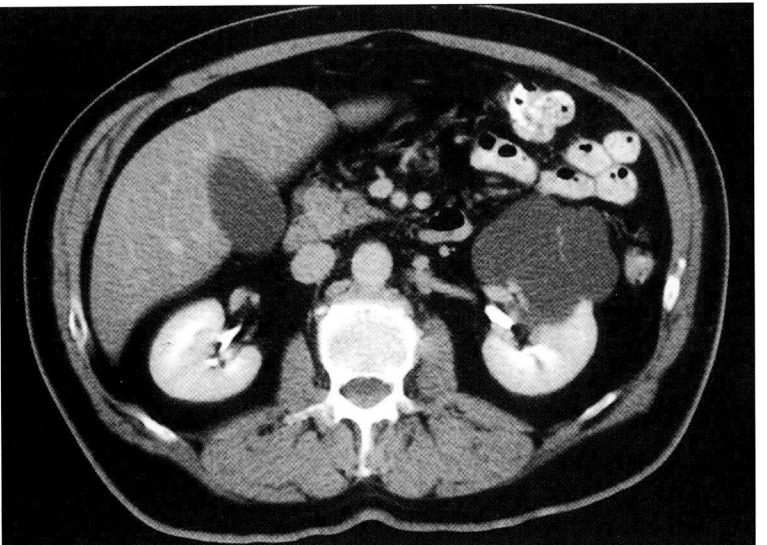

▶ **FIGURE 1-23.** Bosniak category 2 lesion. This CT scan demonstrates a large cystic mass extending from the anterior aspect of the left kidney with low attenuation, homogeneous water density, and the presence of thin septae characteristic of a Bosniak category 2 lesion. More complex or suspicious category 2 lesions are termed 2F and require periodic follow-up imaging, usually at 3 months, 6 months, and 1 year [37,43].

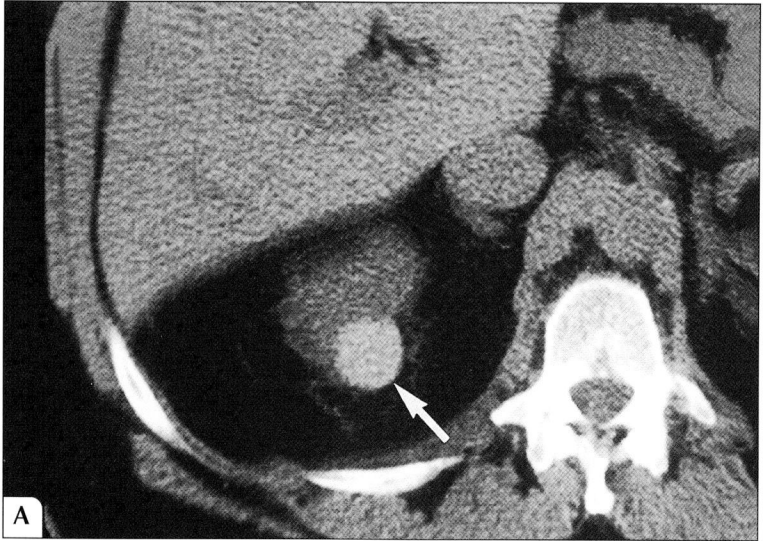 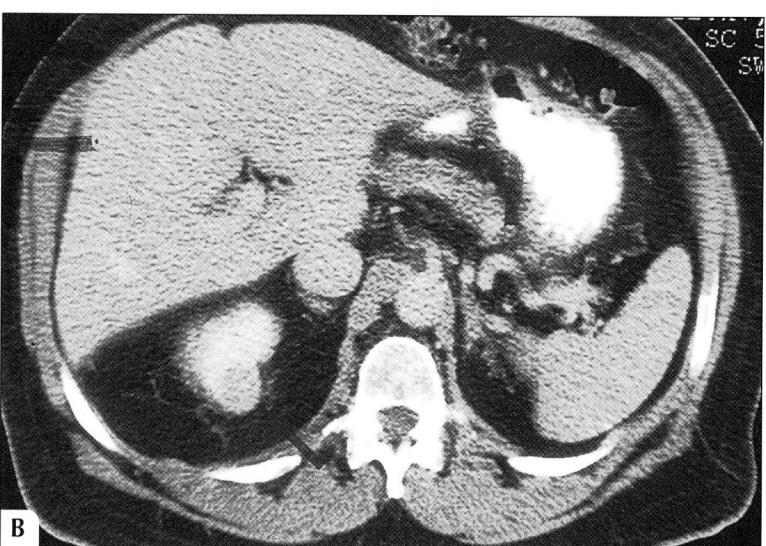

▶ **FIGURE 1-24.** Hyperdense cysts. Hyperdense cysts show density ranging from 40 to 90 Hounsfield units on noncontrast CT because of blood, colloid, iodine, or protein within the cyst [43]. Strict CT criteria for classifying a hyperdense cyst as Bosniak category 2 include all of the following: size (<3.0 cm in diameter), round shape with sharply margined borders, homogeneity, absence of contrast enhancement, and at least one quarter of the lesion lying extrinsic to the parenchyma so that smooth contour can be confirmed [44,45]. **A,** A noncontrast CT scan illustrating a hyperdense cyst (*arrow*) with smooth, round shape, sharply defined borders, and a strong interface with the normal renal parenchyma. **B,** This small (<3.0 cm) lesion did not enhance and thus satisfies all criteria for a benign hyperdense cyst.

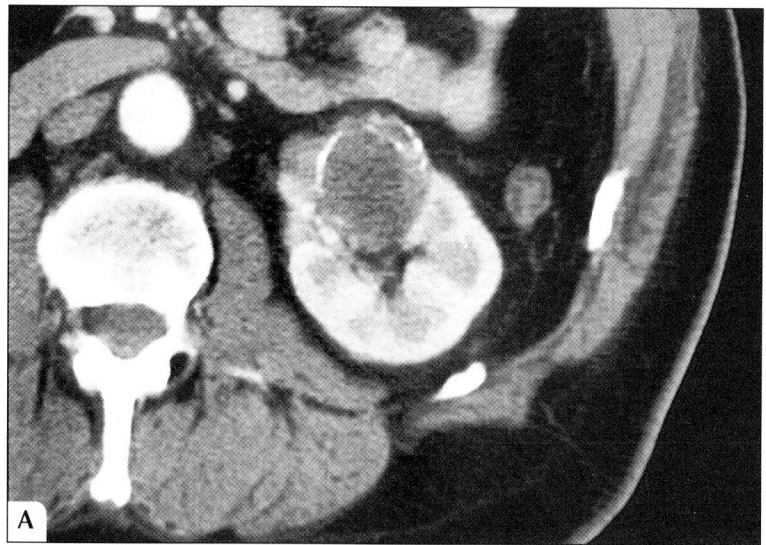 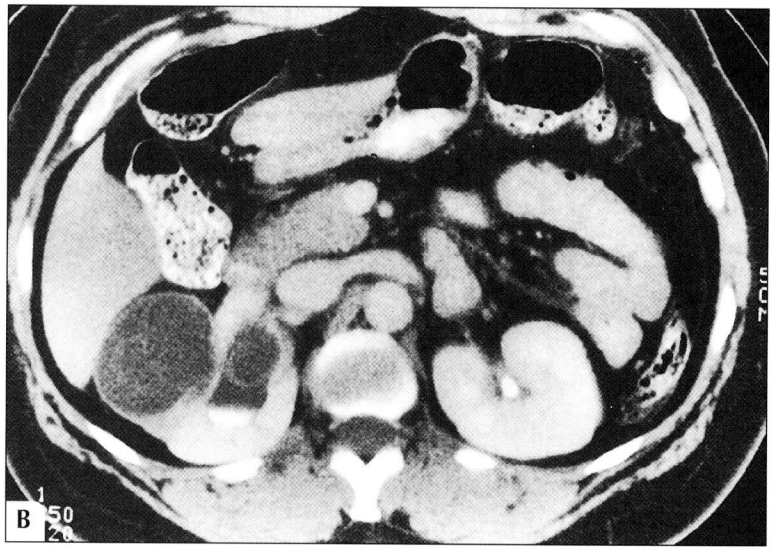

▶ **FIGURE 1-25.** Bosniak category 3 lesions. **A,** A Bosniak category 3 lesion with irregular contour and thickened, non–border-forming calcifications (findings suspicious for malignancy). **B,** However, many of these lesions are benign, including multilocular cystic nephroma with typical CT characteristics such as clustered cysts separated by septae with enhanced walls, with or without calcifications [36]. Unfortunately, this diagnosis cannot be definitively made preoperatively. Roughly one half of Bosniak category 3 lesions are ultimately proved malignant by surgical excision [3,43].

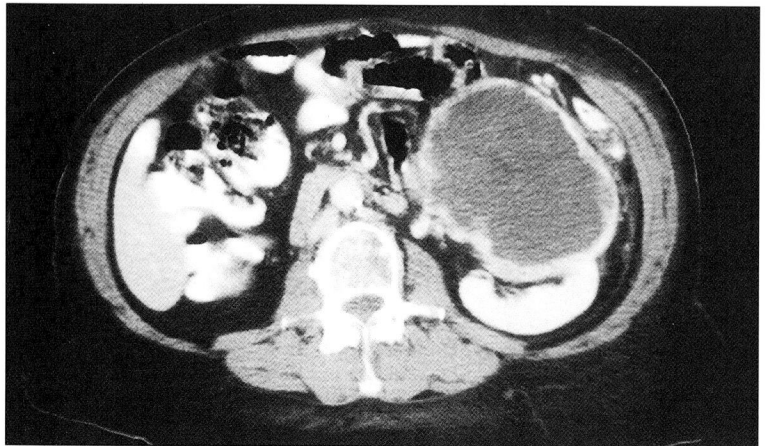

▶ **FIGURE 1-26.** Bosniak category 4 lesion. Bosniak category 4 lesions are frankly malignant with cystic elements due to intrinsic cystic growth, hemorrhage, necrosis, or liquefaction of solid tumor [43]. This CT scan demonstrates a Bosniak category 4 cystic mass of the left kidney with irregular shape, solid components distinct from normal parenchyma, and unequivocal contrast enhancement. Bosniak category 4 lesions are almost always malignant and thus treated with radical or partial nephrectomy.

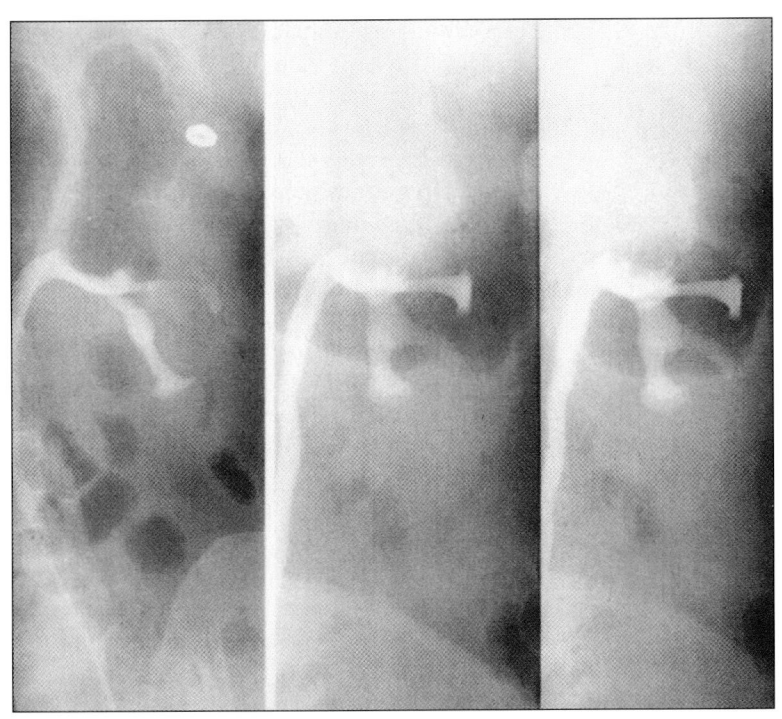

▶ **FIGURE 1-27.** Retrograde pyelography (RPG) study. Tumors of the urothelium account for approximately 6% to 8% of primary malignant renal neoplasms, second only to renal cell carcinoma in frequency. Of these urothelial malignancies, 90% are transitional cell carcinoma (TCC), with squamous cell carcinoma comprising most other cases [4]. Of patients with upper tract TCC, 2% to 4% have bilateral tumors and 50% to 75% will be diagnosed with TCC of the bladder during their lifetimes [1,4]. TCC of the upper tracts is rarely serendipitously discovered because 75% to 95% of patients present with gross hematuria. Another 3% to 11% manifest microscopic hematuria with pain, palpable mass, obstruction, and pyelonephritis accounting for the remainder [1,4]. Intravenous urography (IVU) is the most common initial diagnostic test for upper tract TCC. Most patients display a filling defect on IVU, but nonvisualization of the affected renal unit is occasionally seen due to venous occlusion, parenchymal destruction, or high-grade ureteral obstruction [1,36]. Cystoscopy with retrograde pyelography (RPG) is a reasonable alternative if suspicion of a urothelial tumor is high or if use of intravenous contrast is relatively contraindicated. Meticulously performed RPG is diagnostic in up to 85% of upper tract tumors [1]. The three views of this RPG study performed in a patient with a solitary left kidney who presented with gross hematuria, illustrates distortion of the renal pelvis with complete obliteration of the upper pole collecting system, highly suggestive of TCC.

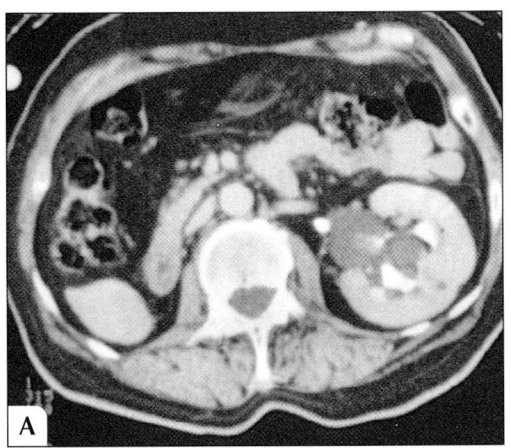

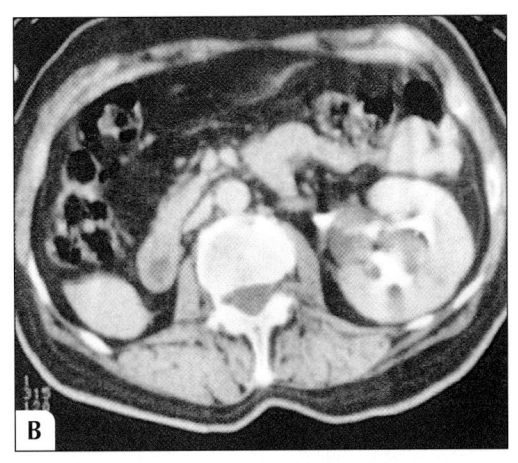

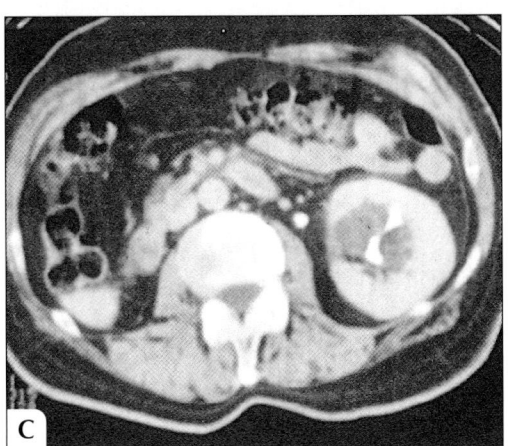

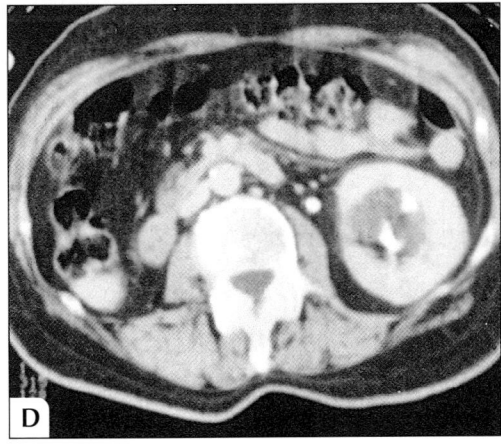

▶ **FIGURE 1-28.** Computed tomographic images of transitional cell carcinoma (TCC). CT has many strengths in evaluating suspected transitional cell carcinoma (TCC) of the upper tracts. It is sensitive for detection of filling defects and can differentiate radiolucent stones from TCC. CT may also help distinguish TCC from renal cell carcinoma because the former is invariably hypovascular. Multiple views (**A–D**) from this study demonstrate the CT characteristics of TCC of the renal pelvis, including a solid hypodense mass with a central location not disturbing normal renal contour, the presence of a polypoid filling defect distorting the renal pelvis and calyces, and lack of contrast enhancement [36,46,47]. Note the absence of the right kidney in this patient with a solitary left kidney and gross hematuria. CT staging has limited utility, with reported accuracy ranging from 40% to 90%. Nonetheless, detection of lymphadenopathy or invasion into the peripelvic fat, renal parenchyma, or adjacent organs provides important staging information for upper tract TCC [46,47].

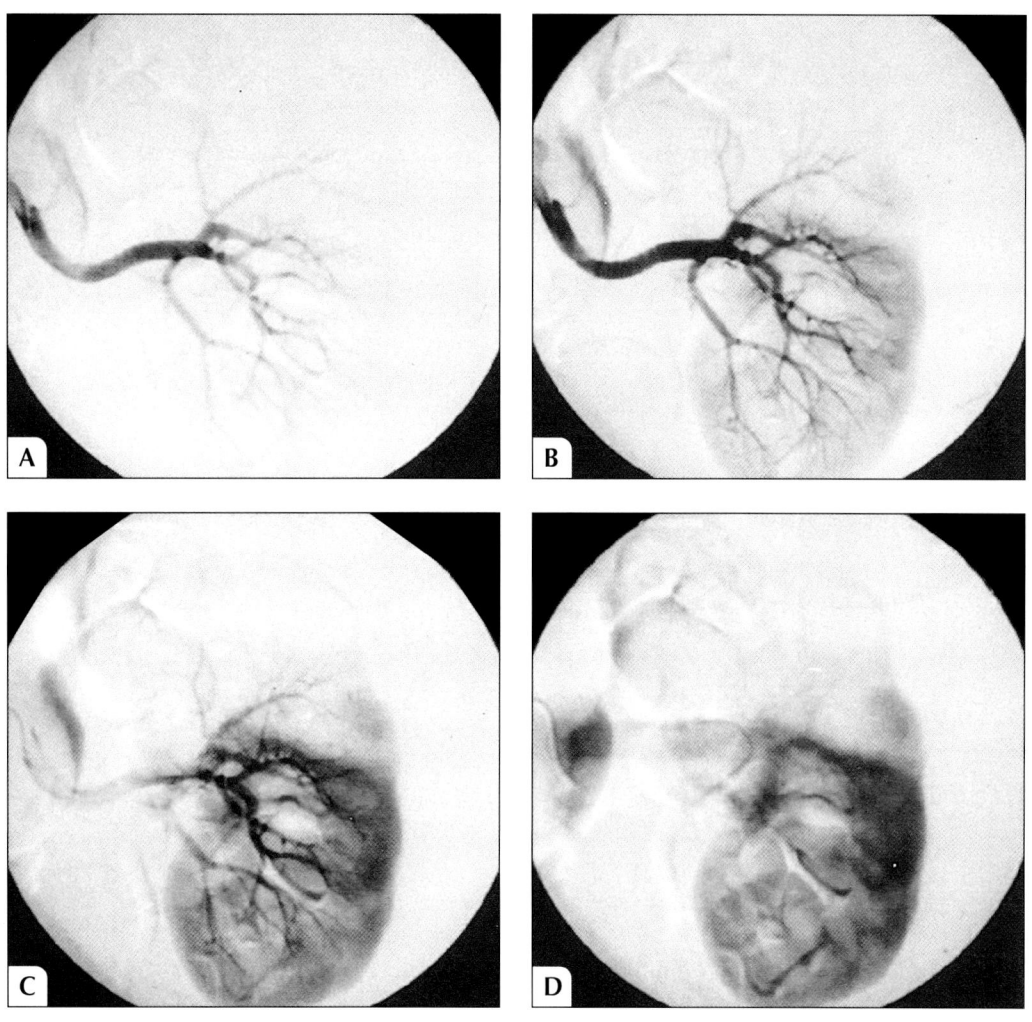

▶ **FIGURE 1-29.** Four views of a selective left renal arteriogram (*panels A–D*). Transitional cell carcinoma (TCC) of the upper tracts is typically hypovascular on angiography but cannot be reliably distinguished from renal cell carcinoma (RCC). TCC may show fine tumor vasculature on magnified views, and RCC is hypovascular in up to 10% of cases [13]. Renal arteriography is rarely performed for TCC but may provide crucial vascular mapping if nephron-sparing surgery is indicated [1]. These four views were obtained for vascular mapping prior to partial nephrectomy in a patient with TCC in a solitary kidney. The study reveals a single left renal artery, with normal vasculature and parenchyma of the lower pole but distinct hypovascularity of the upper pole characteristic of TCC.

RENAL ONCOCYTOMA

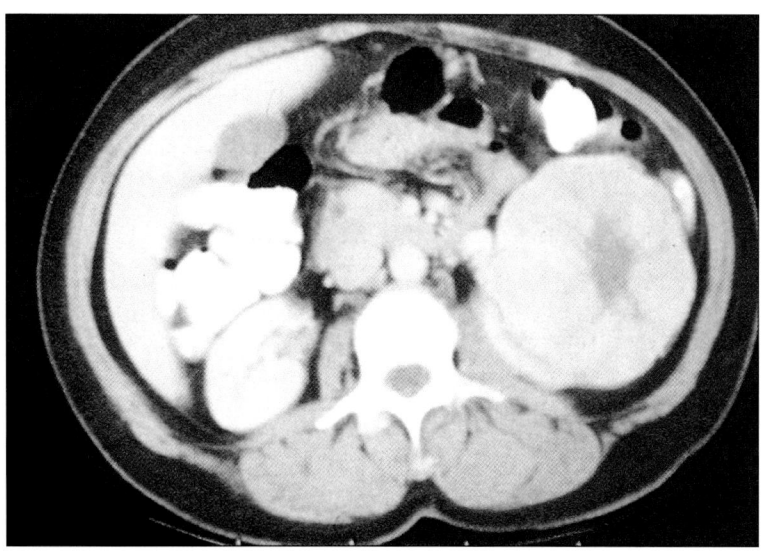

▶ **FIGURE 1-30.** Oncocytoma is a benign solid tumor accounting for 3% to 14% of all renal neoplasms. The demographics of oncocytoma are similar to those of renal cell carcinoma (RCC) with a male to female ratio of 2:1 and peak incidence at 55 years of age [4,48]. Most oncocytomas are incidentally discovered; a minority of patients present with pain, mass, or hematuria usually related to the size of the lesion. Bilateral, multifocal oncocytomas are reported but rare [49,50]. Oncocytoma cannot be distinguished from RCC based on radiologic findings or clinical presentation and is most commonly a pathologic diagnosis [4,48,51]. The "central stellate scar" shown in this CT image of an oncocytoma is now known to be a nonspecific finding. Recent reports suggest that magnetic resonance imaging may improve our ability to detect oncocytoma preoperatively [52].

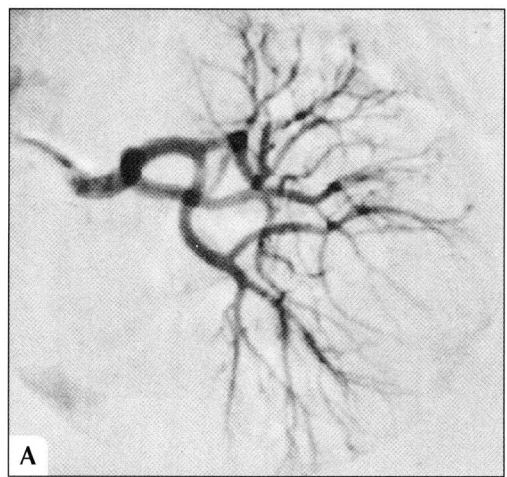

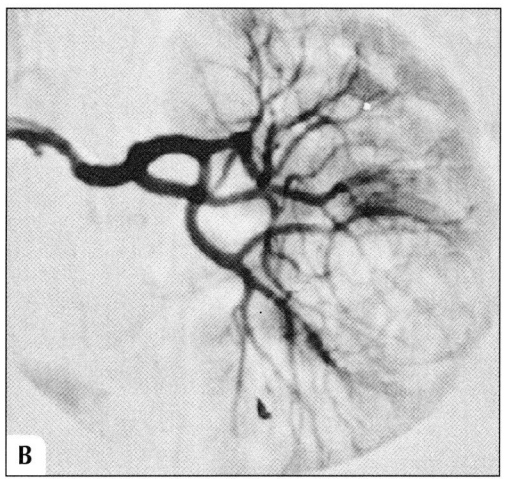

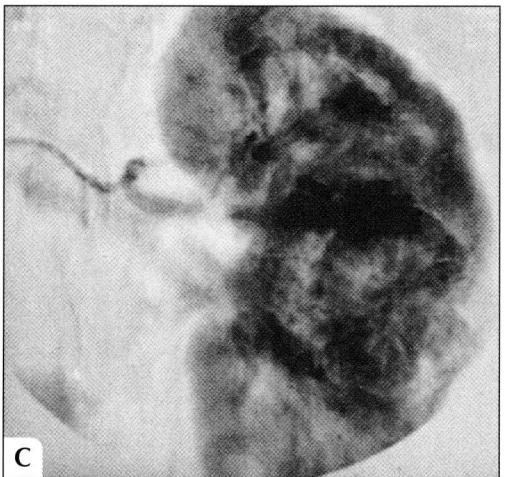

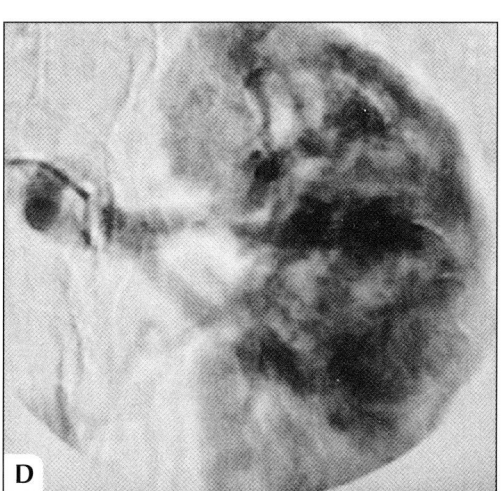

▶ **FIGURE 1-31.** Angiographic images of oncocytoma versus renal cell carcinoma (RCC) **(A–D)**. Angiography is also unreliable in differentiating oncocytoma from renal cell carcinoma (RCC). The classically described "spoke-wheel pattern" demonstrated in this figure is rarely seen and not specific for oncocytoma [48]. Most oncocytomas are hypovascular on angiography, but so are 5% to 10% of RCCs [13]. Preoperative or open surgical biopsy for diagnosis of oncocytoma is unreliable because oncocytoma often coexists with RCC [48].

ANGIOMYOLIPOMA

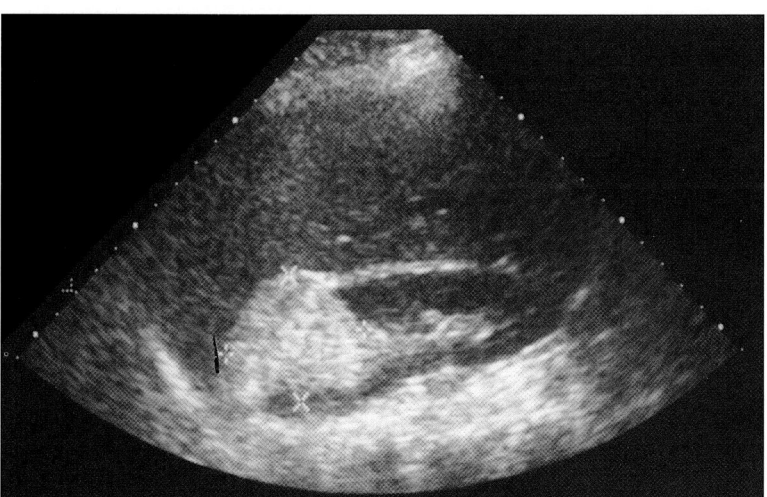

▶ **FIGURE 1-32.** Ultrasonographic characteristics of renal angiomyolipoma (AML). AML is a benign solid tumor characterized by the presence of vascular elements, fat, and muscle in various proportions. A well-defined association exists between tuberous sclerosis and AML; roughly 80% of patients with

tuberous sclerosis manifest AMLs, which are often bilateral and asymptomatic. In patients without tuberous sclerosis, AML is typically unilateral and may present with abdominal or flank pain, mass, hematuria, or retroperitoneal hemorrhage [4]. AML follows a benign clinical course without metastases, but aggressive local behavior is well documented, with reports of extrarenal extension, hilar lymph node involvement, and invasion of the renal vein or inferior vena cava with tumor thrombus [53–55]. Venous or lymphatic involvement represents only local invasion; pathologic examination invariably shows lack of malignant transformation [54]. This renal ultrasonographic image illustrates ultrasonographic characteristics of AML, including a sharply marginated, homogeneous mass with markedly increased echogenicity equivalent to the renal sinus. Ultrasonographic differentiation of AML from hyperechoic renal cell carcinoma (RCC) is difficult; acoustic shadowing suggests AML, whereas a hypoechoic rim or intralesional cysts are suspicious for RCC [56,57]. Recent reports suggest that ultrasonic frequency-dependent attenuation may further help distinguish AML from RCC [58]. However, CT or magnetic resonance imaging must currently be performed for further characterization of echogenic renal masses found on ultrasonography. If a confident diagnosis of AML is rendered, ultrasonography is also reliable in clinical follow-up [59,60].

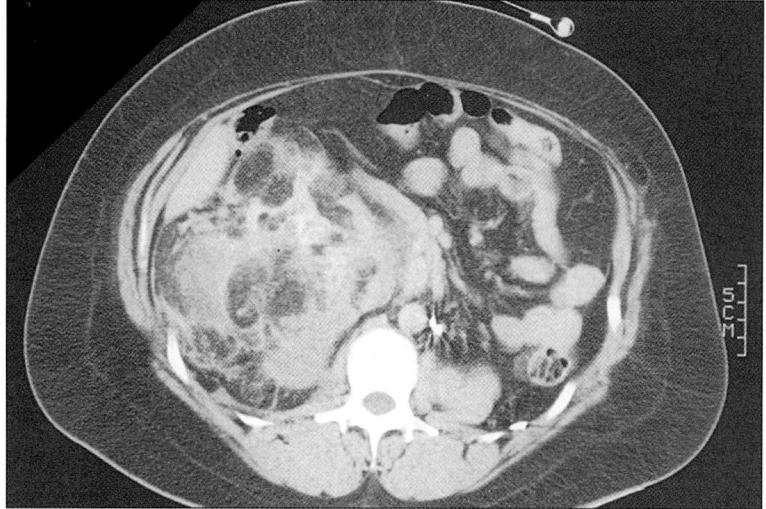

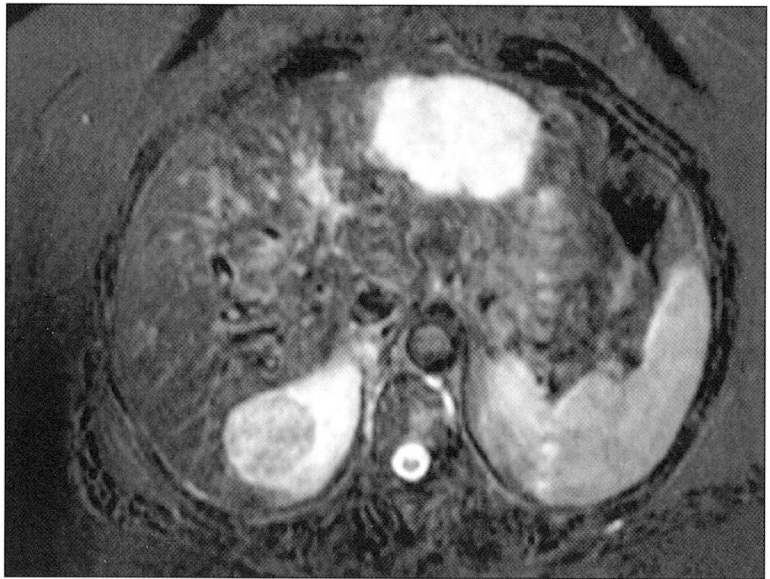

▶ **FIGURE 1-33.** Computed tomographic image of a large, heterogeneous right renal mass with fat density diagnostic for angiomylipoma (AML). Vascular and muscular components give AML a variable appearance on CT, but the presence of fat density (-20 to -80 Hounsfield units) is virtually diagnostic [1,4,13]. The literature describes renal cell carcinoma (RCC) with admixtures of fat density on CT [11,12,61]. However, each case of RCC with fatty elements also had calcifications, which are invariably absent in AML. Therefore, fat density on CT in the absence of calcification essentially excludes RCC from diagnosis. Novel advances in CT show further promise for detection of fat in renal lesions as small as 0.4 cm [62–64].

▶ **FIGURE 1-34.** Fat-suppressed magnetic resonance image. The role of magnetic resonance imaging in the evaluation of angiomyolipoma (AML) is evolving. This image demonstrates a mass of low signal intensity in the right kidney, which is characteristic of AML. Fat suppression techniques are particularly helpful for the diagnosis of AML because the high signal intensity of AML on T_1- and T_2-weighted images is nonspecific, whereas low signal intensity with fat saturation images confirms the presence of fatty components [21].

INFLAMMATORY RENAL MASSES

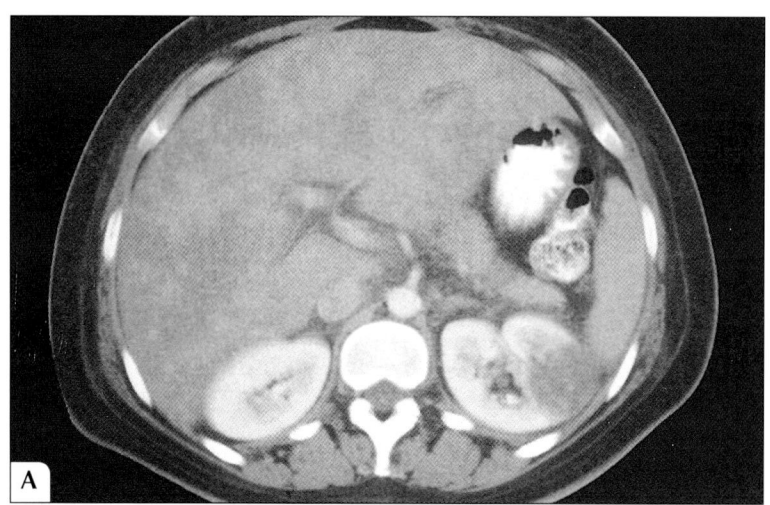

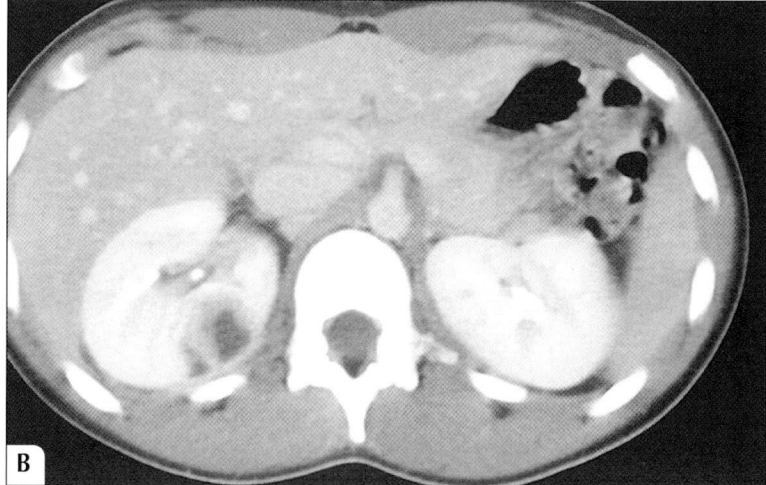

▶ **FIGURE 1-35.** Computed tomographic images of various renal infections. Urinary tract infection (UTI) in the adult is usually a straightforward diagnosis based on clinical presentation and laboratory examination. Imaging for presumed UTI is generally reserved for severely ill or immunocompromised patients, those with infections unresponsive to appropriate antimicrobials, those with suspected obstruction, or those in whom diagnosis remains in question. Inflammatory masses of the kidney include acute focal or diffuse pyelonephritis, renal abscess, emphysematous pyelonephritis, pyonephrosis, and xanthogranulomatous pyelonephritis (XGP) [65,66]. Acute pyelonephritis may be focal or diffuse based on extent of renal involvement. Intravenous urography or ultrasonographic studies are most commonly normal with either the focal or diffuse type [65]. CT characteristics of diffuse pyelonephritis include renal enlargement, poor enhancement and excretion of contrast, and a "striated" nephrogram. **A,** CT findings characteristic of left acute focal pyelonephritis, such as unilateral renal enlargement and focal areas of rounded or wedge-shaped hypodensity [65,66]. In addition, this patient demonstrates heterogeneous hepatic enhancement due to right-sided heart failure. Delayed CT approximately 3 hours after administration of contrast may be helpful to differentiate areas of infection from ischemia or edema [67]. Although focal pyelonephritis is often confidently diagnosed on the basis of clinical and CT findings, follow-up imaging is usually performed after convalescence to prove resolution of the mass. Renal abscess may form with progression of inadequately treated acute pyelonephritis. **B,** CT findings of early renal abscess, including an irregular mass with central low attenuation indicative of liquefaction and necrosis. A zone of diminished enhancement separates the central hypodensity from normal renal architecture and is thought to represent infected parenchyma that is not yet necrotic [65,66]. (*Continued on next page*)

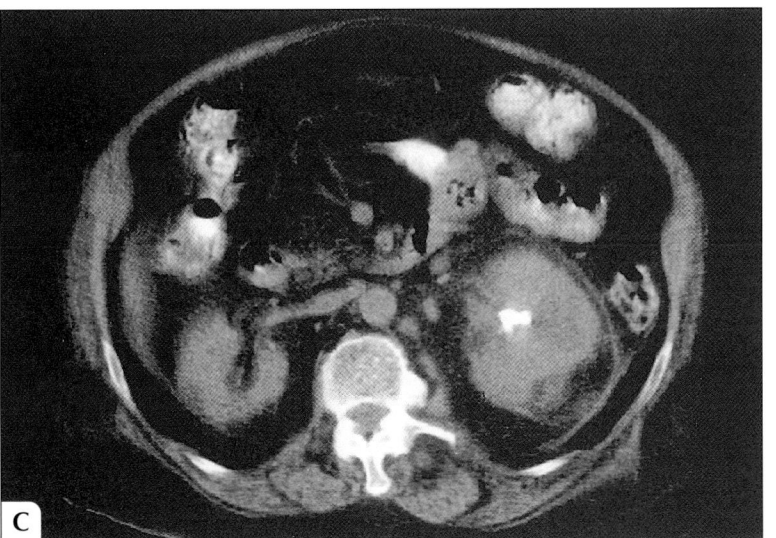

FIGURE 1-35. *Continued* peripheral rim of enhancement or gas formation is occasionally seen with mature renal abscess [65]. Abscess is usually treated with percutaneous drainage and appropriate intravenous antibiotics. XGP is a rare complication of chronic urinary obstruction and infection, usually with *Proteus* or *Escherichia coli* species. Common presentation includes unilateral flank or abdominal pain, fevers, chills, malaise, or weight loss [68]. XGP originally involves the renal pelvis but may spread to the parenchyma with extension into the perinephric space or retroperitoneum [65,66,69]. **C,** Typical CT findings of XGP, such as an enlarged, heterogeneous mass with perinephric stranding and the classic large central calculus [65,66]. Renal calculi are present in up to 80% of cases and are commonly staghorn [65,66,68,69]. Poor ipsilateral renal function is also common. Focal XGP can mimic renal cell carcinoma radiographically, particularly in the absence of renal stones [65]. Antimicrobials alone are ineffective in the treatment of XGP; partial nephrectomy can be considered if technically feasible [68,69].

RENAL LYMPHOMA

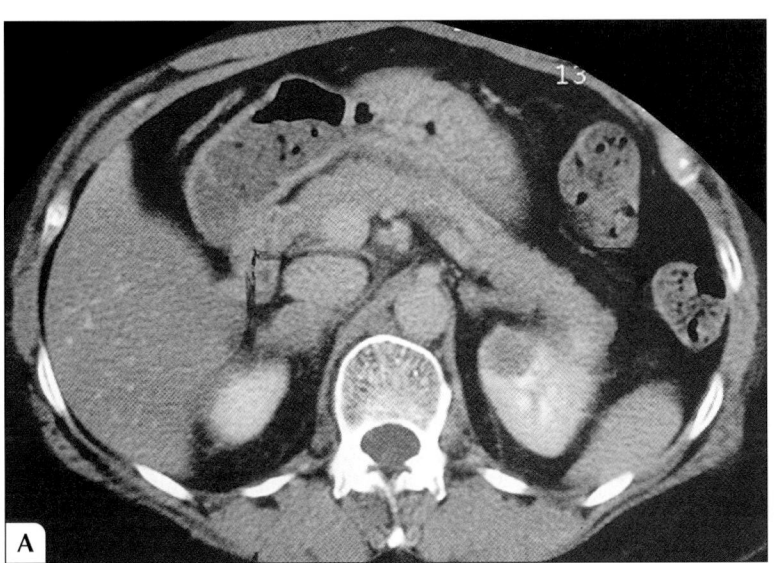

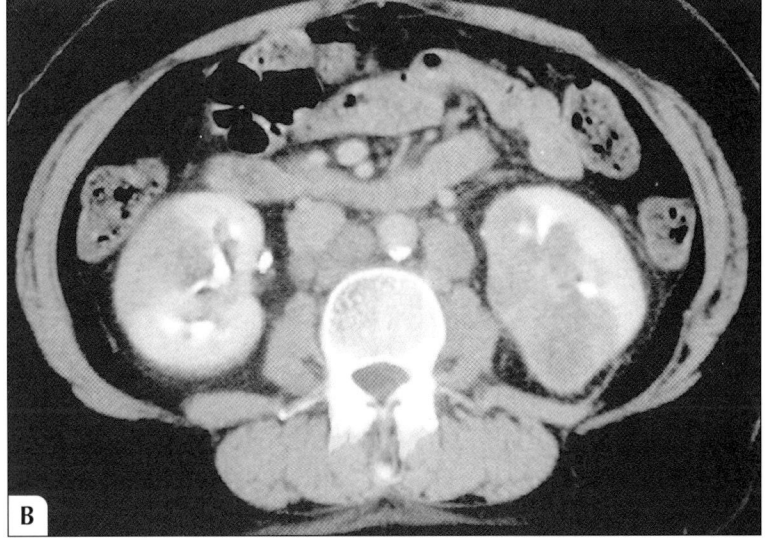

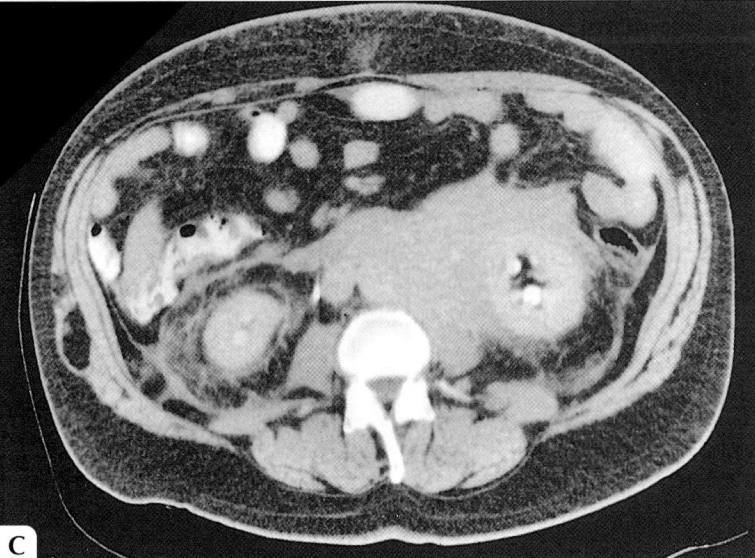

FIGURE 1-36. Images of renal lymphoma. Renal lymphoma most commonly occurs in the setting of systemic disease and is often diagnosed by CT or magnetic resonance imaging of the retroperitoneum [70,71]. Several different patterns of lymphomatous involvement of the kidneys are described. Focal parenchymal disease (**A**) is often misdiagnosed as renal cell carcinoma (RCC) [71], whereas multifocal bilateral renal masses (**B**) are more readily distinguished from RCC. Diffuse bilateral infiltration by lymphoma with nephromegaly is also occasionally present. Finally, massive retroperitoneal lymphadenopathy with engulfment of the kidney (**C**) is highly suggestive of lymphoma [70]. Percutaneous or open surgical biopsy can be performed for definitive diagnosis, with treatment directed systemically toward the primary pathology.

METASTATIC DISEASE TO THE KIDNEY

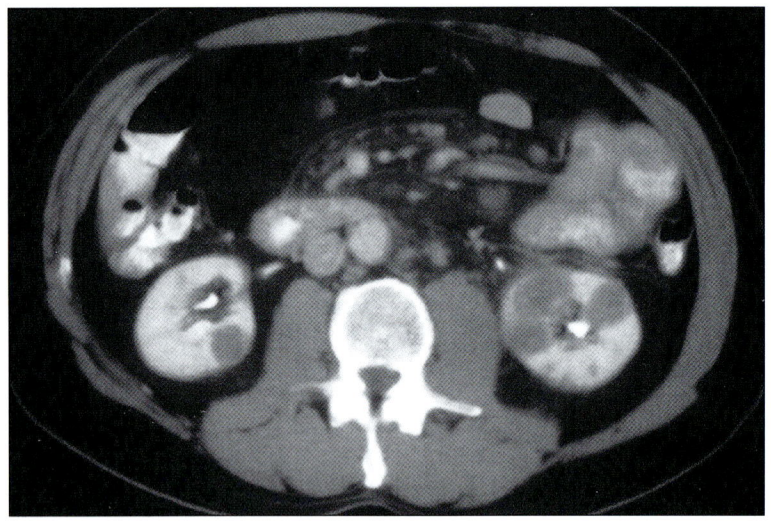

FIGURE 1-37. Multiple malignant lesions in the kidneys. These lesions most commonly indicate diffuse metastatic disease. Renal metastases are found in roughly 12% of autopsies in patients with known malignancy and are most commonly from lung, breast, gastrointestinal, or malignant melanoma primary tumors, in decreasing order of frequency [38]. Renal metastases are most commonly hematogenous [4]; fewer than 10% of cases result from direct invasion or lymphatic spread [38]. This CT scan shows small, multifocal, and bilateral lesions suggestive of renal metastases; bronchogenic carcinoma was confirmed on biopsy.

ARTERIOVENOUS MALFORMATIONS

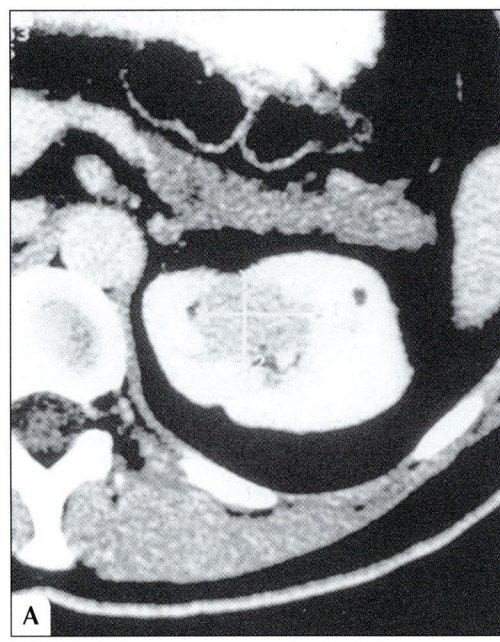

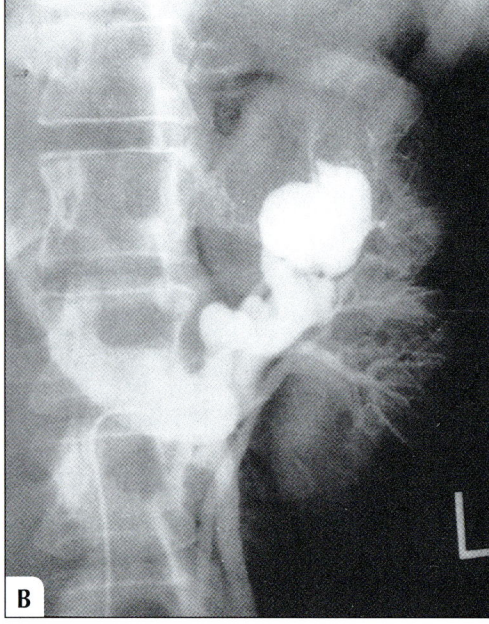

FIGURE 1-38. Renal arteriovenous malformations (AVMs). AVMs can mimic renal cell carcinoma and most commonly manifest in young patients with gross hematuria, although signs and symptoms of congestive heart failure may be present [34]. Intravenous urography is often the initial diagnostic study because of hematuria and may reveal delayed excretion, filling defects, or suspicion of mass. **A,** Contrast-enhanced CT characteristic of AVM with a central or hilar mass that rapidly enhances with contrast. Dilated renal veins or early venous filling may be present. **B,** Arteriography is the gold standard for diagnosing AVM, characterized by simultaneous filling of arteries and veins with contrast [34]. Because treatment consists of partial nephrectomy, angiographic embolization, or simple nephrectomy, based on the size and complexity of the lesion, angiography is also useful for vascular mapping.

REFERENCES

1. Jennings SB, Linehan WM: Renal, perirenal, and ureteral neoplasms. In *Adult and Pediatric Urology*. Edited by Gillenwater JY, Grayhack JT, Howards SS, *et al.* St. Louis: Mosby-Year Book; 1996:643–694.

2. Smith SJ, Bosniak MA, Megibow AJ, *et al.*: Renal cell carcinoma: earlier discovery and increased detection. *Radiology* 1989, 170:699–703.

3. Silverman SG, Bloom DA, Seltzer SE: The radiological evaluation of renal masses: approach, analysis, and new technologies. *AUA Update Series* 1994, 13:1–7.

4. Rodriguez R, Fishman EK, Marshall FF: Differential diagnosis and evaluation of the incidentally discovered renal mass. *Semin Urol Oncol* 1995, 13:246–253.

5. Amendola MA, Bree RL, Pollack HM, *et al.*: Small renal cell carcinomas: resolving a diagnostic dilemma. *Radiology* 1988, 166:637–641.

6. Warshauer DM, McCarthy SM, Street L, *et al.*: Detection of renal masses: sensitivities and specificities of excretory urography/linear tomography, US, and CT. *Radiology* 1988, 169:363–365.

7. Curry NS, Schabel SI, Betsill WL, Jr: Small renal neoplasms: diagnostic imaging, pathologic features, and clinical course. *Radiology* 1986, 158:113–117.

8. Older RA, Kellum CD, Fisher LM, *et al.*: Imaging/excretory urography. In *Adult and Pediatric Urology*. Edited by Gillenwater JY, Grayhack JT, Howards SS, *et al.* St. Louis: Mosby-Year Book, 1997:79–100.

9. Haas CA, Resnick MI: Office-based ultrasound for urologists. *AUA Update Series* 1997, 16:242–247.

10. Coleman BG: Ultrasonography of the upper genitourinary tract. *Urol Clin North Am* 1985, 12:633–644.

11. Strotzer M, Lehner KB, Becker K: Detection of fat in a renal cell carcinoma mimicking angiomyolipoma. *Radiology* 1993, 188:427–428.

12. Helenon O, Chretien Y, Paraf F, *et al.*: Renal cell carcinoma containing fat: demonstration with CT. *Radiology* 1993, 188:429–430.

13. Vogelzang RL: Renal arteriography and computed tomography. In *Adult and Pediatric Urology*. Edited by Gillenwater JY, Grayhack JT, Howards SS, *et al.* St. Louis: Mosby-Year Book; 1996:100–145.

14. Bosniak MA, Rofsky NM: Problems in the detection and characterization of small renal masses. *Radiology* 1996, 198:638–641.

15. Silverman SG, Lee BY, Seltzer SE, *et al.*: Small (<or = 3 cm) renal masses: correlation of spiral CT features and pathologic findings. *AJR Am J Roentgenol* 1994, 163:597–605.

16. Jamis-Dow CA, Choyke PL, Jennings SB, *et al.*: Small (<3 cm) renal masses: detection with CT versus US and pathologic correlation. *Radiology* 1996, 198:785–788.

17. Szolar DH, Kammerhuber F, Altziebler S, *et al.*: Multiphasic helical CT of the kidney: increased conspicuity for detection and characterization of small (F3 cm) renal masses. *Radiology* 1997, 202:211–217.

18. Urban BA: The small renal mass: what is the role of multiphasic helical scanning? *Radiology* 1997, 202:22–23.

19. Chernoff DM, Silverman SG, Kikinis R, *et al.*: Three-dimensional imaging and display of renal tumors using spiral CT: a potential aid to partial nephrectomy. *Urology* 1994, 43:125–129.

20. Choyke PL: Magnetic resonance imaging. In *Adult and Pediatric Urology*. Edited by Gillenwater JY, Grayhack JT, Howards SS, *et al.* St. Louis: Mosby-Year Book; 1996:146–165.

21. King BF Jr, Schnall MD, Levy J: Magnetic resonance imaging (MRI) in urology. *AUA Update Series* 1997, 16:298–303.

22. McClennan BL, Deoye LA: The imaging evaluation of renal cell carcinoma: diagnosis and staging. *Radiol Clin North Am* 1994, 32:55–69.

23. Horan JJ, Robertson CN, Choyke PL, *et al.*: The detection of renal carcinoma extension into the renal vein and inferior vena cava: a prospective comparison of venacavography and magnetic resonance imaging. *J Urol* 1989, 142:943–948.

24. Rofsky NM, Weinreb JC, Bosniak MA, *et al.*: Renal lesion characterization with gadolinium-enhanced MR imaging: efficacy and safety in patients with renal insufficiency. *Radiology* 1991, 180:85–89.

25. Haustein J, Niendorf HP, Krestin G, *et al*: Renal tolerance of gadolinium-DTPA/dimeglumine in patients with chronic renal failure. *Invest Radiol* 1992, 27:153–156.

26. Semelka RC, Hricak H, Stevens SK, *et al.*: Combined gadolinium-enhanced and fat-saturation MR imaging of renal masses. *Radiology* 1991, 178:803–809.

27. Semelka RC, Shoenut JP, Kroeker MA, *et al.*: Renal lesions: controlled comparison between CT and 1.5-T MR imaging with nonenhanced and gadolinium-enhanced fat-suppressed spin-echo and breath-hold FLASH techniques. *Radiology* 1992, 182:425–430.

28. Murray JG, Eustace S, Breatnach E, *et al.*: MR diagnosis of haemorrhagic cystic renal cell carcinoma. *J Comput Assist Tomogr* 1994, 18:68–71.

29. Kirkali Z, Esen AA, Pirnar T, *et al.*: Magnetic resonance imaging in the staging of renal cell carcinoma. *Int Urol Nephrol* 1994, 26:615–619.

30. Choyke PL: Detection and staging of renal cancer. *Magn Reson Imaging Clin North Am* 1997, 5:29–47.

31. Campbell S, Novick A, Streem S, *et al.*: Management of renal cell carcinoma with coexistent renal artery disease. *J Urol* 1993, 150:808–813.

32. Sinsky CA, Dahlberg PJ, O'Connor J: Unilateral acquired renal cystic disease and neoplasia in a patient with renal artery stenosis. *Urology* 1993, 41:287–288.

33. Cooper SG: Renal artery stenosis with contralateral renal cell carcinoma: an indication for prophylactic angioplasty? *AJR Am J Roentgenol* 1995, 165:1553–1554.

34. Vasavada SP, Manion S, Flanigan RC, *et al.*: Renal arteriovenous malformations masquerading as renal cell carcinoma. *Urology* 1995, 46:716–721.

35. Croft BY, Joyce JM, Parekh J, *et al.*: Nuclide studies. In *Adult and Pediatric Urology*. Edited by Gillenwater JY, Grayhack JT, Howards SS, *et al.* St. Louis: Mosby-Year Book; 1996:193–217.

36. Newhouse JH: The radiologic evaluation of the patient with renal cancer. *Urol Clin North Am* 1993, 20:231–246.

37. Bosniak MA: Problems in the radiologic diagnosis of renal parenchymal tumors. *Urol Clin North Am* 1993, 20:217–230.

38. Hauser M, Krestin GP, Hagspiel KD: Bilateral solid multifocal intrarenal and perirenal lesions: differentiation with ultrasonography, computed tomography and magnetic resonance imaging. *Clin Radiol* 1995, 50:288–294.

39. Bosniak MA: The current radiological approach to renal cysts. *Radiology* 1986, 158:1–10.

40. Redman BG, Kawachi M, Schwartz D: Urothelial and kidney cancer. In *Cancer Management: A Multidisciplinary Approach*. Edited by Pazdur R, Coia LR, Hoskins WJ, *et al.* Huntington, NY: PRR, 1998:441–448.

41. Levine E: Renal cell carcinoma: clinical aspects, imaging diagnosis, and staging. *Semin Roentgenol* 1995, 30:128–148.

42. Bechtold RE, Zagoria RJ: Imaging approach to staging of renal cell carcinoma. *Urol Clin North Am* 1997, 24:507–522.

43. Curry NS, Bissada NK: Radiologic evaluation of small and indeterminant renal masses. *Urol Clin North Am* 1997, 24:493–505.

44. Aronson S, Frazier HA, Baluch JD, *et al.*: Cystic renal masses: usefulness of the Bosniak classification. *Urol Radiol* 1991, 13:83–90.

45. Bosniak MA: Difficulties in classifying cystic lesions of the kidney. *Urol Radiol* 1991, 13:91–93.

46. Planz B, George R, Adam G, *et al.*: Computed tomography for detection and staging of transitional cell carcinoma of the upper urinary tract. *Eur Urol* 1995, 27:146–150.

47. Buckley JA, Urban BA, Soyer P, *et al.*: Transitional cell carcinoma of the renal pelvis: a retrospective look at CT staging with pathologic correlation. *Radiology* 1996, 201:194–198.

48. Licht MR: Renal adenoma and oncocytoma. *Semin Urol Oncol* 1995, 13:262–266.

49. Holmes SAV, Rickards D, Kirby RS: Multifocal bilateral oncocytomas. *Br J Urol* 1993, 71:484–491.

50. Fukuzawa S, Oishi K, Takeuchi H, *et al.*: Multifocal renal oncocytoma: a case report. *Acta Urol Jpn* 1993, 39:163–166.

51. Davidson AJ, Hayes WS, Hartman DS, *et al.*: Renal oncocytoma and carcinoma: failure of differentiation with CT. *Radiology* 1993, 186:693–696.

52. Harmon WJ, King BF, Lieber MM: Renal oncocytoma: magnetic resonance imaging characteristics. *J Urol* 1996, 155:863–867.

53. Cittadini G Jr, Mucelli FP, Danza FM, *et al.*: "Aggressive" renal angiomyolipoma. *Acta Radiol* 1996, 37:927–932.

54. Leder RA: Genitourinary case of the day. *AJR Am J Roentgenol* 1995, 165:198–199.

55. Baert J, Vandamme B, Sciot R, *et al.*: Benign angiomyolipoma involving the renal vein and vena cava as a tumor thrombus: case report. *J Urol* 1995, 153:1205–1207.

56. Forman HP, Middleton WD, Melson GL, *et al.*: Hyperechoic renal cell carcinomas: increase in detection at US. *Radiology* 1993, 188:431–434.

57. Siegel CL, Middleton WD, Teefey SA, *et al.*: Angiomyolipoma and renal cell carcinoma: US differentiation. *Radiology* 1996, 198:789–793.

58. Taniguchi N, Itoh K, Nakamura S, *et al*: Differentiation of renal cell carcinomas from angiomyolipomas by ultrasonic frequency dependent attenuation. *J Urol* 1997, 157:1242–1245.

59. Hobarth K, Klingler C, Kuber W, *et al.*: Value of routine sonography in the diagnosis and conservative management of renal angiomyolipoma. *Eur Urol* 1993, 24:239–243.

60. Lemaitre L, Robert Y, Dubrulle F, *et al.*: Renal angiomyolipoma: growth followed up with CT and/or US. *Radiology* 1995, 197:598–602.

61. Henderson RJ, Germany R, Peavy PW, *et al.*: Fat density in renal cell carcinoma: demonstration with computerized tomography. *J Urol* 1997, 157:1347–1348.

62. Silverman SG, Pearson GDN, Seltzer SE, *et al.*: Small (<3 cm) hyperechoic renal masses: comparison of helical and conventional CT for diagnosing angiomyolipoma. *AJR Am J Roentgenol* 1996, 167:877–881.

63. Takahashi K, Honda M, Okubo RS, *et al.*: CT pixel mapping in the diagnosis of small angiomyolipomas of the kidneys. *J Comput Assist Tomog* 1993, 17:98–101.

64. Kurosaki Y, Tanaka Y, Kuramoto K, *et al.*: Improved CT fat detection in small kidney angiomyolipomas using thin sections and single voxel measurements. *J Comput Assist Tomog* 1993, 17:745–748.

65. Baumgarten DA, Baumgartner B: Imaging and radiologic management of upper urinary tract infections. *Uroradiology* 1997, 24:545–569.

66. Rabushka LS, Fishman EK, Goldman SM: Pictorial review: computed tomography of renal inflammatory disease. *Urology* 1994, 44:473–480.

67. Dalla-Palma L, Pozzi-Mucelli F, Pozzi-Mucelli RS: Delayed CT findings in acute renal infection. *Clin Radiol* 1995, 50:364–370.

68. Perez LM, Thrasher JB, Paulson DF: Recurrent urinary tract infections and intermittent left flank pain in young woman. *Urology* 1993, 41:384–386.

69. Morey AF, Leckie R, Adams SD, *et al.*: Extensive retroperitoneal mass. *Urology* 1993, 41:185–188.

70. Semelka RC, Kelekis NL, Burdeny DA, *et al.*: Renal lymphoma: demonstration by MR imaging. *AJR Am J Roentgenol* 1996, 166:823–827.

71. Dimopoulos MA, Moulopoulos LA, Costantinides C, *et al.*: Primary renal lymphoma: a clinical and radiological study. *J Urol* 1996, 155:1865–1867.

Screening, Diagnosis, and Staging of Renal Cell Carcinoma

J. Stuart Wolf, Jr,
James E. Montie

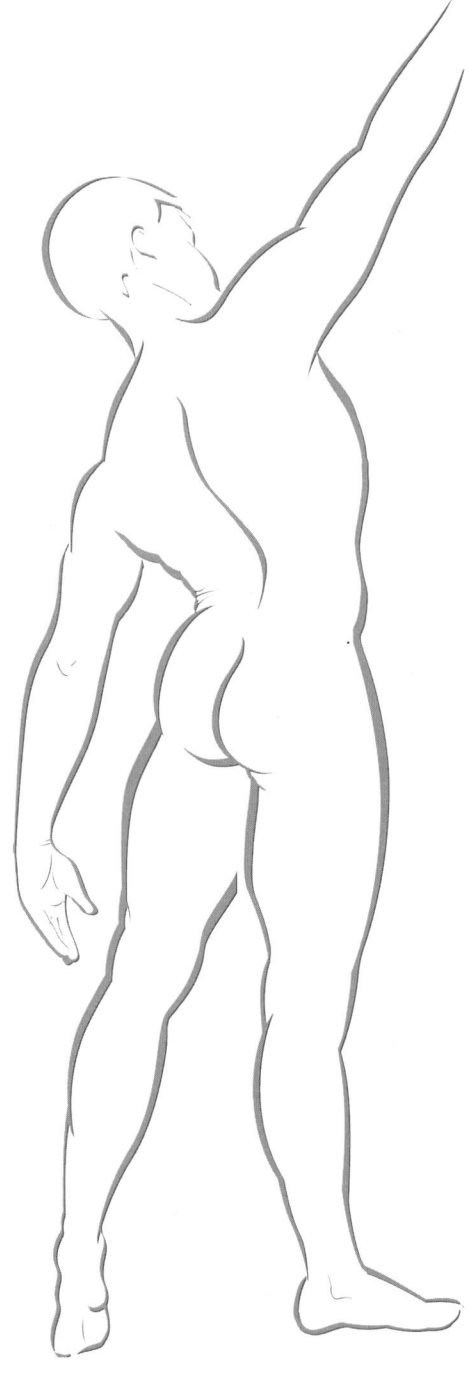

The greater use of imaging modalities such as ultrasonography and CT have contributed to an increase in the number of renal tumors diagnosed. The 1996 estimate for new cases of kidney cancer in the United States was 30,600, with an estimated mortality of 12,000 [1]. For a man 40 years of age the estimated lifetime risk of renal cell carcinoma, which comprises the vast majority of renal tumors, is 1.34% (mortality risk, >0.50%) [2]. More frequent imaging also has resulted in a shift in the stage and size of renal cell carcinoma at time of detection, with 25% of tumors being less than 3 cm and 17% of patients presenting with metastases in the 1980s, compared with 5% and 32%, respectively, in the 1970s [3].

Although screening for renal cell carcinoma is not frequently practiced in the general population in the United States, one study of 6678 men aged 50 to 79 years who were screened with ultrasonography revealed a 0.33% incidence of renal tumors that were pathologically or clinically malignant [4]. The argument for screening is stronger for selected populations. Patients with von Hippel-Lindau disease and tuberous sclerosis have a significantly increased risk of developing renal cell carcinoma and therefore merit routine screening. Although controversial, screening is also often practiced for patients on kidney dialysis.

The diagnosis of renal cell carcinoma revolves around radiographic imaging. The four-part Bosniak classification for cystic renal masses, based on CT, has been helpful in defining an approach to renal lesions that are not completely solid [5]. Bosniak category 1 cystic renal masses have a thin wall, without septations or calcifications, a precontrast density of 0 to 20 Hounsfield units, and no enhancement with intravenous contrast material. Bosniak category 2 cystic renal masses also have thin walls but may have a few thin septations and calcifications. The precontrast density is still 0 to 20 Hounsfield units (except in hyperdense cysts), and there is no enhancement following intravenous administration of contrast material. Bosniak category 3 cystic renal masses have a slightly thickened wall and more numerous or thicker septations and calcifications. The precontrast density of these lesions remains at 0 to 20 Hounsfield units, and there is still no enhancement following the intravenous administration of contrast material. Bosniak category 4 cystic renal masses are characterized by thick or nodular walls, numerous or thick septations, coarse or chunky calcifications, a precontrast density of greater than 20 Hounsfield units (not including hyperdense cysts), enhancement with intravenous contrast material, or any combination of these features.

Solid renal masses are assumed to be malignant renal cell carcinomas unless radiographically definable characteristics or components of the history and physical examination strongly suggest another diagnosis. Invasive tests such as percutaneous biopsy or laparoscopic exploration are indicated for only a minority of lesions. For the patient in whom a renal mass has first been detected on intravenous urography, a renal ultrasonogram is usually the next step because most abnormalities are found to be simple renal cysts. CT, or in selected instances magnetic resonance imaging, is used to evaluate a lesion that on ultrasonographic imaging is not consistent with a simple renal cyst.

Following the diagnosis of renal cell carcinoma by CT scan or magnetic resonance imaging, further staging evaluation is necessary to plan for therapy. Common sites of metastases include the adrenal gland, lung, liver, bones, and brain. Because renal cell carcinoma has the unusual propensity for extension into the renal vein and vena cava, assessment for venous invasion is often an important part of the staging.

DIAGNOSIS AND DIFFERENTIAL DIAGNOSIS

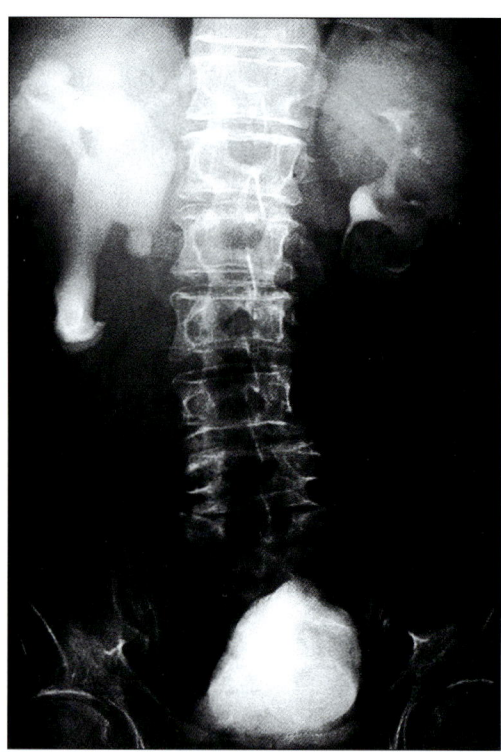

▶ FIGURE 2-1. Right kidney mass. The splaying of the intrarenal collecting system seen in this intravenous urogram indicates the presence of a mass in the right kidney. Findings on intravenous urography that suggest a renal mass include a bulge in the renal outline, displacement or splaying of the calices or infundibula, displacement of the entire kidney or alteration of its axis, and external impression upon the renal pelvis. Although a cyst rather than a solid lesion may be indicated if the interior of the lesion appears radiolucent during the tomographic portion of the intravenous urogram, any urogram suggesting a renal mass effect should be followed by further imaging studies.

Differential Diagnosis of Solid and Cystic Renal Masses

Radiographically probable benign cysts
  Simple cyst (*ie,* Bosniak category 1 cystic renal mass)
  Hyperdense cyst (homogeneous precontrast density >20 Hounsfield units, round and
    smaller than 3 cm, at least some extrarenal wall, and no enhancement with intravenous
    contrast material)
  Minimally complicated cyst (*ie,* Bosniak category 2 cystic renal mass)
  Polycystic kidneys (autosomal dominant and autosomal recessive)
  Infected cyst or renal abscess
Radiographically cystic masses possibly associated with malignancy
  Renal lesions in von Hippel-Lindau disease (cysts, renal cell carcinomas)
  Renal lesions in tuberous sclerosis (cysts, angiomyolipomas, renal cell carcinomas)
  Acquired cystic kidney disease (cysts, renal cell carcinomas)
  Multilocular cystic nephroma
  Truly indeterminate cyst (*ie,* Bosniak category 3 cystic renal mass)
Radiographically definable benign solid masses
  Angiomyolipoma
  Intrarenal or perirenal hematoma
  Anomalous renal tissue (hypertrophied column of Bertin, parenchymal defect or fetal lobulation,
    or dromedary hump)
  Lobar nephronia
  Xanthogranulomatous pyelonephritis
  Renal infarction
Radiographically probable malignant solid masses
  Renal cell carcinoma
  Intrarenal urothelial cell cancer
  Oncocytoma
  Renal lymphoma
  Metastases to kidney
  Other malignant solid masses
  Other benign solid masses

▶ FIGURE 2-2. Differential diagnosis of solid and cystic renal masses. Renal masses are classified according to their radiographic appearance. "Radiographically probable benign cysts" and "radiographically definable benign solid masses" usually can be determined with noninvasive imaging alone. "Radiographically cystic masses possibly associated with malignancy" can present difficult diagnostic dilemmas and often require invasive methods for diagnosis (which is often coexistent with therapy). "Radiographically probable malignant solid masses" usually require invasive diagnostic maneuvers only if a lesion other than renal cell carcinoma is expected.

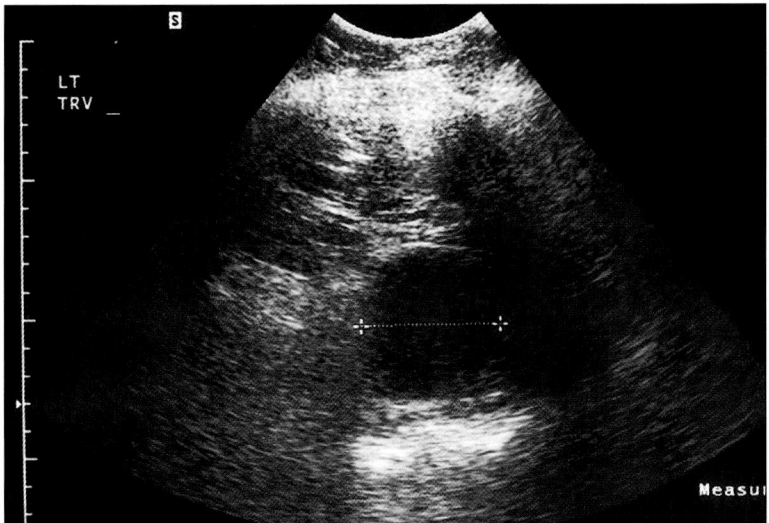

▶ **FIGURE 2-3.** Ultrasonogram of a simple renal cyst. This type of cyst is suggested on ultrasonography by increased through-transmission, an anechoic internal component of the cyst, an imperceptible extrarenal wall, and a sharply demarcated intrarenal wall. All four characteristics must be present to fit the strict definition of an ultrasonographically determined simple renal cyst. When these criteria are not met, further imaging is necessary. LT TRV—left transverse.

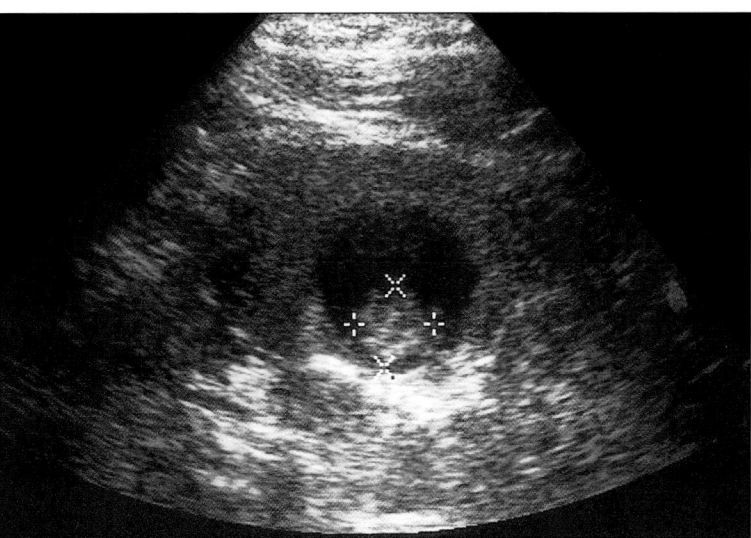

▶ **FIGURE 2-4.** Ultrasonogram of a complicated renal cyst. Echogenic foci in the wall, septa inside the cyst, nodularity of the wall, and a thickened wall all suggest a complicated cyst. A distinct nodule is seen at the base of this cyst. Because the ultrasonogram provides inadequate information about the nature of the lesion, further imaging is required. LT KID—left kidney.

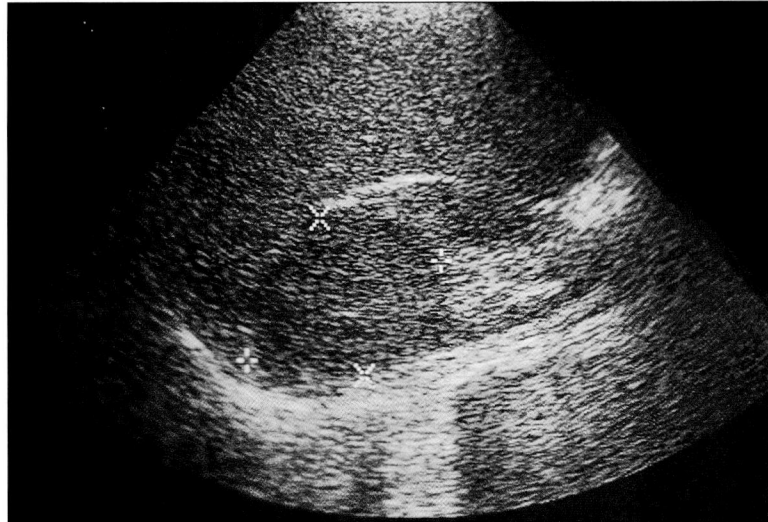

▶ **FIGURE 2-5.** Ultrasonogram of a solid renal mass. Most solid renal cell carcinomas are isoechoic, or slightly hyperechoic or hypoechoic, to the renal parenchyma. There is no increased through-transmission.

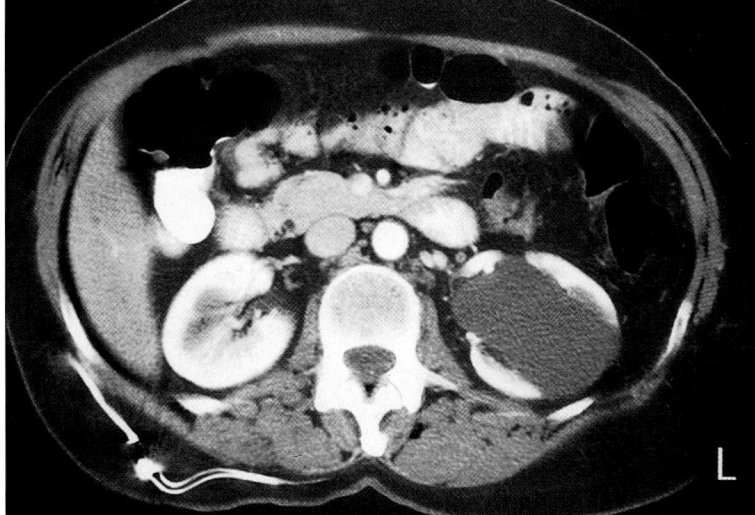

▶ **FIGURE 2-6.** Computed tomographic image of a benign simple cyst. This lesion belongs in the Bosniak category 1 classification of cystic renal masses. The wall is thin, no septations or calcifications are present, the precontrast density is 0 to 20 Hounsfield units, and there is no enhancement with intravenous contrast material. This cyst is highly unlikely ever to harbor a renal cell carcinoma, and follow-up is not necessary in the absence of other signs or symptoms. Such simple renal cysts are found by CT in 25% to 33% of patients older than 50 years of age [6,7]. L—left.

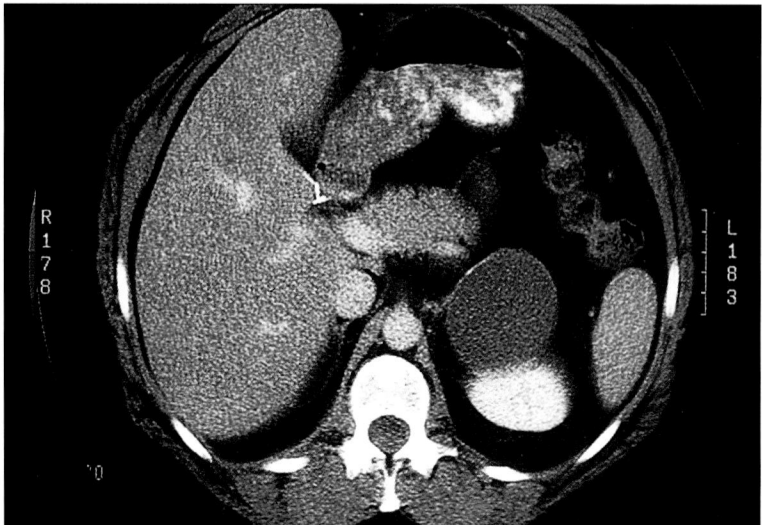

▶ **FIGURE 2-7.** Computed tomographic image of a minimally complicated renal cyst. At the anteromedial aspect of this cyst is a bright spot,
which was present on the precontrast scan as well. This spot represents a
peripheral calcification that excludes the cyst from consideration as a benign
simple cyst and places it into the Bosniak category 2 classification of cystic
renal masses. Lesions in this category have thin walls and may have a few
thin septations and calcifications. The precontrast density is still 0 to 20
Hounsfield units (except in hyperdense cysts), and there is no enhancement
following intravenous administration of contrast material. A hyperdense
cyst, also classified in Bosniak category 2, meets the criteria for a Bosniak
category 1 cystic renal mass except that the precontrast density is greater
than 20 Hounsfield units. Cystic renal masses in this category usually
require radiographic follow-up.

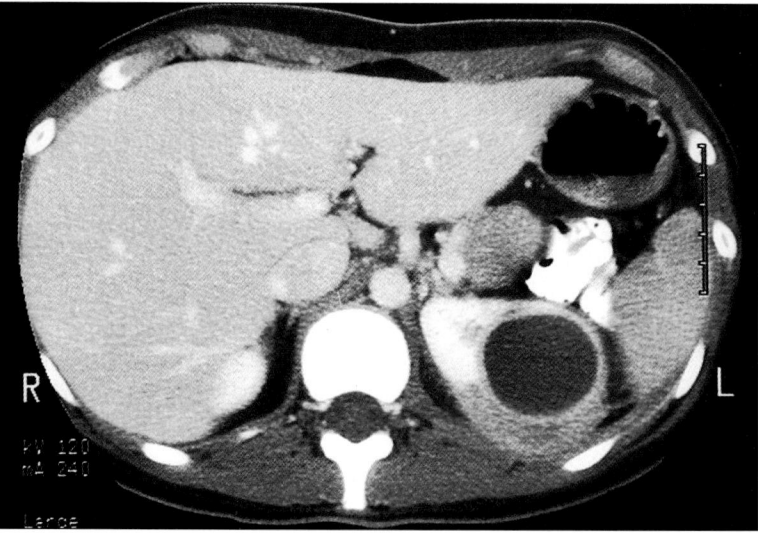

▶ **FIGURE 2-8.** Computed tomographic image of an indeterminate
renal cyst. This lesion has a thickened wall on the postcontrast CT. Such
lesions are placed in the Bosniak category 3 classification of cystic renal
masses, which includes those with a slightly thickened wall and more
numerous or thicker septations and calcifications. The precontrast density
of these lesions remains at 0 to 20 Hounsfield units, and there is still no
enhancement following the intravenous administration of contrast material. The incidence of malignancy in such lesions is approximately 50%.
L—left; R—right.

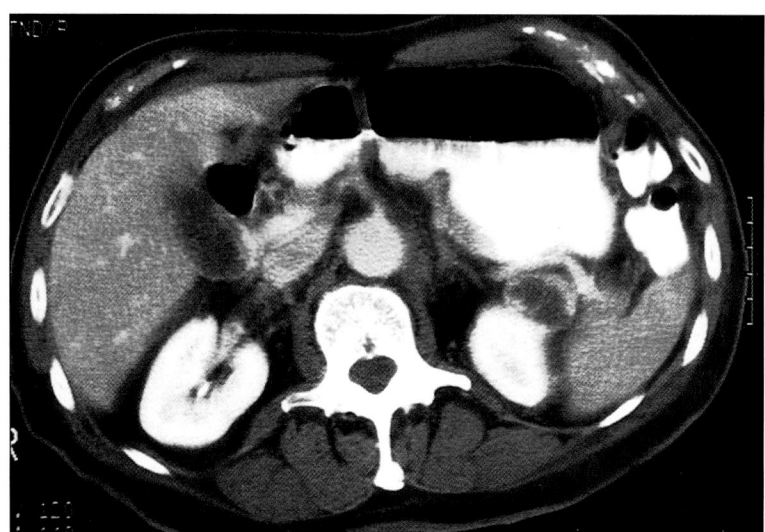

▶ **FIGURE 2-9.** Computed tomographic image of complicated cystic renal
mass. This and other Bosniak category 4 cystic renal masses are characterized
by thick or nodular walls, numerous or thick septations, coarse or chunky
calcifications, a precontrast density of greater than 20 Hounsfield units
(not including hyperdense cysts; *see* Fig. 2-7), enhancement with intravenous contrast material, or any combination of these features. These
Bosniak category 4 lesions are presumed malignant.

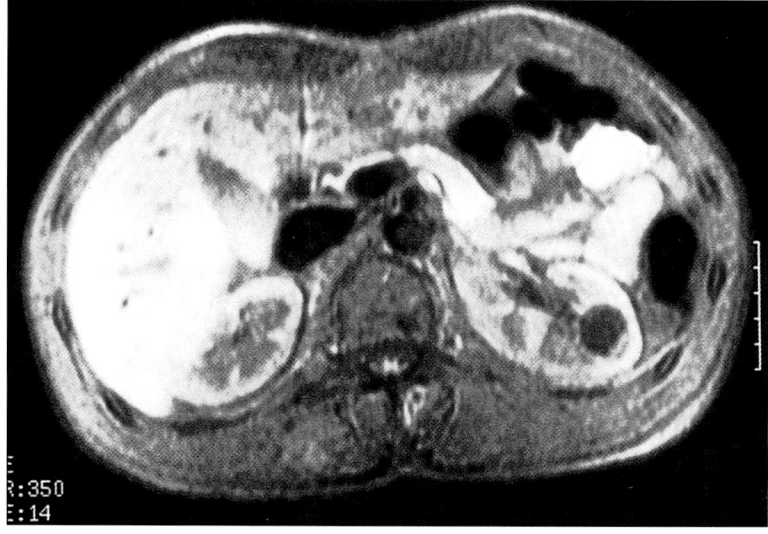

▶ **FIGURE 2-10.** Magnetic resonance image of cystic renal mass. Note
the brighter material lining the posterolateral aspect of the dark cyst in the
left kidney. Occasionally, magnetic resonance imaging provides superior
delineation of cyst characteristics, but it is most commonly used instead of
CT in patients with contrast material allergy, an elevated serum creatinine
level, or a hyperdense renal cyst in which the intercystic aspect of the wall
cannot be identified on CT. Images before and after intravenous administration of gadolinium-DTPA (diethylenetriaminepenta-acetic acid) are
recommended.

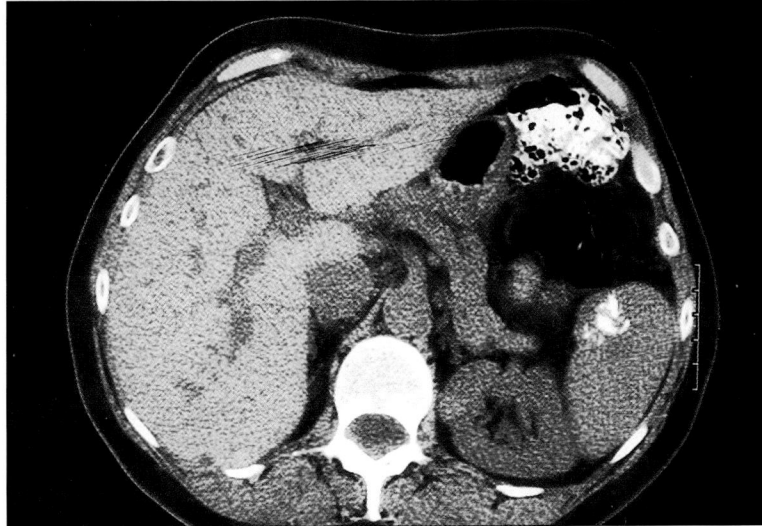

▶ **FIGURE 2-11.** Precontrast CT of a small renal cell carcinoma. The first part of a renal protocol CT consists of precontrast images obtained at 5-mm intervals and thicknesses. At the University of Michigan we currently use a helical scanner for all dedicated renal protocol scans because the entire abdomen can be imaged in one breath hold, which minimizes motion artifact. The volume of data in a helical CT can be reconstructed in any plane.

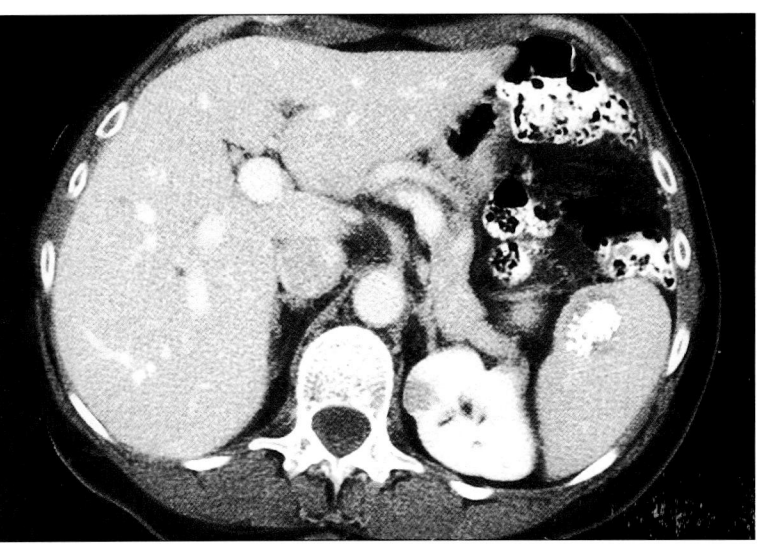

▶ **FIGURE 2-12.** Postcontrast CT of the same small renal cell carcinoma as in Figure 2-11. Following intravenous administration of contrast material, a small mass in the anteromedial aspect of the left kidney that enhances less than the surrounding parenchyma is visualized. Very little contour disruption is noted on the precontrast scan in Figure 2-11. For renal protocol CT, the postcontrast scan is obtained no less than 100 seconds after intravenous administration of contrast material to allow sufficient uptake by the renal parenchyma. Most renal cancers do enhance with contrast material, but somewhat less so than the surrounding normal renal parenchyma.

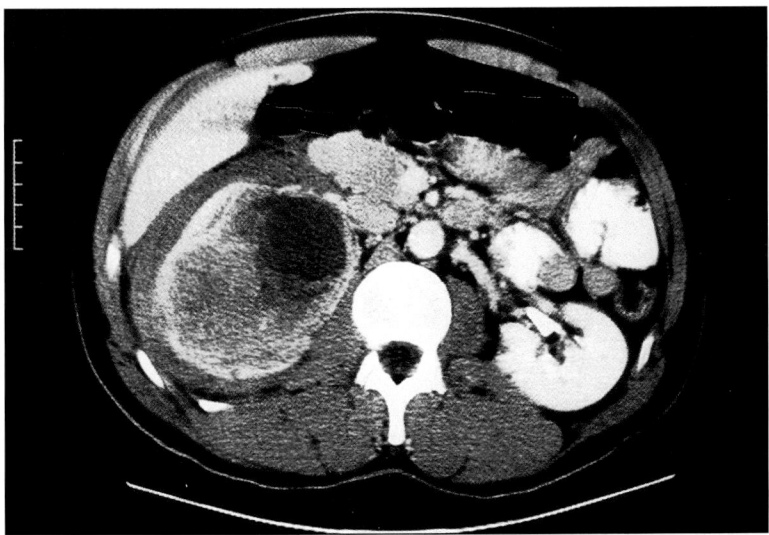

▶ **FIGURE 2-13.** Computed tomographic image of a large hemorrhagic renal cell carcinoma. In contrast to the small renal cell carcinoma in Figures 2-11 and 2-12, this large hemorrhagic renal cell carcinoma is easily visualized in the right kidney. Hemorrhagic necrosis is common in large renal cell carcinomas.

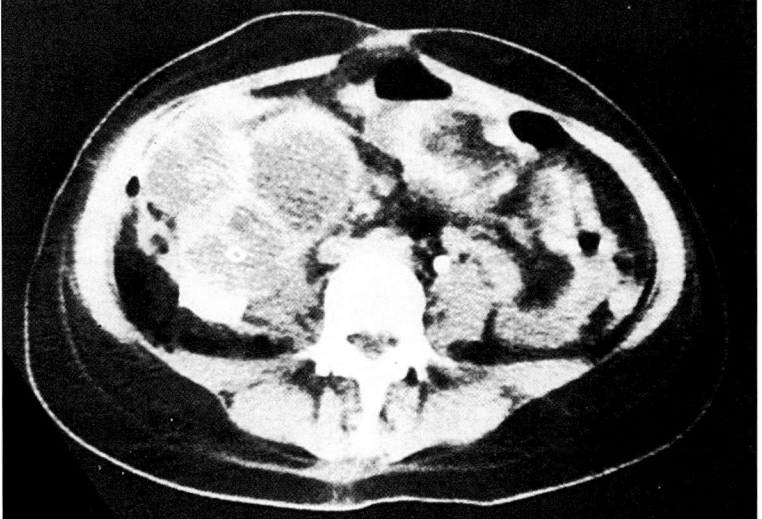

▶ **FIGURE 2-14.** Computed tomographic image of xanthogranulomatous pyelonephritis. A complex cystic mass displaying contrast enhancement and significant nodularity is seen to involve the right kidney. Because the patient had a fever and urinary tract infection, it was suspected that this lesion might represent xanthogranulomatous pyelonephritis instead of renal cell carcinoma, which can have an equally cystic and nodular appearance. Because of the severity of the patient's condition, nephrectomy was performed, and pathologic analysis confirmed the diagnosis of xanthogranulomatous pyelonephritis.

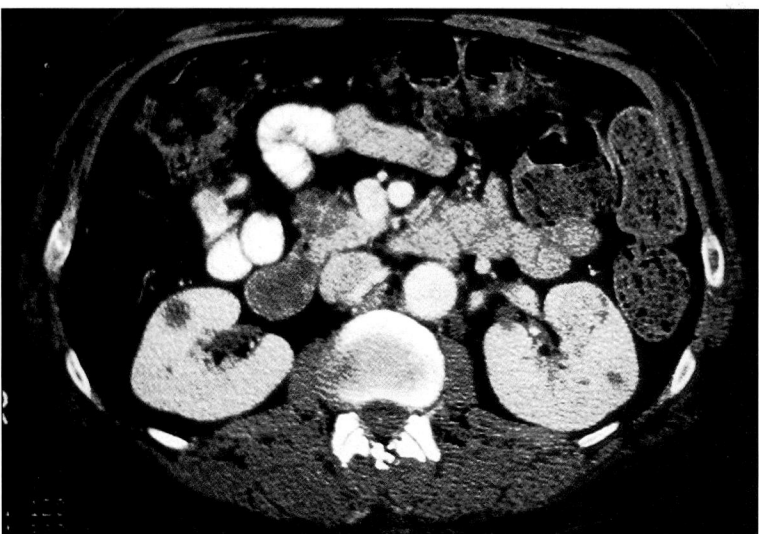

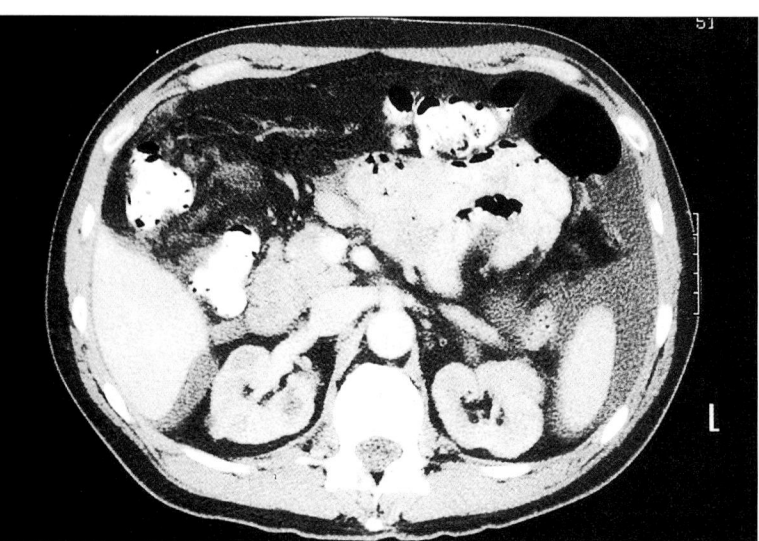

▶ **FIGURE 2-15.** Computed tomographic image of a renal cell carcinoma in the anteromedial portion of the left (L) kidney of a patient with von Hippel-Lindau disease. Renal lesions in von Hippel-Lindau disease include renal cysts and renal cell carcinomas. The latter often occur in the walls of cysts and may be highly difficult to diagnose. The sensitivity of CT for renal cell carcinomas smaller than 2 cm in patients with von Hippel-Lindau disease is 47% to 100%, compared with that of ultrasonography, which is 0% to 58% [8]. Small renal cell carcinomas complicating renal cysts may also occur in patients with tuberous sclerosis.

▶ **FIGURE 2-16.** Computed tomographic image demonstrating a small renal cell carcinoma in the lateral aspect of the right (R) kidney. This hemodialysis patient has acquired cystic disease of the kidney; note the multiple small cysts in both kidneys, including one adjacent to the small renal cell carcinoma. After 5 to 10 years of dialysis, up to 90% of patients with end-stage renal disease have acquired renal cystic disease. Renal cell carcinoma may develop in association with cysts in 1% to 2% of patients [9]. This prevalence of renal cell carcinoma appears to be greater than that seen in screening or autopsy studies, but the clinical usefulness of screening is debated [10,11]. L—left.

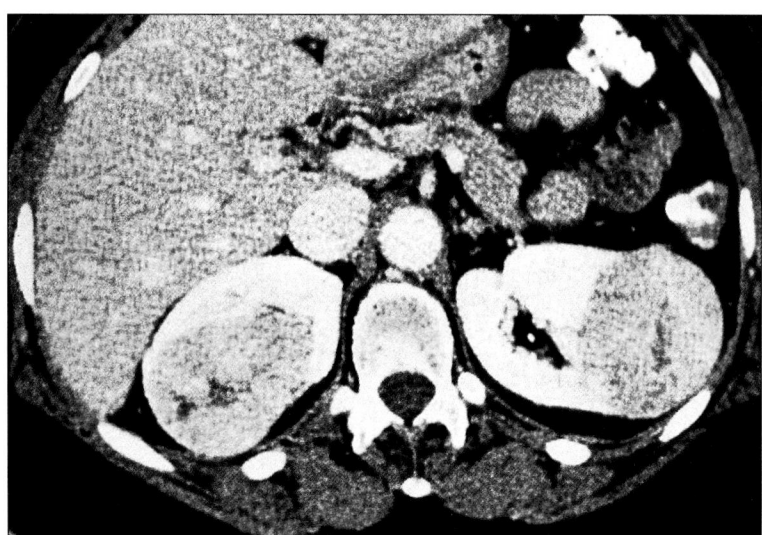

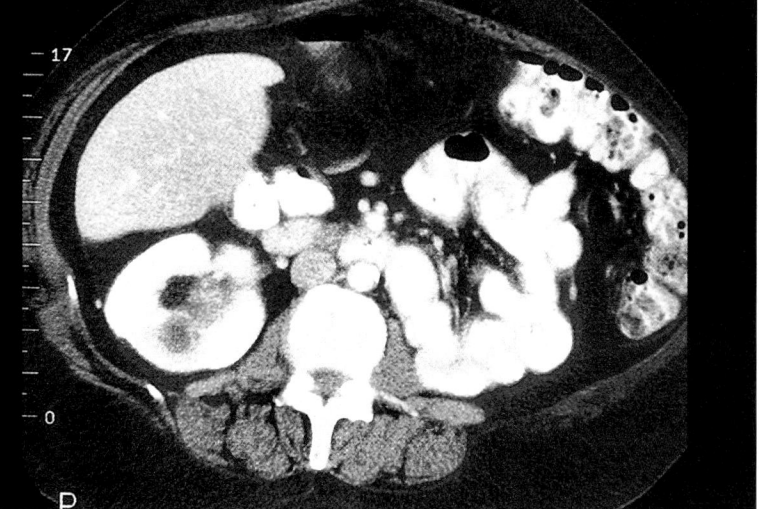

▶ **FIGURE 2-17.** Computed tomographic image of bilateral oncocytomas. Classically, oncocytomas on CT have "central scars," as seen in both of these lesions. This appearance, however, may be noted in renal cell carcinomas as well. To be considered an oncocytoma histologically, the neoplastic renal cells must be large epithelial cells with finely granular eosinophilic cytoplasm and a cytologic appearance consistent with a grade 1 neoplasm. More aggressive-appearing cells should prompt the diagnosis of an oncocytic renal neoplasm rather than oncocytoma. Whereas the latter lesions are uniformly benign, the former may be associated with metastases.

▶ **FIGURE 2-18.** Computed tomographic image of coexisting intrarenal pelvic and parenchymal lesions in the right kidney. When a mass in the collecting system is noted together with a parenchymal renal lesion, renal cell carcinoma invading the collecting system must be distinguished from transitional cell carcinoma invading the renal parenchyma. Cytologic and ureteroscopic studies are useful in making the distinction.

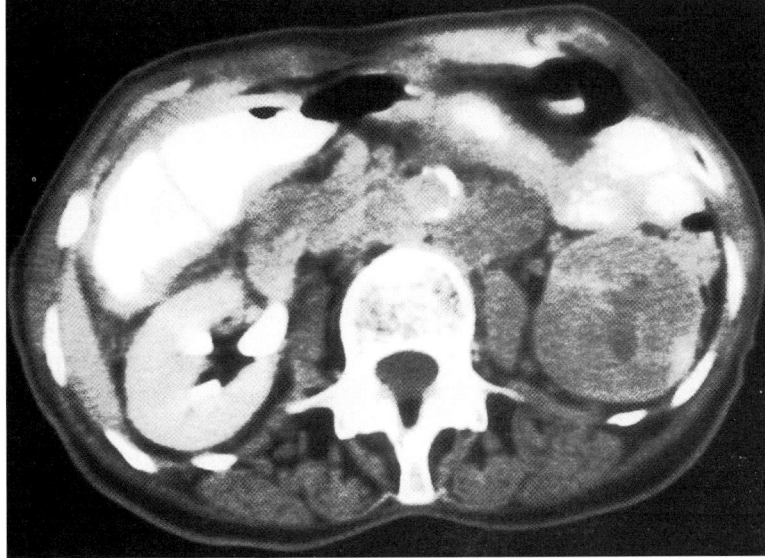

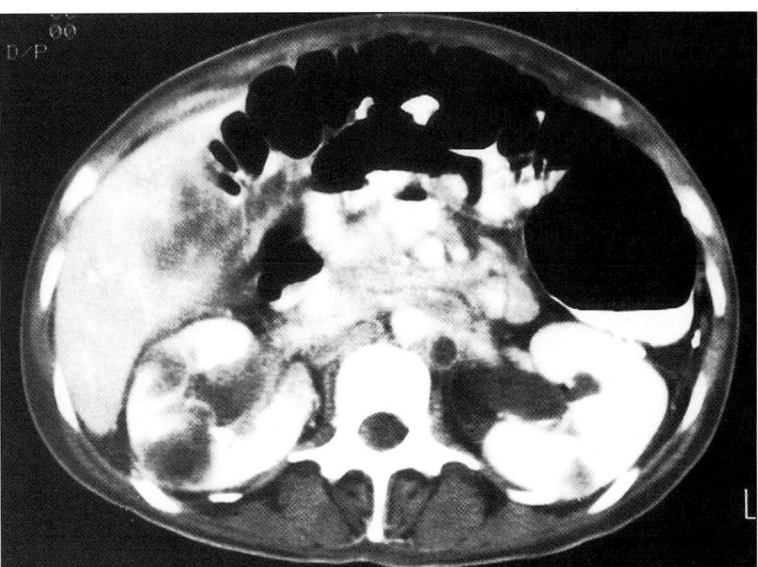

▶ **FIGURE 2-19.** Computed tomographic image of a left renal lymphoma. Approximately 5% of patients with lymphoma are noted to have renal involvement. The radiographic appearance may be of multiple or solitary nodular lesions or of diffuse lymphomatous infiltrates within the kidney, as in this patient. In this scan, adenopathy coexists in the left retroperitoneum, which aids in the diagnosis. Percutaneous renal biopsy may be required if lymphoma has not already been documented at another site.

▶ **FIGURE 2-20.** Computed tomographic image of liver metastases and bilateral renal metastases. Multiple abnormal foci within the kidney, especially in a patient with a known other primary cancer, raise the suspicion of metastases to the kidney. This patient had metastatic colon cancer with involvement of the liver, both kidneys, and the lung. Metastases to the kidney are usually isodense to the kidney on the precontrast scan and enhance only slightly with the intravenous administration of contrast material. L—left. (*Courtesy of* R. Cohan, MD.)

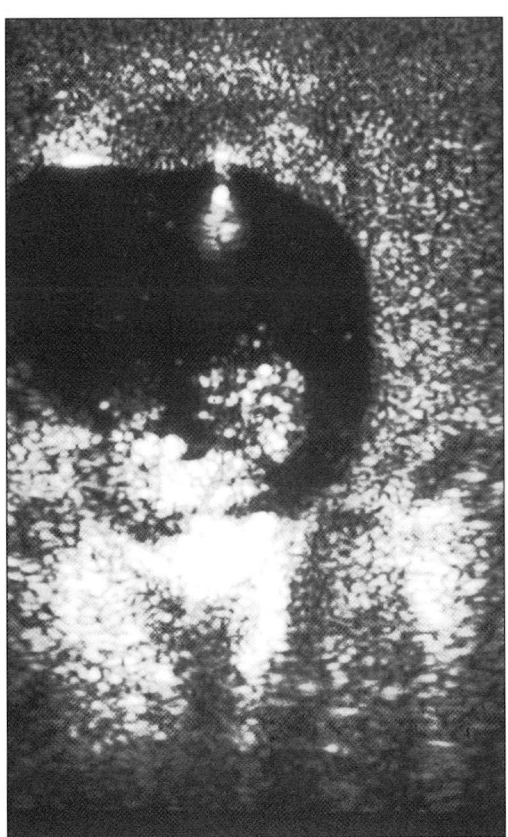

▶ **FIGURE 2-21.** Intraoperative ultrasonogram of a complicated renal cyst. Intraoperative ultrasonography is particularly useful in the assessment of an indeterminate cystic renal mass, in planning for partial nephrectomy, or in patients with multiple renal lesions (such as those with von Hippel-Lindau disease). Compared with transcutaneous ultrasonography, intraoperative ultrasonography demonstrates lesions with greatly increased clarity. Compare the appearance of this study with that of the same patient in Figure 2-4.

Histologic Classification of Renal Cell Tumors

Renal carcinoma
  Clear cell
  Chromophil
    Eosinophil
    Basophil
  Chromophobe
    Typical
    Eosinophil
Carcinoma of Bellini's collecting ducts
Renal oncocytoma

▶ **FIGURE 2-22.** Histologic classification of renal cell tumors. Also to be considered are renal adenomas. Although defined in the past as tumors less than 3 cm in diameter that have the histologic appearance of renal cell carcinoma, currently many uropathologists favor the term *renal epithelial tumor of low malignant potential* for renal cell neoplasms less than 3 cm in diameter only if the cells are cytologically within normal limits. (*Adapted from* Eble [12].)

Staging of Suspected Renal Cell Carcinoma

Required studies
  CT or magnetic resonance imaging of abdomen
  Chest radiograph
Preferred studies
  Required studies plus the following
  Complete blood count
  Serum creatinine level
  Serum calcium level
  Liver function tests
Optional studies
  Required studies, preferred studies, plus the following
    Venous imaging if tumor thrombus is suspected
    Bone scintigraphy if serum alkaline phosphatase level is elevated or if musculoskeletal
      symptoms are present
    Magnetic resonance imaging or coned-down radiographs of any suspicious sites on
      bone scintigraphy
    CT of head if neurologic symptoms are present
    CT of chest if abnormalities are present on chest radiograph
    Percutaneous renal biopsy or aspiration if lymphoma, metastasis to kidney, or infection
      is suspected; for confirmation of histology in patient with metastatic disease; or for a
      questionable lesion in a patient with poor surgical risk

▶ FIGURE 2-23. Staging of suspected renal cell carcinoma. The required tests are the minimum necessary to allow appropriate treatment of renal cell carcinoma. These tests would be sufficient in a patient with a small peripheral renal cell carcinoma in whom metastases or venous invasion would be extremely unlikely. These, plus the preferred tests, constitute the staging work-up in most patients. The complete blood count is used to screen for polycythemia or anemia, the serum creatinine level provides an indication of renal function, and serum calcium levels and liver function tests are used to screen for paraneoplastic syndrome, which is associated with renal cell carcinoma. Tests listed as optional are required for further staging in selected patients.

TNM Classification of Renal Cell Carcinoma (1997)

Primary tumor (T)
  TX   Primary tumor cannot be assessed
  T0   No evidence of primary tumor
  T1   Tumor ≤7 cm in greatest dimension, limited to the kidney
  T2   Tumor ≥7 cm in greatest dimension, limited to the kidney
  T3   Tumor extends into major veins or invades the adrenal gland or perinephric tissues,
       but not beyond Gerota's fascia
  T3a Tumor invades the adrenal gland or perinephric tissues, but not beyond Gerota's fascia
  T3b Tumor grossly extends into the renal vein(s) or vena cava below the diaphragm
  T3c Tumor grossly extends into the renal vein(s) or vena cava above the diaphragm
  T4   Tumor invades beyond Gerota's fascia
Regional lymph nodes (N)*
  NX   Regional lymph nodes cannot be assessed
  N0   No regional lymph node metastases
  N1   Metastasis in a single regional lymph node
  N2   Metastases in more than one regional lymph node
Distant metastases (M)
  MX   Distant metastases cannot be assessed
  M0   No distant metastases
  M1   Distant metastases
Stage grouping

	T	N	M
Stage I	T1	N0	M0
Stage II	T2	N0	M0
Stage III	T1–2	N1	M0
	T3	N0–1	M0
Stage IV	T4	N0–1	M0
	Any	N2	M0
	Any	Any	M1

*Not affected by laterality. Regional lymph nodes include renal hilar, paracaval, aortic (para-aortic), periaortic, lateral aortic), and NOS retroperitoneal.

▶ FIGURE 2-24. Tumor, nodes, and metastases (TNM) classification of renal parenchymal tumors [13]. Preoperative and postoperative staging of tumors using the TNM system is encouraged. NOS–not otherwise specified.

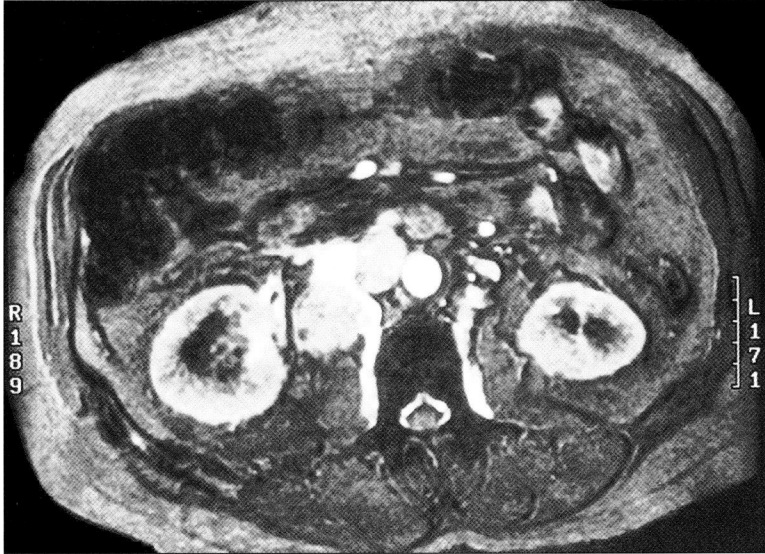

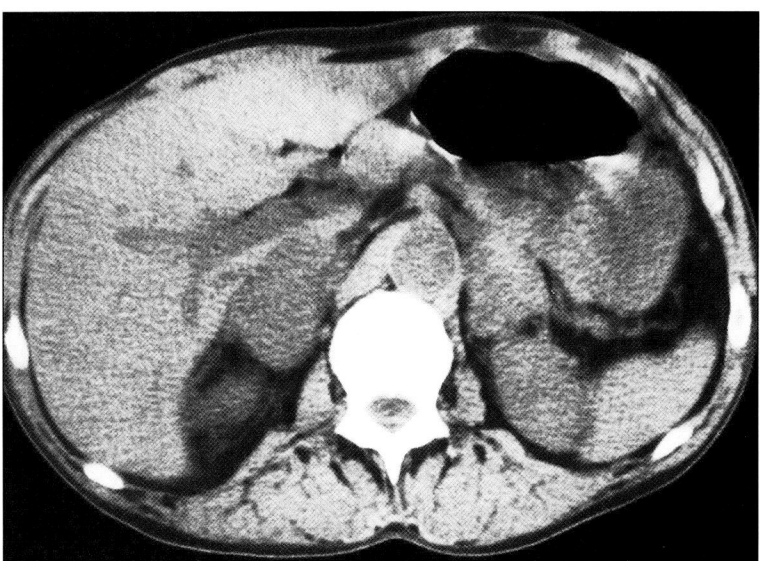

▶ **FIGURE 2-25.** Magnetic resonance image demonstrating nodal metastases from renal cell carcinoma. A large retrocaval lymph node is seen adjacent to the right kidney, which shows involvement by renal cell carcinoma. CT and magnetic resonance imaging usually can clearly define adenopathy in excess of 1 cm.

▶ **FIGURE 2-26.** Computed tomographic image demonstrating large bilateral adrenal metastases from renal cell carcinoma. The ipsilateral adrenal gland, which is contained within Gerota's fascia along with the kidney, is the most common site of extranodal organ involvement by renal cell carcinoma.

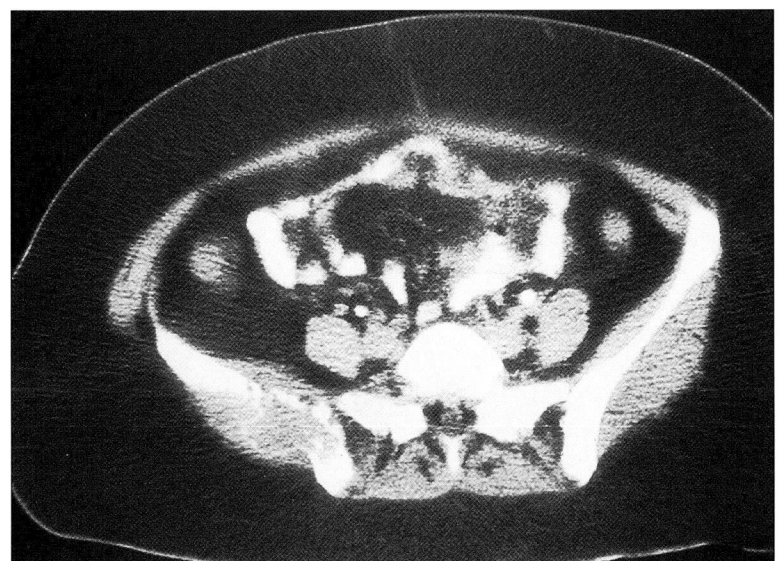

▶ **FIGURE 2-27.** Computed tomographic image demonstrating an osteolytic lesion in the right ileum that represents bone metastases from renal cell carcinoma. This scan was obtained for other reasons; bone staging in renal cell carcinoma is usually performed with bone scintigraphy initially if the serum alkaline phosphatase level is elevated or if musculoskeletal symptoms are present. Magnetic resonance imaging studies or coned-down radiographs of any suspicious sites on bone scan are subsequently obtained.

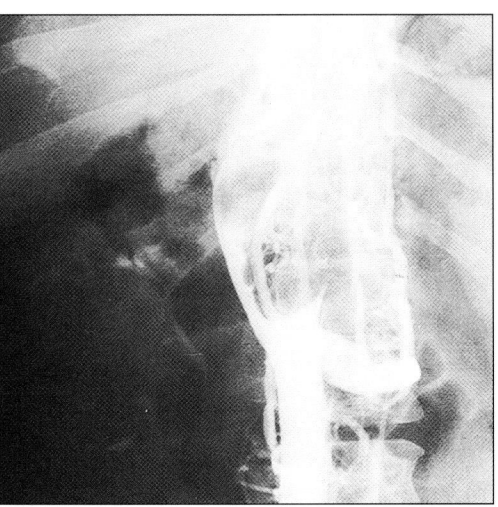

▶ **FIGURE 2-28.** Venogram showing venous tumor thrombus. For many years venography has been the standard method of assessing for venous invasion by renal cell carcinoma, but the use of other modalities has reduced its role. The tumor thrombus appears as a filling defect in the contrast-filled inferior vena cava.

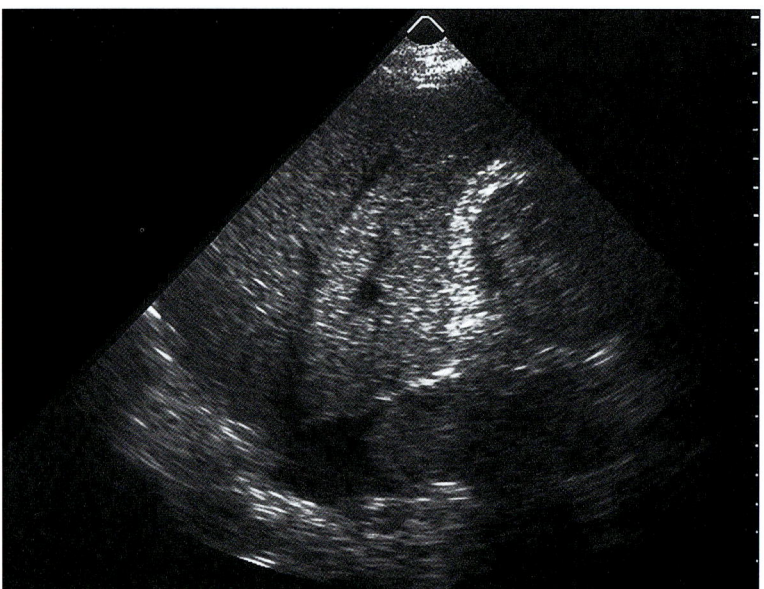

▶ **FIGURE 2-29.** Ultrasonogram revealing a venous tumor thrombus extending to the level of the liver (tissue density within the otherwise anechoic vena cava). Transcutaneous ultrasonography can be used to assess the suprarenal inferior vena cava (IVC), and transesophageal echocardiography can detect supradiaphragmatic extension of the tumor thrombus. The use of Doppler ultrasonography to determine blood flow may increase the sensitivity of detecting venous tumor thrombus.

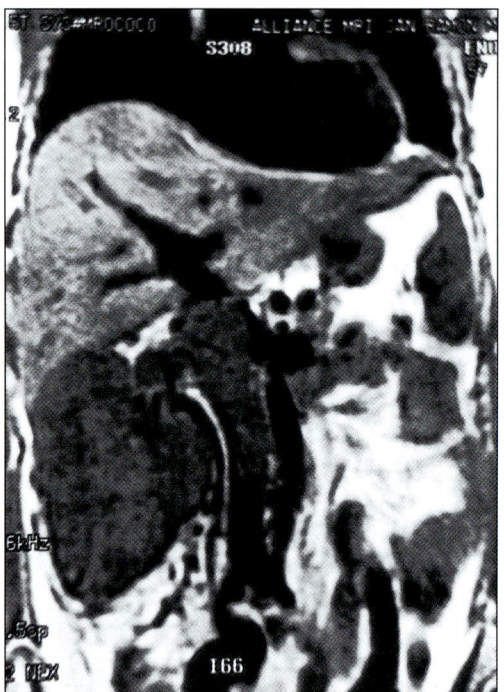

▶ **FIGURE 2-30.** Magnetic resonance image demonstrating tumor thrombus extending into the liver. Magnetic resonance imaging provides very sensitive contrast between the flowing venous blood and a stationary intraluminal mass, without the use of contrast material. On a standard T_1-weighted image, as shown here, flowing blood appears black. In this image, the thrombus from the right kidney extends upward to just below the level of the liver. Renal vein involvement by renal cell carcinoma may be noted in up to 39% of patients, with as many as 25% having caval extension of the tumor thrombus [14].

REFERENCES

1. Parker SL, Tong T, Bolden S, Wingo PA: Cancer statistics, 1996. *CA Cancer J Clin* 1996, 65:5–27.

2. Ries LA, Kosary CK, Hankey BF, *et al.*: SEER Cancer Statistics Review, 1973–1994. NIH Publication No. 97-2789. Bethesda, MD: National Cancer Institute, P. 222, 1997.

3. Smith SJ, Bosniak MA, Megibow AJ, *et al.*: Renal cell carcinoma: earlier discovery and increased detection. *Radiology* 1989, 170:699–703.

4. Koeneman KS, Cote WL, Martin DJ, *et al.*: Renal screening in an older population with pathologic correlation [abstract 1276]. *J Urol* 1997, 157(suppl):327.

5. Bosniak MA: The current radiographic approach to renal cysts. *Radiology* 1986, 158:1–10.

6. Laucks SP Jr, McLachlan MSF: Aging and simple cysts of the kidney. *Br J Radiol* 1981, 54:12–14.

7. Tada S, Yamagishi J, Kobayashi H, *et al.*: The incidence of simple renal cyst by computed tomography. *Clin Radiol* 1983, 34:437–439.

8. Jamis-Dow CA, Choyke PL, Jennings SB, *et al.*: Small (≤3 cm) renal masses: detection with CT versus US and pathologic correlation. *Radiology* 1996, 198:785–788.

9. Matson MA, Cohen EP: Acquired cystic kidney disease: occurrence, prevalence, and renal cancers. *Medicine* 1990, 69:217–226.

10. Chandhoke PS, Torrence RJ, Clayman RV, Rothstein M: Acquired cystic disease of the kidney: a management dilemma. *J Urol* 1992, 147:969–974.

11. Ishikawa I: Re: Acquired cystic disease of the kidney: a management dilemma [letter]. *J Urol* 1993, 149:1148.

12. Eble JN: Neoplasms of the kidney. In *Urologic Surgical Pathology*. Edited by Bostwick DG, Eble JN. St. Louis: Mosby; 1997:82–147.

13. *AJCC Cancer Staging Manual*, edn 5. Edited by Fleming ID, Cooper JS, Henson DE, *et al.* Philadelphia: Lippincott-Raven; 1997:1–294.

14. Horan JJ, Robertson CN, Choyke PL, *et al.*: The detection of renal carcinoma extension into the renal vein and inferior vena cava: a prospective comparison of venacavography and magnetic resonance imaging. *J Urol* 1989, 142:943–948.

Molecular Genetics of Sporadic and Familial Renal Cell Carcinoma

W. Marston Linehan

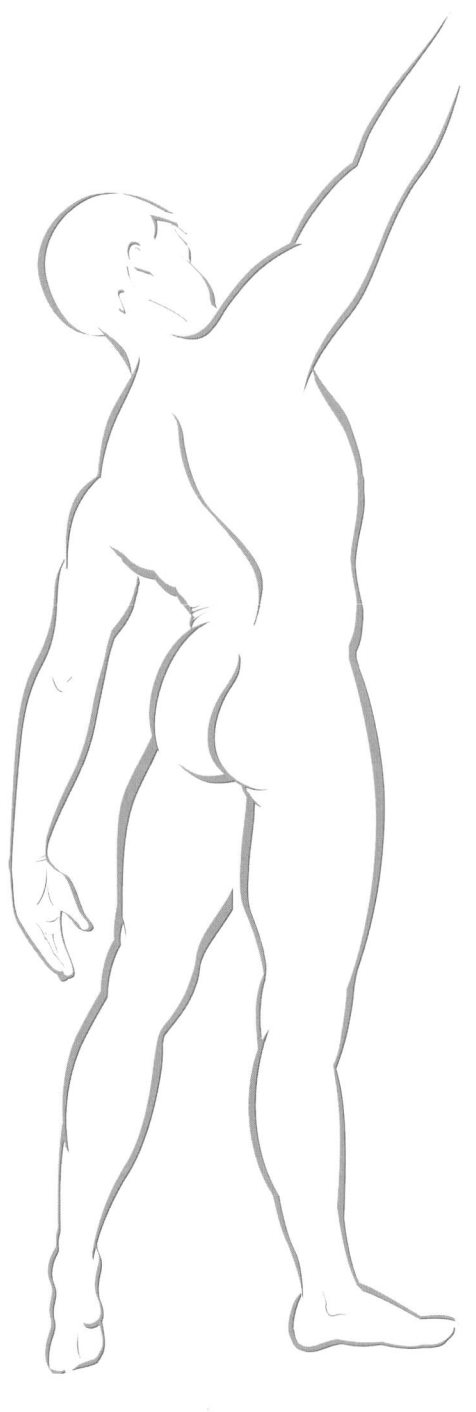

Kidney cancer affects nearly 28,000 Americans each year and is responsible for 12,000 deaths annually in the United States. Kidney cancer can occur as localized, locally advanced, or advanced disease. Little is known about the specific cause of kidney cancer, although as with smoking, a number of associations have been noted. Kidney cancer can occur in both a hereditary as well as a nonhereditary sporadic form [1]. When two or more members of the same family are found to have kidney cancer, screening of other at-risk individuals in the family is recommended.

Studies to locate the site of a potential kidney cancer gene detected a consistent segment loss on chromosome 3 in tumor tissue from patients with clear-cell kidney cancer. Further analysis detected a potential location of a kidney cancer gene on chromosome 3 [2].

To localize the gene for clear-cell kidney cancer further, scientists initiated studies of a hereditary form of renal carcinoma associated with von Hippel-Lindau (VHL) disease [3,4]. Genetic linkage analysis was used to localize the *VHL* gene to the short arm of chromosome 3. Subsequent genetic and physical mapping identified the *VHL* gene at the 3p25 locus on chromosome 3 [5]. Inactivating mutations in the *VHL* gene have been detected in the germline of affected individuals [6,7].

The *VHL* gene mutations were detected in a high percentage of tumors from patients with clear-cell renal carcinoma [8,9]. *VHL* gene abnormalities have not been detected in papillary renal carcinoma. These findings provide the basis for a molecular genetic classification of kidney cancer (*ie*, papillary vs clear-cell), with clear-cell renal carcinoma being characterized by a mutation in the *VHL* gene. In addition, *VHL* gene abnormalities have been detected in formalin-fixed tissues and in tissue aspirates [10,11].

Hereditary papillary renal carcinoma (HPRC) is an autosomal-dominant hereditary cancer syndrome in which patients inherit a predisposition to develop bilateral, multifocal papillary renal carcinoma [12,13].

Genetic linkage studies performed at the National Cancer Institute identified a locus on the long arm of chromosome 7 as the site for the *HPRC* gene. Subsequently, the *MET* gene was identified as the *HPRC* gene. Although the *VHL* gene has the characteristics of a classic tumor-suppressor gene of the Knudson model, the *MET* gene fits the characteristics of an oncogene. Mutations in the tyrosine kinase domain of the *MET* gene have been detected in the germline of affected individuals [14]. It is thought that mutations in the *MET* gene, which is the receptor for the ligand hepatocyte growth factor, result in the development of the papillary renal carcinomas detected in these patients.

Recently, five families have been identified in which two or more members are affected with renal oncocytoma. Affected individuals, who may be asymptomatic, are likely to develop bilateral, multifocal oncocytoma. These findings raise the possibility that there may be a genetic basis for the predisposition to develop renal oncocytoma [15]. Studies are currently in progress to identify such a genetic basis for familial renal oncocytoma.

CANCER GENES

Hereditary Forms of Kidney Tumors

VHL
HPRC
FRO

▶ **FIGURE 3-1.** Hereditary forms of kidney tumors. Kidney cancer, like prostate cancer, bladder cancer, colon cancer, and breast cancer, occurs in both a hereditary and a nonhereditary sporadic form. There are three forms of hereditary renal cancer: von Hippel-Lindau (VHL), hereditary papillary renal carcinoma (HPRC), and familial renal oncocytoma (FRO) [1,12,15].

Cancer Genes

Tumor suppressor gene
  "Two-hit" hypothesis
  Inactivation of *both* copies
  Resulting in loss of growth inhibition
Oncogene
  "Single" hit
  Activating mutation
  Resulting in gain of growth advantage

▶ **FIGURE 3-2.** Cancer genes. There are two basic types of cancer genes, both of which are found in kidney cancer. A tumor-suppressor gene is a cancer gene in which transformation (cancer) may occur after both copies of the tumor-suppressor gene are inactivated. Inactivation of both copies of a tumor-suppressor gene results in loss of growth inhibition (*ie*, unregulated growth). This is the basis of the Knudson "two-hit" model in which both copies of a gene, such as the retinoblastoma gene or the von Hippel-Lindau gene, are inactivated in retinoblastoma or clear-cell kidney cancer, respectively [16,17]. An oncogene is a dominantly acting gene in which a "single hit" mutation activates the gene, resulting in a gain of growth advantage that is characteristic of a cancer cell.

Kidney Cancer Genes

VHL gene
  Tumor suppressor gene (loss of function)
  VHL, HRCC
  Sporadic clear-cell renal carcinoma
MET gene
  Proto-oncogene (gain of function)
  HPRC
  Sporadic papillary renal carcinoma

▶ **FIGURE 3-3.** Kidney cancer genes. The *VHL* gene is a tumor-suppressor gene of the classic Knudson model. *VHL* gene mutations are found in the germline of affected individuals with von Hippel-Lindau disease and in nonhereditary, sporadic clear-cell renal carcinoma [1,9,18]. The *MET* gene is a dominantly acting (gain of function) oncogene that is mutated in the germline of patients with hereditary papillary renal carcinoma and in some forms of sporadic papillary renal carcinoma [14]. HPRC—hereditary papillary renal carcinoma; HRCC—hereditary renal cell carcinoma.

Clinical Features of von Hippel-Lindau Disease

Bilateral kidney tumors, cysts
Cerebellar or spinal hemangioblastomas
Retinal angiomas
ELST
Pancreatic cyst, tumors
Pheochromocytoma
Epididymal cystadenoma

▶ **FIGURE 3-4.** Clinical features of von Hippel-Lindau (VHL) disease. VHL disease is a hereditary cancer syndrome in which affected individuals are at risk for developing bilateral, multifocal, early-onset renal tumors. Affected individuals are also at risk for developing tumors in a number of organs including cerebellar or spinal hemangioblastomas, retinal angiomas, endolymphatic sac tumors (in the inner ear), pancreatic cysts and tumors, pheochromocytomas, and epididymal cystadenomas [19]. ELST—endolymphatic sac tumors.

Clinical Evaluation of von Hippel-Lindau Disease

MRI of the brain and spine
Abdominal CT and ultrasound
Ophthalmologic evaluation
Audiometric and ENT evaluation
Testicular ultrasound
Metabolic evaluation (pheochromocytoma)

▶ **FIGURE 3-5.** Clinical evaluation of von Hippel-Lindau (VHL) disease. This evaluation includes magnetic resonance imaging (MRI) of the brain and spine; abdominal CT and ultrasound; ophthalmologic evaluation; audiometric and ear, nose, and throat (ENT) evaluation; testicular ultrasound; and metabolic evaluation to rule out the presence of pheochromocytoma [19]. MEN—multiple endocrine neoplasia type II.

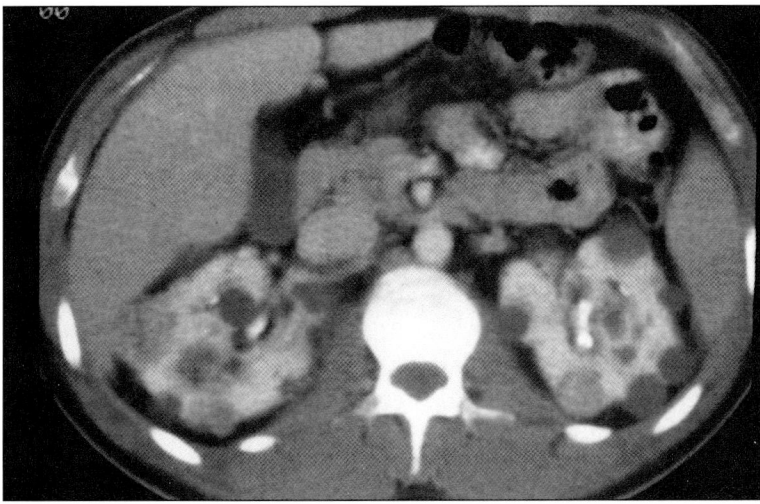

▶ **FIGURE 3-6.** Abdominal CT image of patient with von Hippel-Lindau (VHL) disease. Patients with VHL disease often develop bilateral, multifocal, early-onset renal tumors and cysts. Clinical evaluation includes abdominal CT and renal ultrasound. Nephron-sparing surgery is often recommended when possible to preserve as much normal renal parenchyma as possible [20]. In some patients there may be hundreds of microscopic renal tumors [21]. Renal tumors in patients with VHL may occur as early as the teenage years. (*From* Linehan and Klausner [22]; with permission.)

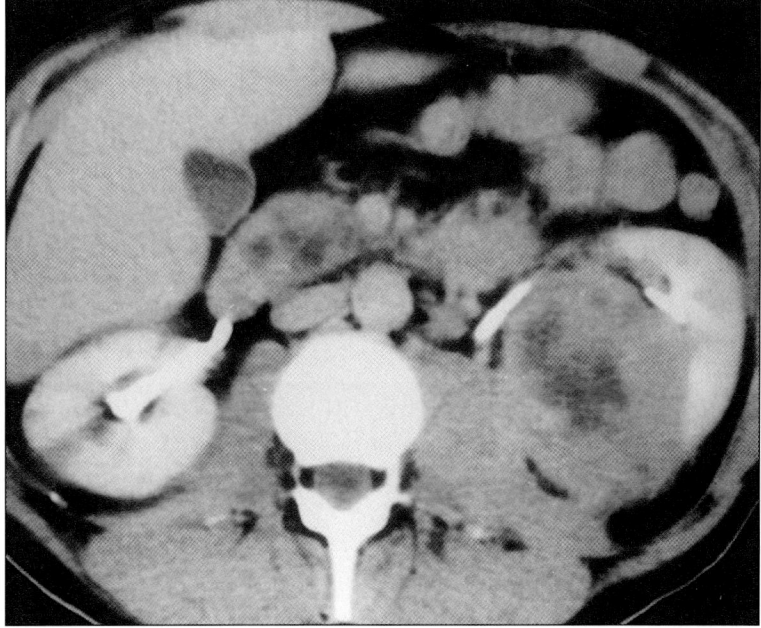

▶ **FIGURE 3-7.** Tumor illustrated by CT. The renal tumors in patients with von Hippel-Lindau (VHL) disease are malignant and can be large. These renal tumors are uniformly clear-cell renal carcinoma [23]. Historically, 35% to 45% of patients with VHL died of metastatic renal cell carcinoma when it was not diagnosed and treated early [19]. (*From* Linehan and Klausner [22]; with permission.)

▶ **FIGURE 3-8.** Neuroendocrine tumor. Patients with von Hippel-Lindau (VHL) disease are at risk for developing pancreatic cysts and tumors [24]. The pancreatic manifestations in VHL include pancreatic cysts, microcystic adenoma, and neuroendocrine tumors. The neuroendocrine tumors are solid, vascular, malignant, and can metastasize. Surgical resection is often recommended when the solid pancreatic tumors reach 3 cm in size. (*From* Linehan and Klausner [22]; with permission.)

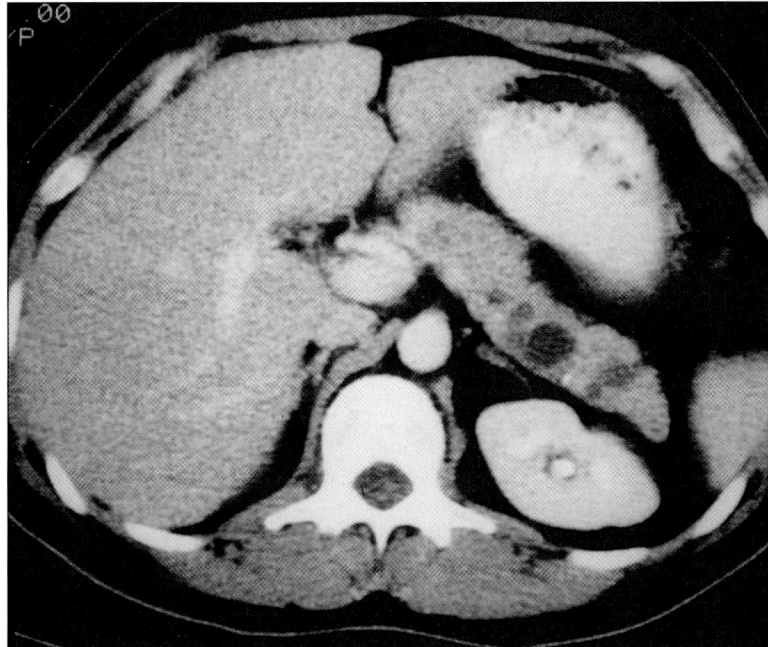

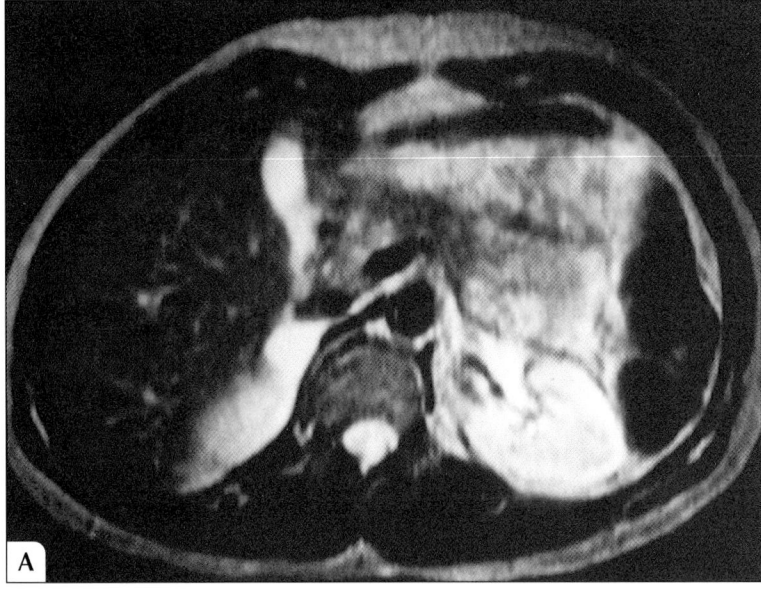 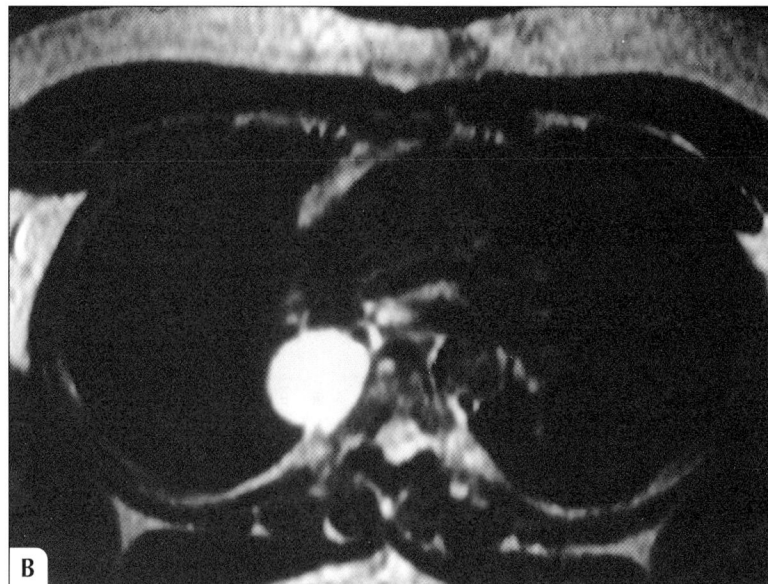

▶ **FIGURE 3-9.** Tumors in the adrenal medulla. Patients with von Hippel-Lindau (VHL) disease are at risk for developing tumors in the adrenal medulla (pheochromocytoma). These adrenal tumors can be bilateral (**A**) or extra-adrenal (**B**) [19]. Clinical evaluation of patients with VHL disease involves measurement of serum and urinary catecholamine levels. Clonidine suppression or glucagon stimulation tests may be used in patients in whom the diagnosis or metabolic activity of an adrenal mass is indeterminant [25,26]. Treatment of metabolically active pheochromocytomas involves surgical resection of the tumor. Recently, laparoscopic adrenalectomy has been found to be a useful method for surgical management of VHL-associated pheochromocytomas in selected individuals [27]. Because pheochromocytomas can occur in patients with VHL disease before the age of 10, early screening of at-risk individuals is encouraged [19]. (*From* Linehan and Klausner [22]; with permission.)

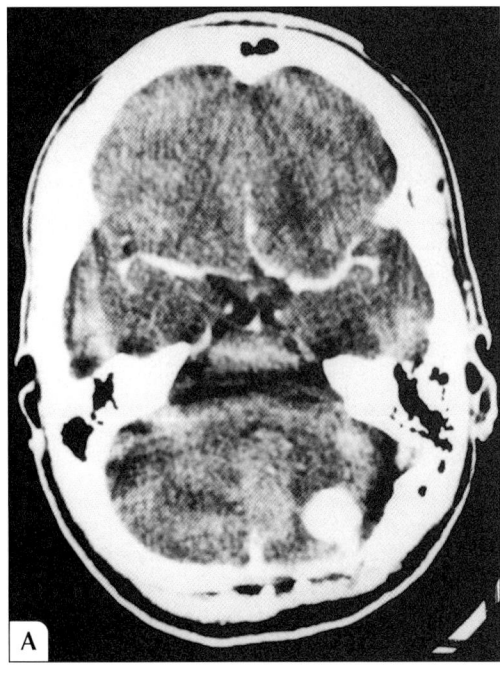 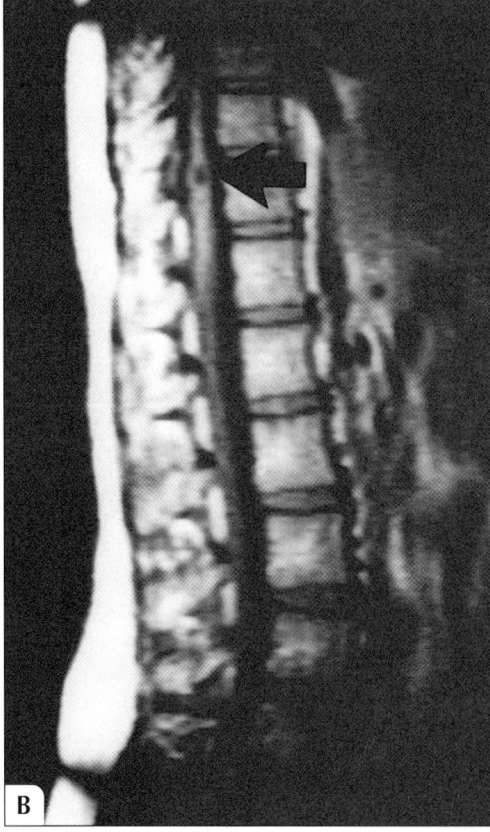

▶ **FIGURE 3-10.** Hemangioblastomas in patients with von Hippel-Lindau (VHL) disease. Patients with VHL disease are at risk for developing hemangioblastomas in the cerebellum (**A**) and spine (**B**). These hemangioblastomas can be solitary or multiple. The hemangioblastomas of the central nervous system (CNS) are benign vascular tumors that can be associated with significant morbidity [28]. Surgical resection of the hemangioblastoma is often recommended for treatment of VHL-associated CNS hemangioblastomas. These tumors may occur at a young age, appearing in some individuals before the age of 10. (*From* Linehan and Klausner [22]; with permission.)

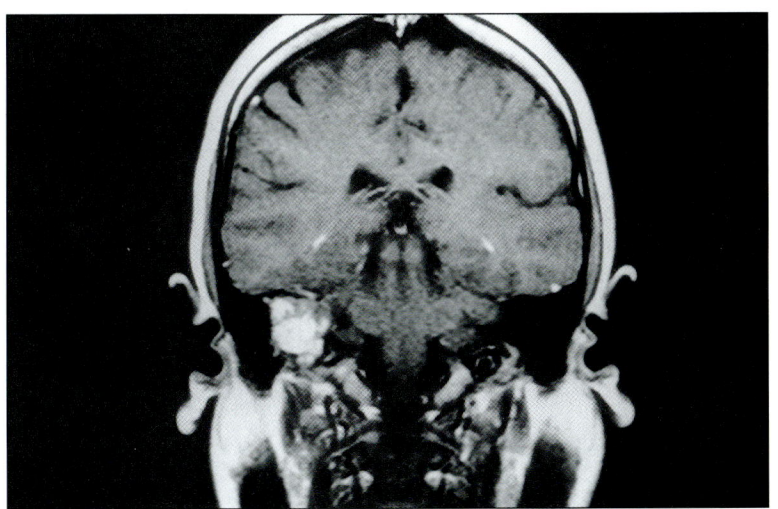

▶ **FIGURE 3-11.** Radiograph of a low-grade malignant tumor in the inner ear. A recently recognized manifestation of von Hippel-Lindau (VHL) disease is the development of a low-grade malignant tumor in the inner ear, in the endolymphatic sac canal. This tumor, referred to as an endolymphatic sac tumor (ELST), is a low-grade malignant tumor that is unlikely to metastasize but that can be associated with significant morbidity. ELST tumors may be detected in up to 12% of patients with VHL [29]. (*From* Vortmeyer *et al.* [30]; with permission.)

GENETIC PATTERN

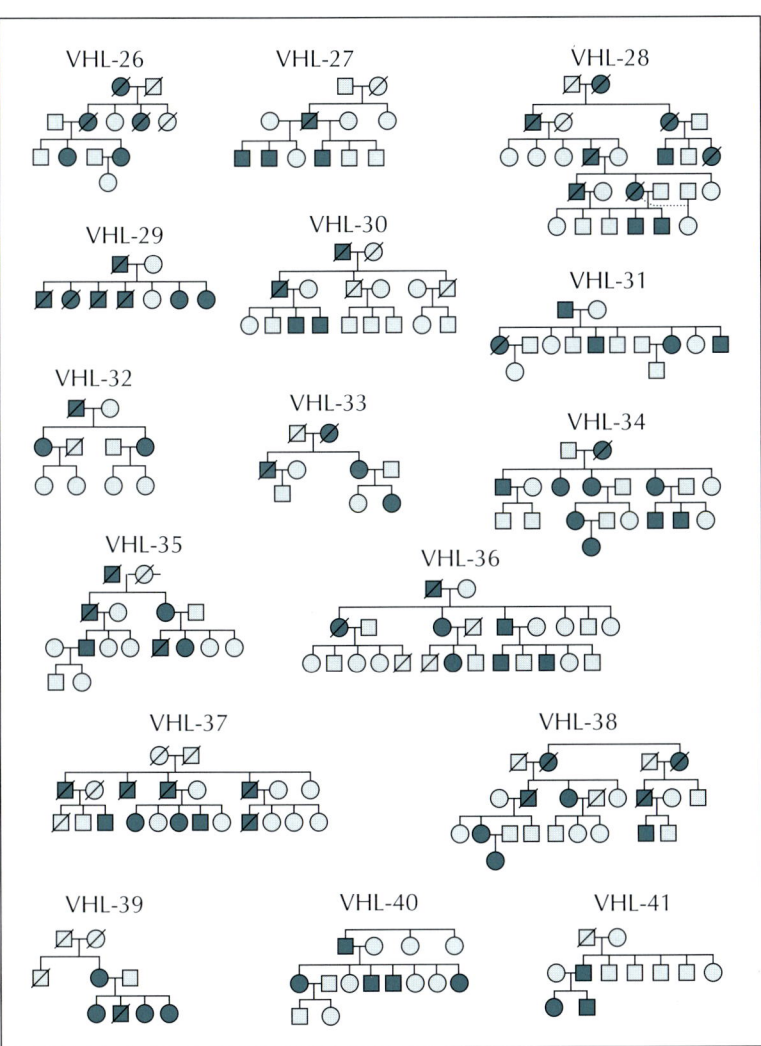

▶ **FIGURE 3-12.** Pattern of von Hippel-Lindau (VHL) disease in 16 families. VHL disease is characterized by an autosomal-dominant inheritance pattern. This means that each offspring has a 50% likelihood of carrying the genetic predisposition for developing VHL disease. The *dark boxes* represent affected individuals. To localize the *VHL* gene, these families underwent a comprehensive clinical evaluation to determine which individuals were affected and which were not. Genetic linkage analysis was used to narrow the region of the *VHL* gene to a small area on the short arm of chromosome 3 [1,31]. (*From* Linehan *et al.* [32].)

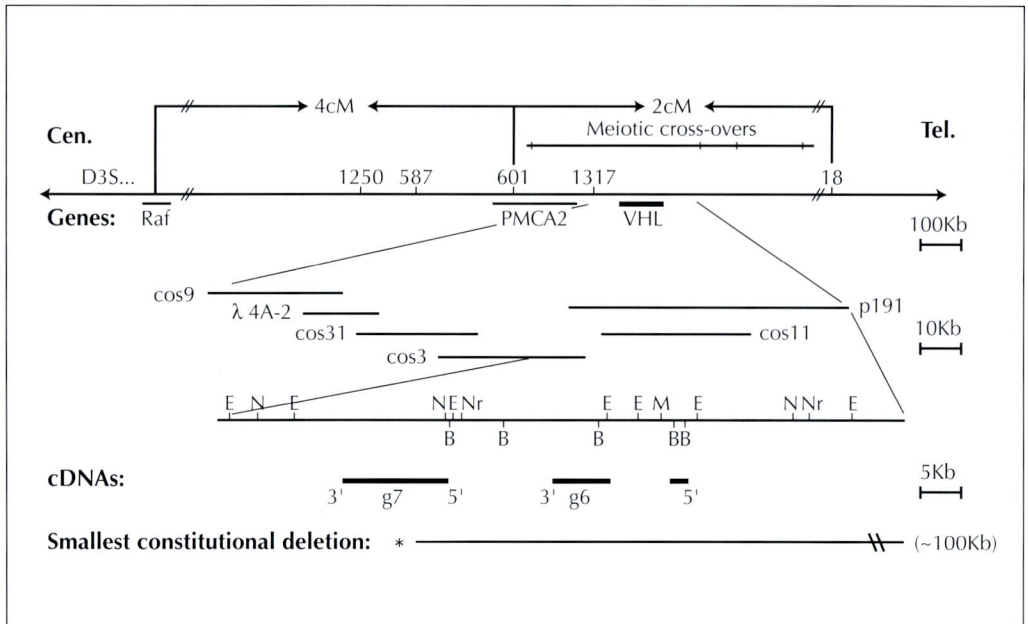

FIGURE 3-13. Genetic and physical maps to identify the gene for von Hippel-Lindau (VHL) disease [5]. A significant clue to the location of the *VHL* gene came when Yao *et al.* [33] identified germline deletions in the area of chromosome 3p in three unrelated families with VHL. This identification enabled the researchers to focus on a specific area of the 3p region of interest. Latif *et al.* [18] were then able to identify a candidate gene, referred to initially as *G7*, which turned out to be the *VHL* gene. The crucial evidence that *G7* was indeed the *VHL* gene was the identification of frequent rearrangements of the constitutional DNA in a large number of VHL kindreds and, finally, the detection of intragenic mutations of the gene that segregated with the disease (*ie*, that were detected in those found to be affected with VHL). (*Adapted from* Latif *et al.* [5].)

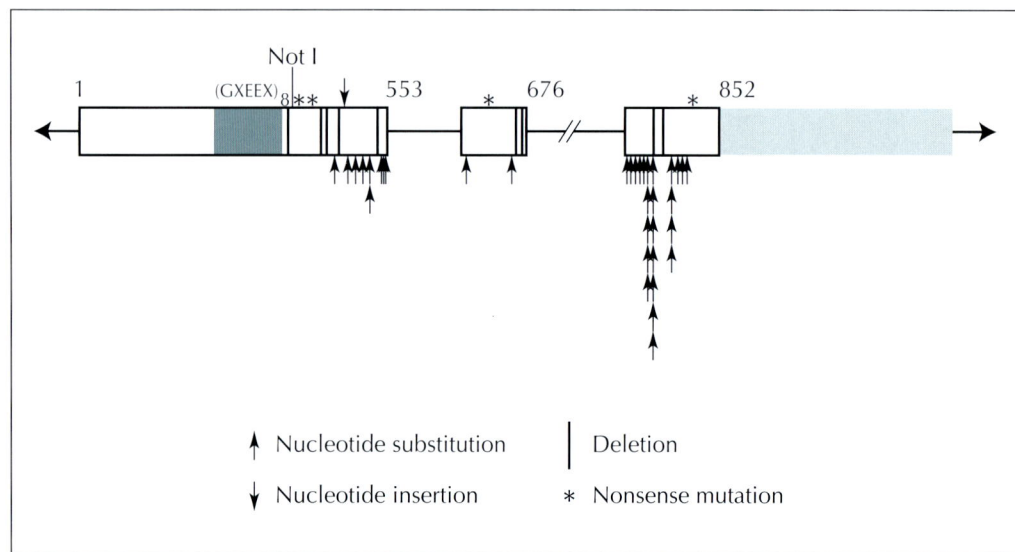

FIGURE 3-14. Intragenic mutations. The *VHL* gene, which contains 852 nucleotides, has three exons (coding regions) and codes for a protein of 213 amino acids [5]. Each *arrow, line,* and *star* indicate a specific type of mutation of the gene in an individual family [7]. In many instances, this method of identification enables physicians to make the diagnosis of von Hippel-Lindau (VHL) disease early in life and to determine which at-risk individuals carry the gene and which do not. Analysis by Chen *et al.* [7] of the correlation between germline mutations in the *VHL* tumor-suppressor gene and the phenotype (clinical manifestations of VHL) has enabled clinicians to make some predictions about which organs are likely to be at risk for tumor development. For example, VHL has been divided into two subtypes (I and II). Type II families are characterized by the presence of pheochromocytoma. The study performed by Chen *et al.* [7] revealed that 96% of the germline mutations in VHL type II families were of a certain type (*ie*, were missense mutations).

Clinical Applications for Germline von Hippel-Lindau Analysis

Early detection in at-risk individuals
   Germline testing recommended at 1 year of age
Accurate diagnosis
   VHL versus MEN II
Ability to predict organs at risk
   Missense mutation codon 238: *VHL* type II

▶ **FIGURE 3-15.** Clinical applications for germline von Hippel-Lindau (VHL) analysis. There are a number of potential clinical applications of the identification of the *VHL* gene. In many instances, early detection in at-risk individuals is possible. Many clinicians recommend germline testing at 1 year

of age because it is important to identify manifestations early in life. In some instances, the retinal manifestations of VHL can occur at a young age and it is possible that early intervention can preserve vision. Pheochromocytomas and hemangioblastomas of the central nervous system, which can be morbid or lethal if not detected and treated, can occur before 10 years of age. It can be difficult for clinicians to differentiate between patients with VHL manifestations and patients with multiple endocrine neoplasia type II (MEN II). In both hereditary cancer syndromes, patients can present with pheochromocytomas; the availability of germline testing for VHL or MEN II can often assist in making the correct diagnosis. Finally, knowledge of the location and the type of VHL mutation can sometimes provide the clinician with the ability to predict which organs are at risk for tumorigenesis [34–36]. For example, in a family in which there is a missense VHL mutation at VHL codon 238, pheochromocytoma is highly likely to be present in affected individuals. This type of information can be useful when counseling and treating such patients.

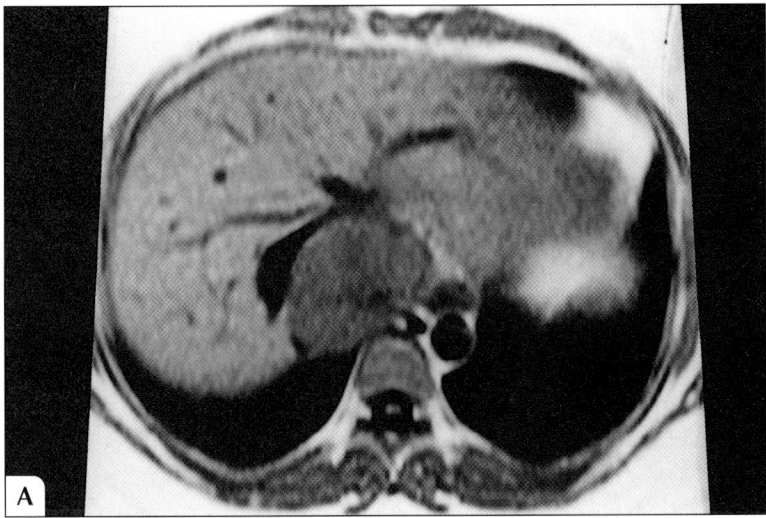
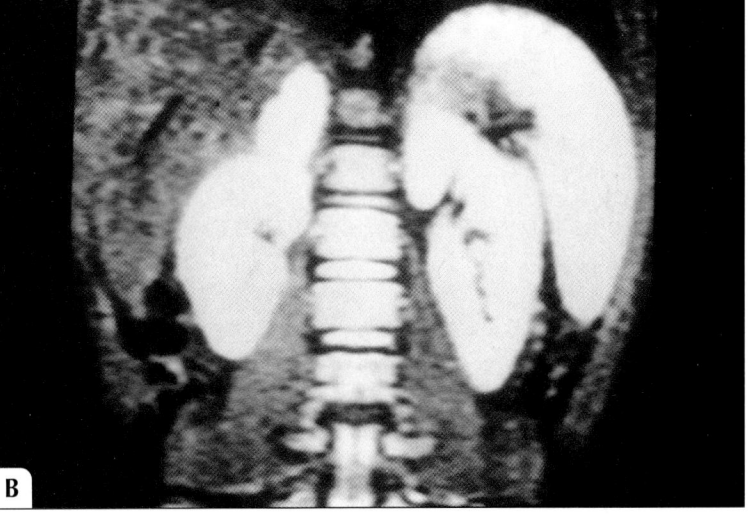

▶ **FIGURE 3-16.** Examples of von Hippel-Lindau (VHL) disease. **A,** Abdominal scan of a 24-year-old woman with a large retroperitoneal mass and a pheochromocytoma. **B,** Magnetic resonance image of the abdomen of a 9-year-old boy with a right-sided pheochromocytoma. In both instances it was initially thought that the most likely diagnosis was multiple endocrine neoplasia type II (MEN II). However, after compre-

hensive clinical evaluation performed in association with *VHL* germline testing, both patients were found to have VHL disease. This information also provided clinicians with a method for presymptomatic germline testing in other at-risk family members. (*From* Linehan and Klausner [22]; with permission.)

VHL Gene Sporadic Renal Cell Carcinoma

Tumor tissues from patients with renal carcinoma were evaluated for:
VHL gene mutation
VHL gene deletion (loss)

▶ **FIGURE 3-17.** *VHL* gene sporadic renal cell carcinoma. Tissue and cell line evaluations from patients with no family history of renal carcinoma were conducted to determine if the *VHL* gene is associated with the nonhereditary, sporadic form of renal carcinoma.

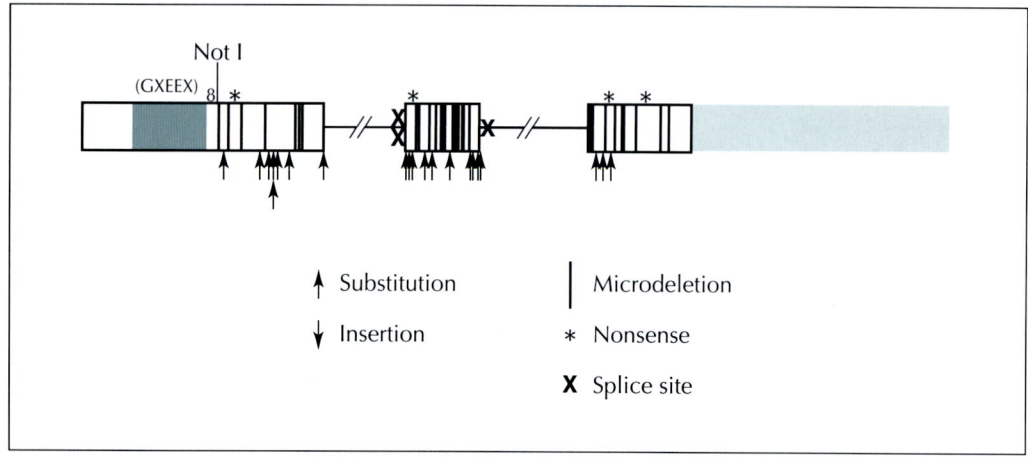

FIGURE 3-18. *VHL* gene mutations in sporadic clear-cell renal carcinoma. Gene mutations in patients with von Hippel-Lindau disease have been found in a high percentage of tumors from patients with clear-cell renal carcinoma [9,37]. *VHL* gene deletion (loss of the second copy of the *VHL* gene) has also been detected in a high percentage of tumors from patients with clear-cell renal carcinoma. *VHL* gene mutation and deletion have been detected in patients with early, small renal carcinomas as well as in tumors from patients with advanced disease. These results demonstrated that inactivation of the *VHL* gene is an early event in tumorigenesis of clear-cell renal carcinoma.

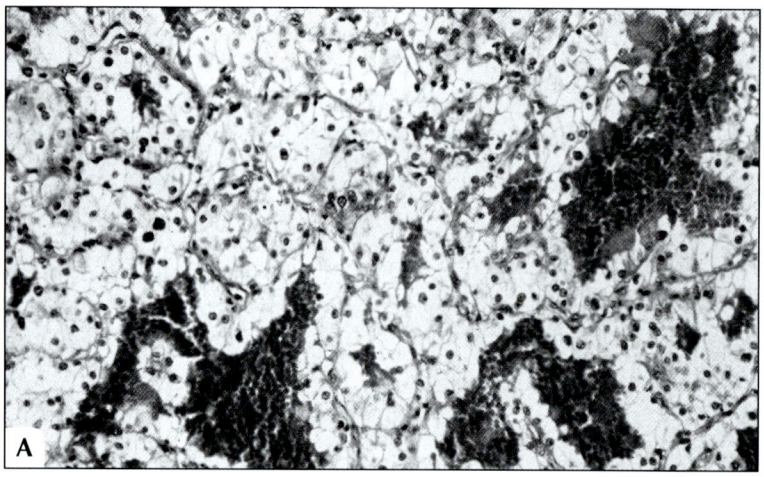

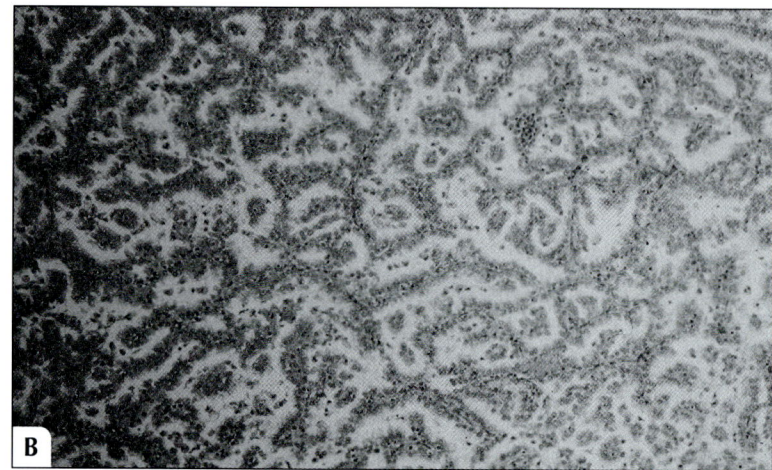

FIGURE 3-19. (*See* Color Plate) *VHL* gene mutation analysis in tumor tissue. Gene mutations in patients with von Hippel-Lindau (VHL) disease have been detected in tumor tissue from patients with clear-cell renal carcinoma (**A**), but are not found in tumor tissue from patients with papillary renal carcinoma (**B**). This distinction provides the basis for a molecular genetic classification of renal carcinoma (*ie*, clear-cell vs papillary), with clear-cell renal carcinoma being characterized by mutation of the VHL gene.

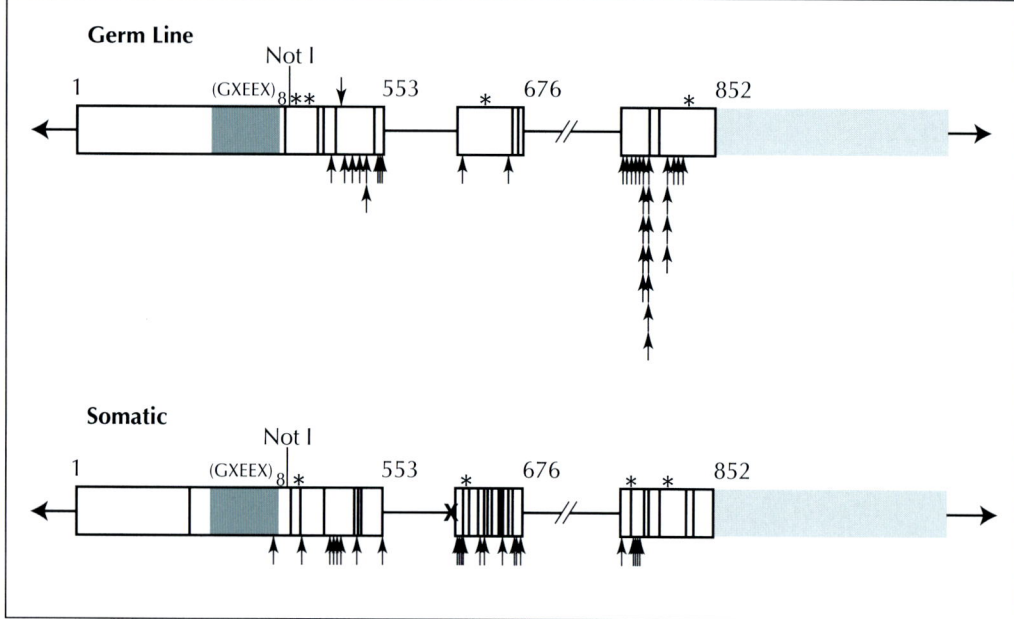

FIGURE 3-20. Gene mutations. The *VHL* gene is the gene for the familial form of renal cell carcinoma associated with von Hippel-Lindau disease. Mutation of this gene is an early event in the most common form of renal carcinoma: clear-cell renal carcinoma. The *VHL* gene has the characteristics of a classic tumor-suppressor gene of the Knudson model (*ie*, in tumor tissue both copies of the gene are inactivated by either mutation or DNA sequence deletion) [16,17]. (*Adapted from* Gnarra *et al.* [9].)

Clinical Application of *VHL* Gene Analysis

Detection of *VHL* gene mutation in
  Formalin-fixed tissues
  Tissue aspirates
Early diagnosis
  Circulating cells
  Urine

▶ **FIGURE 3-21.** Clinical application of *VHL* gene analysis. There are a number of potential clinical applications of gene analysis findings. Zhuang *et al.* [10] have shown that *VHL* gene mutations can be detected in formalin-fixed tissue from tumor material from patients with sporadic clear-cell renal carcinoma. This distinction provides the potential to improve diagnosis of diseases in tissues removed from patients in which the histologic result is uncertain. Beaty *et al.* [11] have recently shown that *VHL* gene abnormalities can be detected in material from tissue aspirates, providing a potential method for determining whether a renal mass is clear-cell renal carcinoma or whether a lesion in another organ is a metastatic site from a primary renal carcinoma. Studies are underway to determine whether *VHL* gene mutations can be detected in circulating cells in the serum or urine as a potential method for early diagnosis or monitoring of recurrence of this disease.

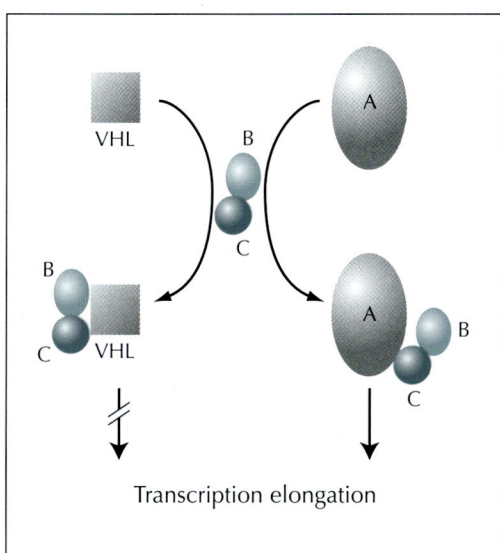

Transcription elongation

▶ **FIGURE 3-22.** Example of the *VHL* gene. The identification of the *VHL* gene provides a method for early identification of at-risk individuals in von Hippel-Lindau (VHL) disease kindreds and may provide a method for early diagnosis of sporadic renal cell carcinoma. It is hoped that understanding the function of the *VHL* gene will lead to potential strategies for the development of methods of treatment for VHL as well as sporadic renal carcinoma. To understand the function of the *VHL* gene, Duan *et al.* [38] performed studies to identify the proteins that interact with the VHL protein. These studies lead to the determination that the cellular transcription factor, elongin (SIII), is a functional target of the VHL protein. The VHL protein forms a trimeric complex with elongin B and C, which are two regulator subunits of the elongin complex [38]. It is not yet known whether the binding of the VHL protein with elongin B and C has an effect on transcription; however, these types of studies will ultimately characterize the cellular function of the VHL kidney cancer tumor-suppressor gene. It is hoped that understanding of the VHL kidney cancer tumor-suppressor gene pathway will lead to the identification of potential therapeutic targets in the treatment of these diseases. (*Adapted from* Duan *et al.* [38].)

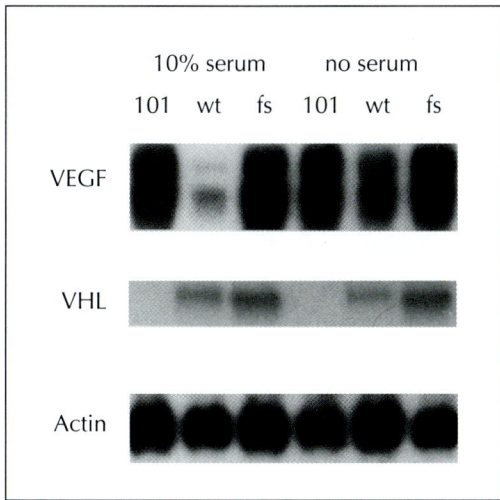

▶ **FIGURE 3-23.** A *VHL* gene mutation. Basic studies of the *VHL* gene have also contributed to understanding the downstream effects of a mutation of the *VHL* gene. The tumors that arise in patients with von Hippel-Lindau (VHL) disease (kidney cancer, pheochromocytoma, pancreatic neuroendocrine tumors, hemangioblastomas of the central nervous system, and retinal angiomas) as well as sporadic clear-cell renal carcinoma are characterized by marked and profound angiogenesis. One of the tumor-produced factors that is thought to play a significant role in angiogenesis is vascular endothelial growth factor (VEGF). Scientists studying clear-cell renal carcinomas have determined that the *VHL* gene regulates messenger RNA levels of VEGF in a posttranscriptional fashion. As shown in this figure, when VEGF message levels are measured (lane 101) in a cell line with a mutant *VHL* gene (*ie*, as in clear-cell renal carcinoma), there is a significant amount of VEGF messenger RNA. However, when the VEGF level is measured in cells in which there is a wild-type (normal) *VHL* gene, there is a significant and profound decrease in the message [39,40]. These and related findings have suggested that angiogenesis might be a potential therapeutic target for patients with VHL as well as patients with advanced renal cell carcinoma. (*Adapted from* Gnarra *et al.* [39].)

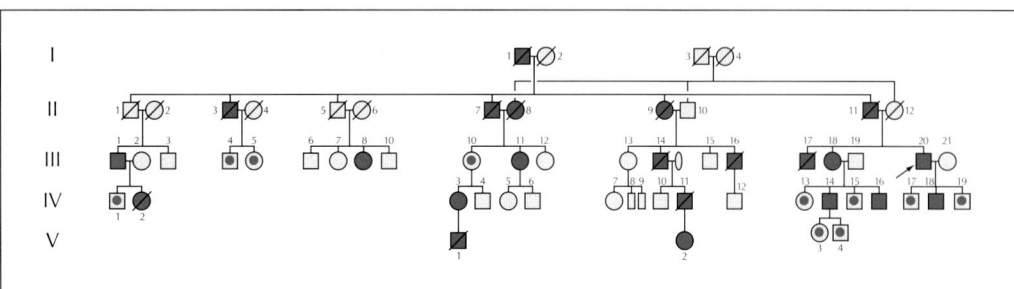

Kindred diagram of hereditary papillary renal carcinoma (HPRC). This new form of hereditary renal cell carcinoma recently has been identified. HPRC is an autosomal-dominant hereditary cancer syndrome in which affected individuals are at risk for developing bilateral, multifocal papillary renal carcinoma [12,13]. This hereditary cancer syndrome is distinct from von Hippel-Lindau (VHL) disease. Patients with VHL are at risk for developing clear-cell renal carcinoma as well as tumors in a number of other organs, including the brain, pancreas, adrenal gland, brain, spine, and eye. In the kindred diagram, *dark boxes* represent patients affected with HPRC.

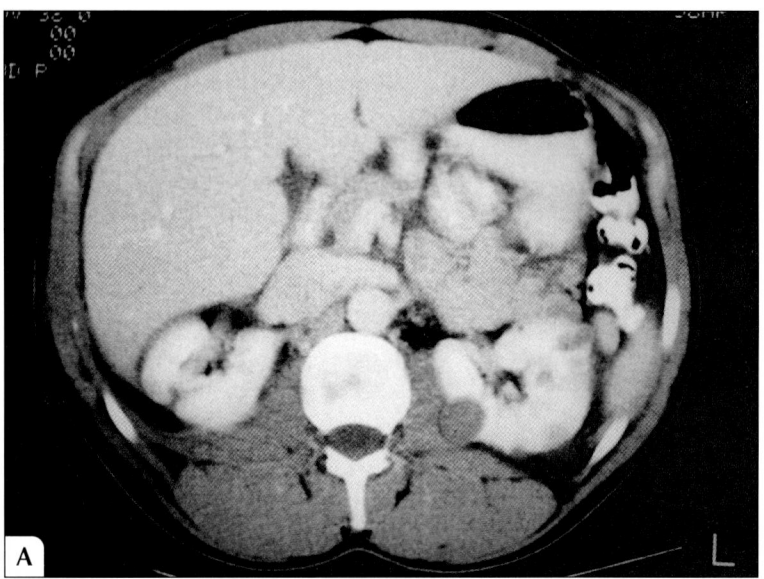

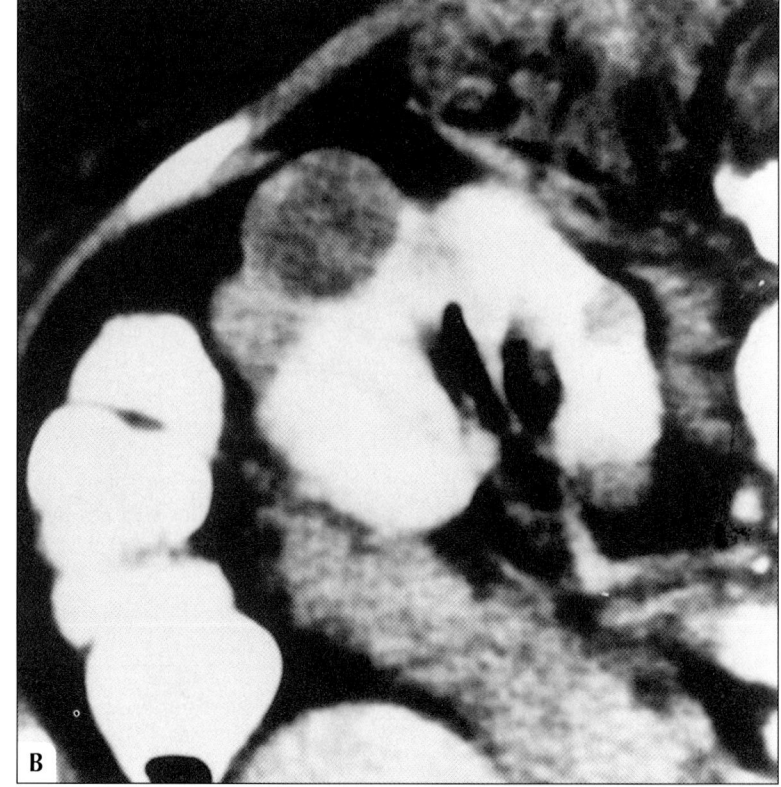

▶ **FIGURE 3-25.** Abdominal CT scans of two affected individuals (**A** and **B**) who are kindreds of a patient with hereditary papillary renal carcinoma (HPRC). Affected individuals are at risk for developing bilateral multifocal papillary renal carcinoma. The tumors in the kidney can be hard to detect by ultrasound because the density of the papillary renal carcinoma can be very similar to that of the surrounding normal renal parenchyma [12,13]. Schmidt *et al.* [14] recently performed genetic linkage analysis in HPRC kindreds and localized the *HPRC* gene to a region on the long arm of chromosome 7. Subsequent analysis has determined that the gene for HPRC is the *MET* gene. Mutations in the *MET* gene have been detected in the germline of affected HPRC individuals [14]. (*From* Zbar *et al.* [12]; with permission.)

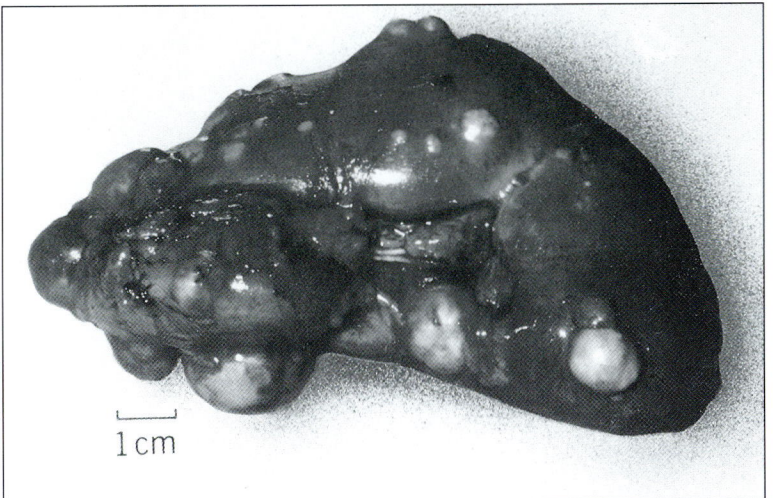

FIGURE 3-26. (*See* Color Plate) Kidney of hereditary papillary renal carcinoma (HPRC) kindred patient. The renal tumors in these patients often develop during the fifth or sixth decade of life. These tumors are malignant and they can metastasize. Many clinicians recommend nephron-sparing surgery to save as much normal renal parenchyma as possible and to preserve the best quality of life for the patient [20]. Recent studies of HPRC kindreds have detected tumors in organs other than the kidney, such as the bile duct, pancreas, and stomach. Further studies of HPRC kindreds will be needed to determine whether HPRC represents a hereditary cancer syndrome in which multiple organs are at risk for the development of tumors. (*From* Zbar *et al.* [12]; with permission.)

REFERENCES

1. Linehan WM, Lerman MI, Zbar B: Identification of the VHL gene: its role in renal carcinoma. *JAMA* 1995, 273:564–570.

2. Zbar B, Brauch H, Talmadge C, Linehan WM: Loss of alleles of loci on the short arm of chromosome 3 in renal cell carcinoma. *Nature* 1987, 327:721–724.

3. Seizinger BR, Rouleau GA, Ozelius LJ, *et al.*: Von Hippel-Lindau disease maps to the region of chromosome 3 associated with renal cell carcinoma. *Nature* 1988, 332:268–269.

4. Hosoe S, Brauch H, Latif F, *et al.*: Localization of the von Hippel-Lindau disease gene to a small region of chromosome 3. *Genomics* 1990, 8:634–640.

5. Latif F, Tory K, Gnarra J, *et al.*: Identification of the von Hippel-Lindau disease tumor suppressor gene. *Science* 1993, 260:1317–1320.

6. Crossey PA, Richards FM, Foster K, *et al.*: Identification of intragenic mutations in the von Hippel-Lindau disease tumor suppressor gene and correlation with disease phenotype. *Hum Mol Genet* 1994, 3:1303–1308.

7. Chen F, Kishida T, Yao M, *et al.*: Germline mutations in the von Hippel-Lindau disease tumor suppressor gene: correlation with phenotype. *Hum Mutat* 1995, 5:66–75.

8. Shuin T, Kondo K, Torigoe S, *et al.*: Frequent somatic mutations and loss of heterozygosity of the von Hippel-Lindau tumor suppressor gene in primary human renal cell carcinomas. *Cancer Res* 1994, 54:2852–2855.

9. Gnarra JR, Tory K, Weng Y, *et al.*: Mutation of the VHL tumor suppressor gene in renal carcinoma. *Nature Genet* 1994, 7:85–90.

10. Zhuang Z, Gnarra J, Zbar B, *et al.*: Detection of the von Hippel-Lindau disease gene mutation by PCR and SSCP in sporadic renal cell carcinoma in paraffin-embedded tissue [abstract]. *Modern Pathology* 1994, 7:86.

11. Beaty MW, Zhuang Z, Park WS, *et al.*: Fine-needle aspiration of metastatic clear cell carcinoma of the kidney. *Cancer/Cancer Cytopathology* 1997, 81:180–186.

12. Zbar B, Tory K, Merino M, *et al.*: Hereditary papillary renal cell carcinoma. *J Urol* 1994, 151:561–566.

13. Zbar B, Glenn G, Lubensky IA, *et al.*: Hereditary papillary renal cell carcinoma: clinical studies in 10 families. *J Urol* 1995, 153:907–912.

14. Schmidt L, Duh F-M, Chen F, *et al.*: Germline and somatic mutations in the tyrosine kinase domain of the MET proto-oncogene in papillary renal carcinomas. *Nature Genet* 1997, 16:68–73.

15. Walther MM, Johnson B, Culley D, *et al.*: Serum interleukin-6 levels in metastatic renal cell carcinoma before treatment with interleukin-2 correlates with paraneoplastic syndromes but not patient survival. *J Urol* 1998, 159:718–722.

16. Knudson AG, Jr.: Mutation and cancer: statistical study of retinoblastoma. *Proc Natl Acad Sci U S A* 1971, 68:820–823.

17. Knudson AG: VHL gene mutation and clear-cell renal carcinomas. *Cancer J* 1995, 1:180–181.

18. Latif F, Duh FM, Gnarra J, *et al.*: Von Hippel-Lindau syndrome: cloning and identification of the plasma membrane Ca transporting ATPase isoform 2 gene that resides in the von Hippel-Lindau gene region. *Cancer Res* 1993, 53:861–867.

19. Glenn GM, Choyke PL, Zbar B, Linehan WM: Von Hippel-Lindau disease: clinical review and molecular genetics. In *Problems in Urologic Surgery: Benign and Malignant Tumors of the Kidney*. Edited by Anderson EE. Philadelphia: JB Lippincott; 1990:312–330.

20. Walther MM, Choyke PL, Weiss G, *et al.*: Parenchymal sparing surgery in patients with hereditary renal cell carcinoma. *J Urol* 1995, 153:913–916.

21. Walther MM, Lubensky IA, Venzon D, *et al.*: Prevalence of microscopic lesions in grossly normal renal parenchyma from patients with von Hippel-Lindau disease, sporadic renal cell carcinoma and no renal disease: clinical implications. *J Urol* 1995, 154:2010–2015.

22. Linehan WM, Klausner RD: Renal carcinoma. In *The Genetic Basis of Human Cancer*, edn 1. Edited by Vogelstein B, Kinzler K. New York: McGraw-Hill; 1997:455–473.

23. Poston CD, Jaffe GS, Lubensky, *et al.*: Characterization of the renal pathology of a familial form of renal cell carcinoma associated with von Hippel-Lindau disease: clinical and molecular genetic implications. *J Urol* 1995, 153:22–26.

24. Vortmeyer AO, Lubensky IA, Fogt F, *et al.*: Allelic deletion and mutation of the VHL tumor suppressor gene in pancreatic microcystic adenomas. *Am J Pathol* 1997, 151:951–956.

25. Keiser HR, Doppman JL, Robertson CN, *et al.*: Diagnosis, localization and management of pheochromocytoma. In *Pathology of the Adrenal Gland*, edn 14. Edited by Lack EE. New York: Churchill-Livingston; 1990:237–255.

26. Maurea S, Cuocolo A, Reynolds JC, *et al.*: Iodine-313-Metaiodobenzylguanidine scintigraphy in preoperative and postoperative evaluation of paragangliomas: comparison with CT and MRI. *J Nucl Med* 1993, 34:173–179.

27. Vargas HI, Kavoussi LR, Bartlett DL, *et al.*: Laparoscopic adrenalectomy: a new standard of care. *Urology* 1997, 49:673–678.

28. Filling-Katz MR, Choyke PL, Oldfield E, *et al.*: Central nervous system involvement in von Hippel Lindau disease. *Neurology* 1991, 41:41–46.

29. Manski TJ, Heffner DK, Glenn GM, *et al.*: Endolymphatic sac tumors: a source of morbid hearing loss in von Hippel-Lindau disease. *JAMA* 1997, 277:1461–1466.

30. Vortmeyer AO, Choo D, Pack SD, *et al.*: von Hippel-Lindau disease gene alterations associated with endolymphatic sac tumor. *J Natl Cancer Inst* 1997, 89:970–972.

31. Glenn GM, Linehan WM, Hosoe S, *et al.*: Screening for von Hippel-Lindau disease by DNA-polymorphism analysis. *JAMA* 1992, 267:1226–1231.

32. Linehan WM, Gnarra JR, Latif F, *et al.*: Genetic basis of renal cell cancer. In *Important Advances in Oncology 1993*. Edited by DeVita VT, Hellman S, Rosenberg SA. Philadelphia: JB Lippincott; 1993:47–70.

33. Yao M, Latif F, Kuzmin I, *et al.*: Von Hippel-Lindau disease: identification of deletion mutations by pulsed field gel electrophoresis. *Hum Genet* 1993, 92:605–614.

34. Brauch H, Kishida T, Glavac D, *et al.*: Von Hippel Lindau (VHL) disease with pheochromocytoma in the Black forest region of Germany: evidence for a founder effect. *Hum Genet* 1995, 95:551–556.

35. Zbar B, Kishida T, Chen F, *et al.*: Germline mutations in the von Hippel-Lindau disease (VHL) gene in families from North America, Europe and Japan. *Hum Mutat* 1996, 8:348–357.

36. Kanno H, Shuin T, Kondo K, *et al.* Molecular genetic diagnosis of von Hippel-Lindau disease: analysis of five Japanese families. *Jpn J Cancer Res* 1996, 87:423–428.

37. Shuin T, Kondo K, Torigoe S, *et al.*: Frequent somatic mutations and loss of heterozygosity of the von Hippel-Lindau tumor suppressor gene in primary human renal cell carcinomas. *Cancer Res* 1994, 54:2852–2855.

38. Duan DR, Pause A, Burgess WH, *et al.*: Inhibition of transcription elongation by the VHL tumor suppressor protein. *Science* 1995, 269:1402–1406.

39. Gnarra JR, Zhou S, Merrill MJ, *et al.*: Post-transcriptional regulation of vascular endothelial growth factor mRNA by the product of the VHL tumor suppressor gene. *Proc Natl Acad Sci U S A* 1996, 93:10589–10594.

40. Iliopoulos O, Jiang C, Levy AP, *et al.*: Negative regulation of hypoxia-inducible genes by the von Hippel-Lindau protein. *Proc Natl Acad Sci U S A* 1996, 93:10595–10599.

Nephron-Sparing Surgery for Renal Cell Carcinoma

Andrew C. Novick

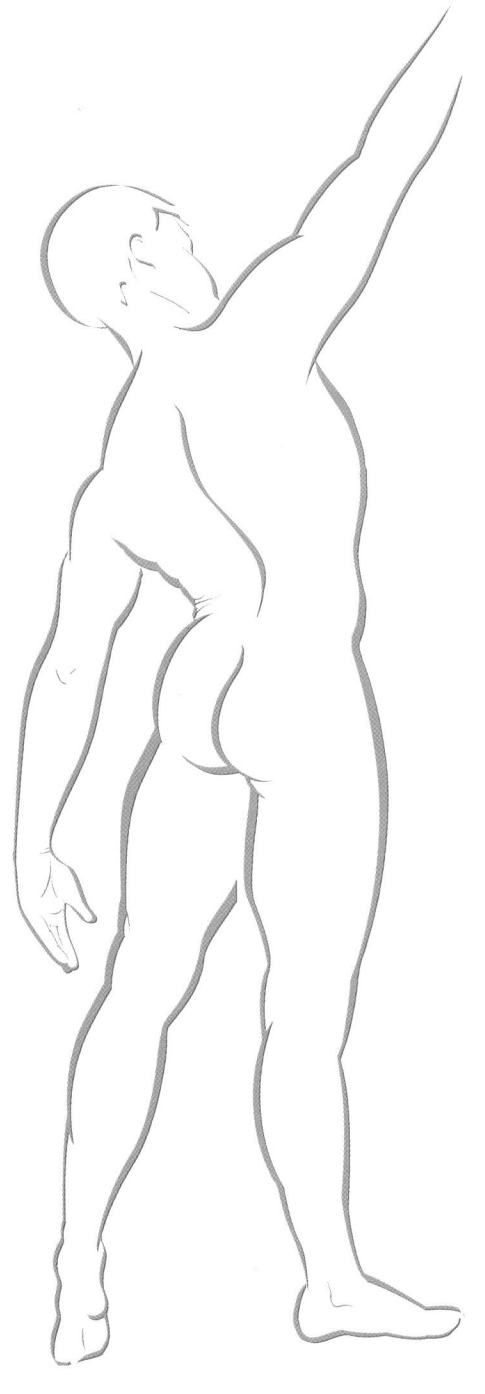

Recent interest in nephron-sparing surgery for renal cell carcinoma has been stimulated by advances in renal imaging, improved surgical techniques, the increasing number of incidentally discovered low-stage renal cell carcinomas and good long-term survival in patients undergoing this form of treatment [1]. Nephron-sparing surgery entails complete local excision of a renal tumor while leaving the largest possible amount of normal functioning parenchyma in the involved kidney.

Accepted indications for nephron-sparing surgery include situations in which radical nephrectomy would render the patient anephric with subsequent immediate need for dialysis. This encompasses patients with bilateral renal cell carcinoma or renal cell carcinoma involving a solitary functioning kidney. The latter circumstance may be present due to unilateral renal agenesis, prior removal of the contralateral kidney, or irreversible impairment of contralateral renal function. Nephron-sparing surgery is also indicated in patients with unilateral renal cell carcinoma and a functioning opposite kidney when the opposite kidney is affected by a condition that might threaten its future function, (*ie*, calculus disease, chronic pyelonephritis, renal artery stenosis, ureteral reflux, or systemic diseases such as diabetes and nephrosclerosis).

Recent studies have clarified the role of nephron-sparing surgery in patients with localized unilateral renal cell carcinoma and a normal contralateral kidney. The data indicate that radical nephrectomy and nephron-sparing surgery provide equally effective curative treatment for such patients who present with a single, small (< 4 cm), and clearly localized renal cell carcinoma. The results of nephron-sparing surgery are less satisfactory in patients with larger (> 4 cm) or multiple localized renal cell carcinomas, and radical nephrectomy remains the treatment of choice in such cases when the opposite kidney is normal.

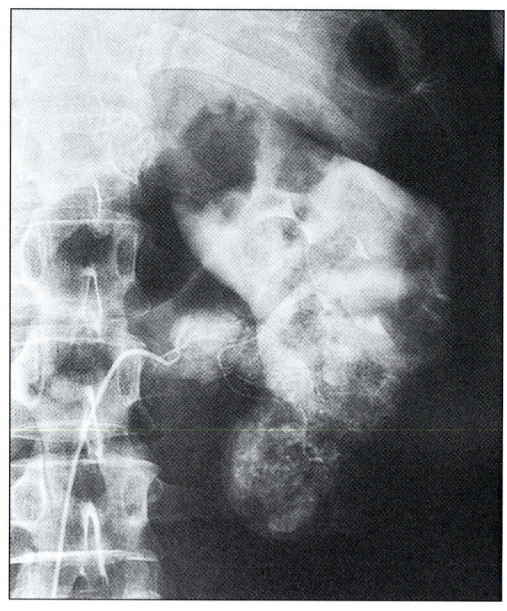

▶ **FIGURE 4-1.** Arteriography of a large vascular tumor. The tumor involves the lower portion of a solitary left kidney. For patients with large tumors who are candidates for nephron-sparing surgery, preoperative renal arteriography to delineate the intrarenal vasculature aids in excising the tumor with minimal blood loss and damage to adjacent normal parenchyma. Arteriography can be deferred in patients with small peripheral tumors.

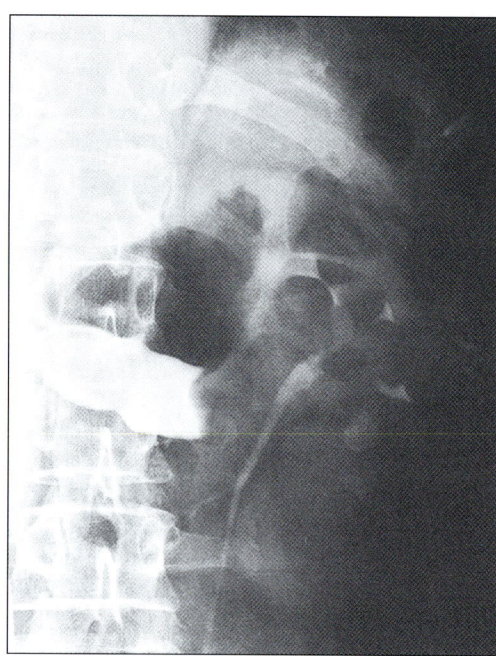

▶ **FIGURE 4-2.** Renal venogram. There is an occlusion of the left main renal vein, near the renal hilus, from an intramural malignant thrombus (same patient as in Fig. 4-1). Selective renal venography is performed in patients with large or centrally located tumors to evaluate for intrarenal venous thrombosis secondary to malignancy. The latter, if present, implies a more advanced local tumor stage and also increases the technical complexity of tumor excision.

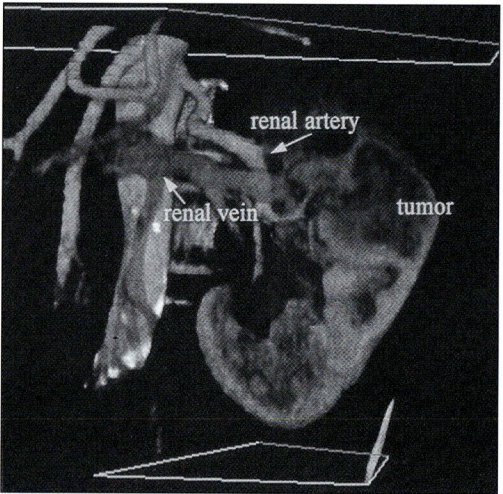

▶ **FIGURE 4-3.** (*See* Color plate) Spiral CT scan. This three-dimensional, or spiral, CT scan provides a detailed view of intrarenal arterial and venous anatomy in relation to the tumor. It is anticipated that this new noninvasive imaging modality will likely supplant the need for formal catheter angiography in the preoperative evaluation of patient candidates for nephron-sparing surgery.

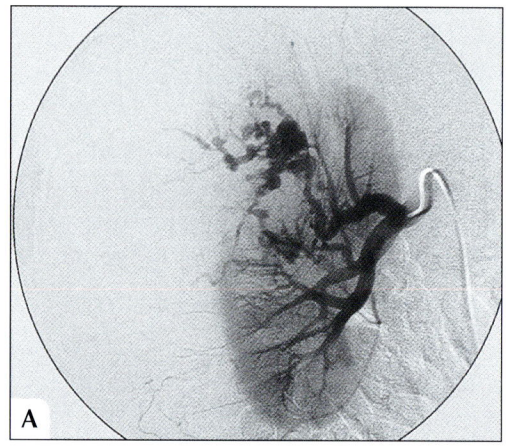

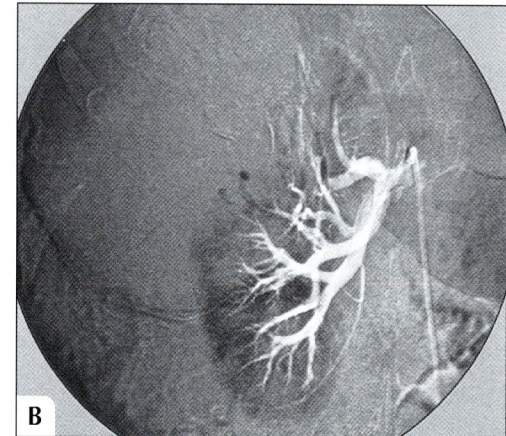

▶ **FIGURE 4-4.** Arteriograms in a patient who had a large vascular tumor. In selected patients with a large tumor supplied by a discrete branch of the renal artery, preoperative segmental angioinfarction of the tumor may reduce its size and vascularity, and thereby aid in its operative excision. **A,** Arteriogram demonstrating a large vascular tumor involving the upper portion of a solitary right kidney. The tumor is supplied exclusively by a superior branch of the renal artery. **B,** Arteriogram following embolization of the segmental arterial branch supplying the tumor, demonstrating that the arterial supply has been obliterated.

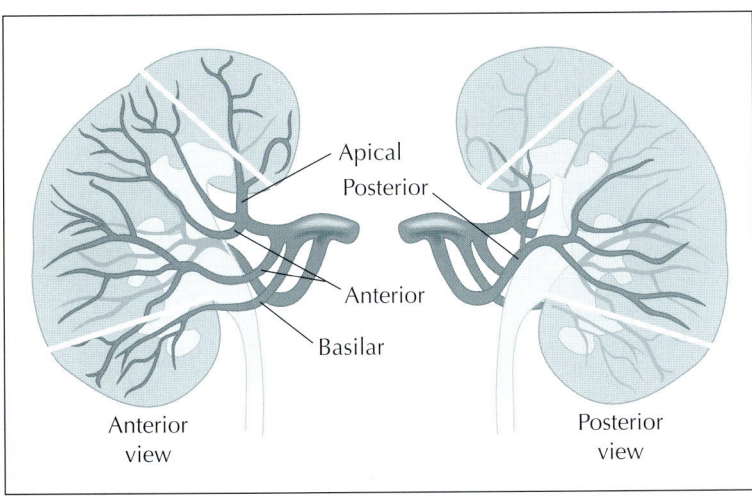

▶ **FIGURE 4-5.** Normal renal arterial blood supply. The kidney has four constant vascular segments: apical, inferior, posterior, and basilar. Each of these segments is supplied by one or more major arterial branches. Although the origin of the branches supplying these segments may vary, the anatomic position of the segments is constant. All segmental arteries are end-arteries with no collateral circulation; therefore, all branches supplying tumor-free parenchyma must be preserved when performing nephron-sparing surgery to avoid devitalization of functioning renal tissue.

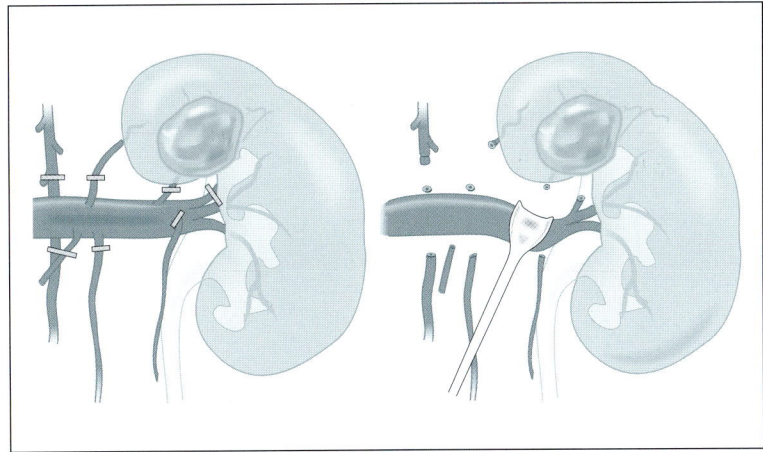

▶ **FIGURE 4-6.** Mobilization of the renal vein. The renal venous drainage system differs significantly from the arterial blood supply in that the intrarenal venous branches intercommunicate freely between the various renal segments. Ligation of a branch of the renal vein, therefore, does not result in segmental infarction of the kidney because collateral venous blood supply provides adequate drainage. This ligation is important clinically because it enables one to obtain surgical access to tumors safely in the renal hilus by ligating and dividing small, adjacent, or overlying venous branches. The main renal vein can then be completely mobilized and freely retracted in either direction to expose the tumor with no vascular compromise of uninvolved parenchyma.

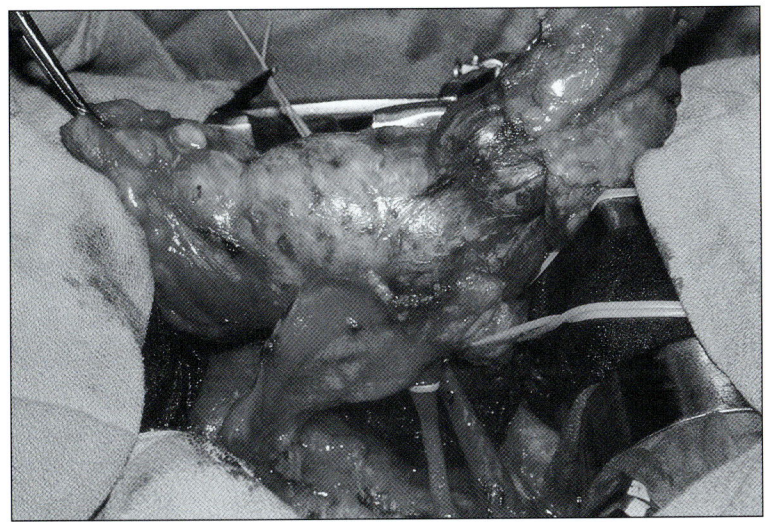

▶ **FIGURE 4-7.** (*See* Color Plate) Tumors in a kidney that involve the upper and lower renal poles although the midportion of the kidney is free of disease. It is usually possible to perform nephron-sparing surgery for malignancy in situ by using an operative approach that optimizes exposure of the kidney and by combining meticulous surgical technique with an understanding of the renal vascular anatomy in relation to the tumor. An extraperitoneal flank incision is employed through the bed of the 11th or 12th rib for almost all of these operations; occasionally, a thoracoabdominal incision is used for very large tumors involving the upper portion of the kidney. The kidney is completely mobilized within Gerota's fascia so that it is only attached by the renal artery, the renal vein, and the ureter. The mobilized kidney can then be elevated almost to skin level, as shown here, yielding excellent exposure for the performance of nephron-sparing surgery. The perirenal fat is usually left on the tumor but removed from the healthy portion of the kidney.

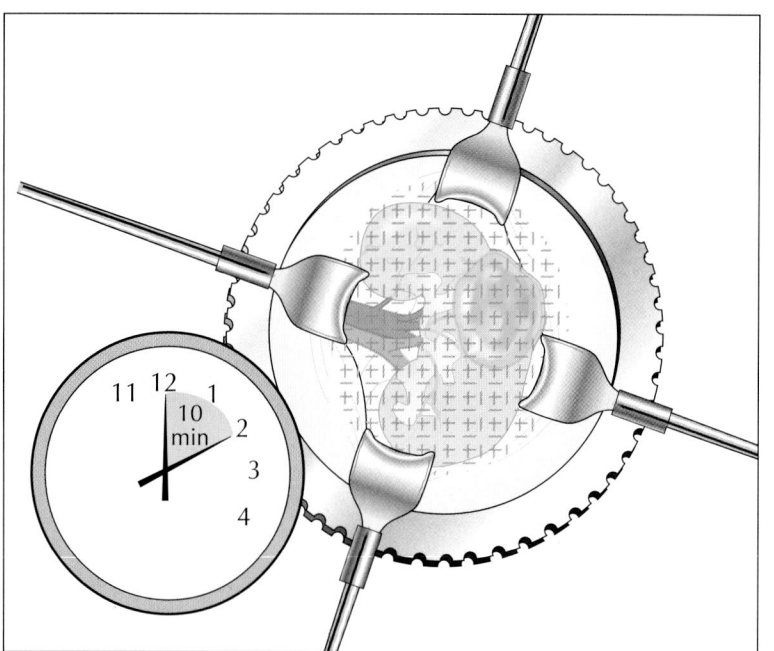

▶ **FIGURE 4-8.** Renal cooling. For small peripheral renal tumors, it is not necessary to control the renal artery. In most other cases, however, nephron-sparing surgery is most effectively performed after temporary renal arterial occlusion. This measure not only limits intraoperative bleeding but, by reducing renal tissue turgor, also improves access to intrarenal structures. In patients with centrally located tumors, it is also necessary to occlude the renal vein temporarily to minimize intraoperative bleeding from transected major venous branches. When the renal circulation is temporarily interrupted, in situ surface renal hypothermia with ice slush is used. This technique allows up to 3 hours of safe ischemia without permanent renal injury. An important caveat with this method is to keep the entire kidney covered with ice slush for 10 to 15 minutes immediately after occluding the renal artery and before commencing the nephron-sparing operation. This amount of time is needed to obtain core renal cooling to a temperature ($\approx 20°C$) that optimizes in situ renal preservation. During excision of the tumor, invariably large portions of the kidney are no longer covered with ice slush and, in the absence of adequate prior renal cooling, rapid rewarming and ischemic renal injury can occur.

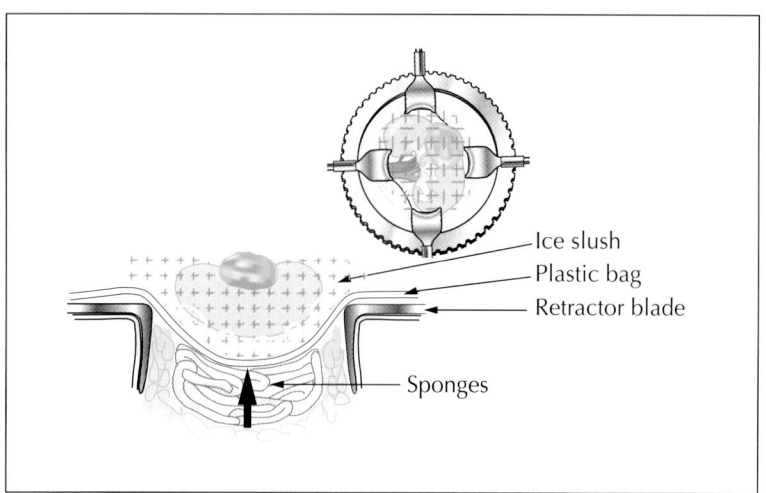

▶ **FIGURE 4-9.** The mobilized kidney surrounded by a plastic bag containing ice slush and elevated to skin level by placing several sponges under the plastic bag. Exposure of the operative field is maintained by a self-retaining ring retractor.

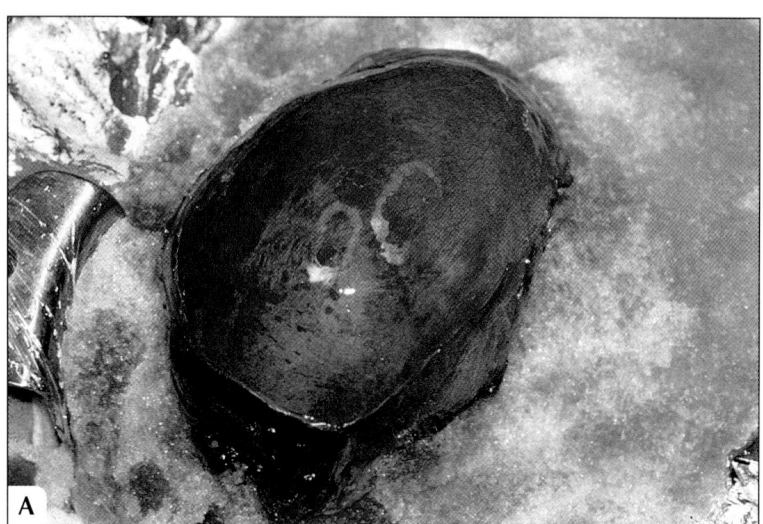

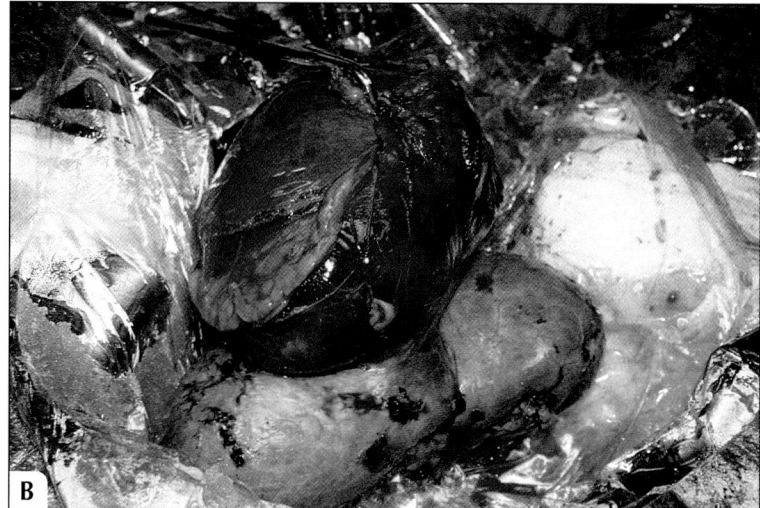

▶ **FIGURE 4-10.** (*See* Color Plate) Kidney mobilization. **A**, A solitary kidney with a large central tumor mobilized, contained within a plastic bag, and elevated to skin level. **B**, The renal artery is temporarily occluded and, hence, the kidney appears pale. The entire non–tumor-bearing portion of the kidney is covered with ice slush, which is left in place for 10 to 15 minutes before excision of the tumor is initiated.

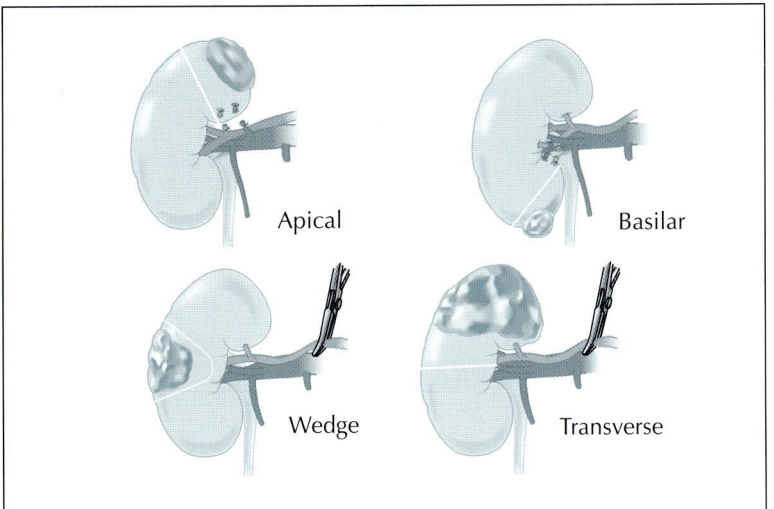

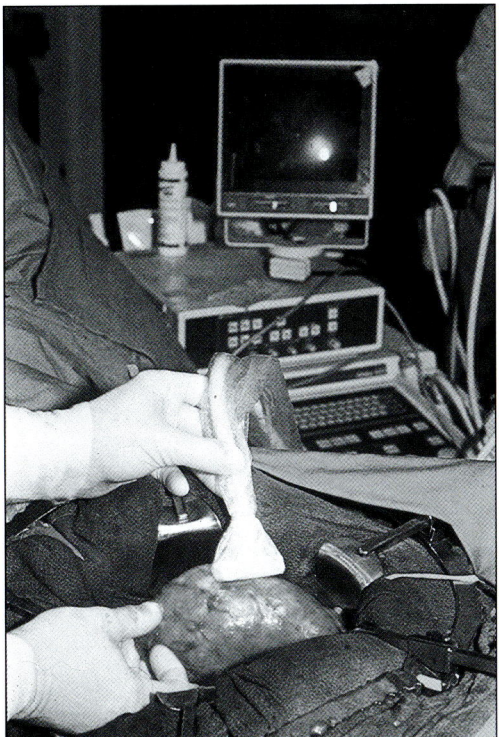

▶ **FIGURE 4-12.** (*See* Color Plate) Intraoperative ultrasound, which is very helpful in achieving accurate tumor localization particularly for intrarenal lesions that are not visible or palpable from the external surface of the kidney [2]. Intraoperative ultrasound is of no added value in detecting occult multicentric tumors elsewhere in the kidney. Preoperative CT scanning combined with intraoperative gross inspection of the kidney remain the most accurate assessments for detecting additional tumors in the involved kidney.

▶ **FIGURE 4-11.** Surgical techniques used for performing partial nephrectomy in patients with a malignancy. These techniques include polar (apical or basilar) segmental nephrectomy, wedge resection, and transverse resection. All of these techniques require adherence to basic principles of early vascular control, avoidance of ischemic renal damage, complete tumor excision with free margins, precise closure of the collecting system, careful hemostasis, and closure or coverage of the renal defect with adjacent fat, fascia, peritoneum, or oxidized cellulose. Regardless of the technique employed, the tumor is removed with a small surrounding margin of grossly normal renal parenchyma.

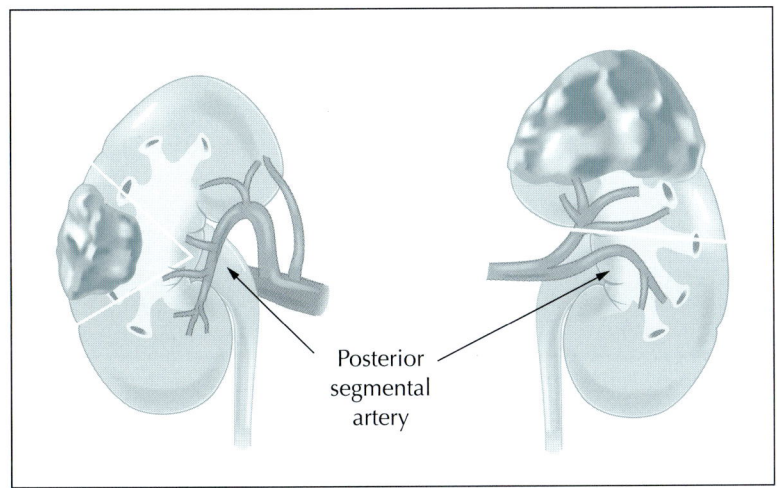

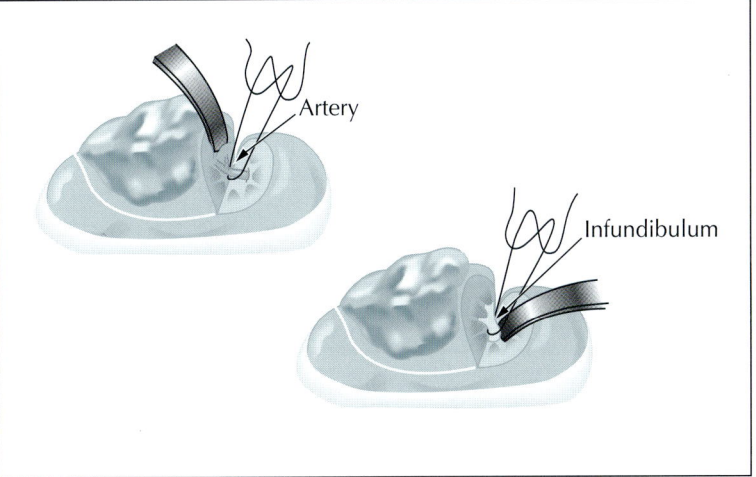

▶ **FIGURE 4-13.** Posterior segmental renal artery. When performing a transverse resection of the upper part of the kidney, care must be taken to avoid injury to the posterior segmental renal arterial branch, which may also occasionally supply the basilar renal segment. Preoperative selective renal arteriography with oblique views is integral to identifying and preserving the posterior segmental artery at surgery, and to thereby avoid devascularizing a major portion of the healthy remnant kidney. Midrenal resections may also be particularly complicated because the arterial supply comprises branches of anterior and posterior renal artery divisions, and the calices often enter the same infundibula as those draining the upper and lower poles.

▶ **FIGURE 4-14.** Ligation of arteries and infundibula. The parenchyma around the tumor is divided with a combination of sharp and blunt dissections regardless of the nephron-sparing technique employed. In many cases, the tumor extends deeply into the kidney and the collecting system. Often, renal arterial and venous branches supplying the tumor can be identified as the parenchyma is being incised, and these should be directly sutured and ligated at that time, while they are most visible. Similarly, in many cases, direct entry into the collecting system may be avoided by isolating and ligating major infundibula that drain the tumor-bearing renal segment as the incision into the parenchyma is developed.

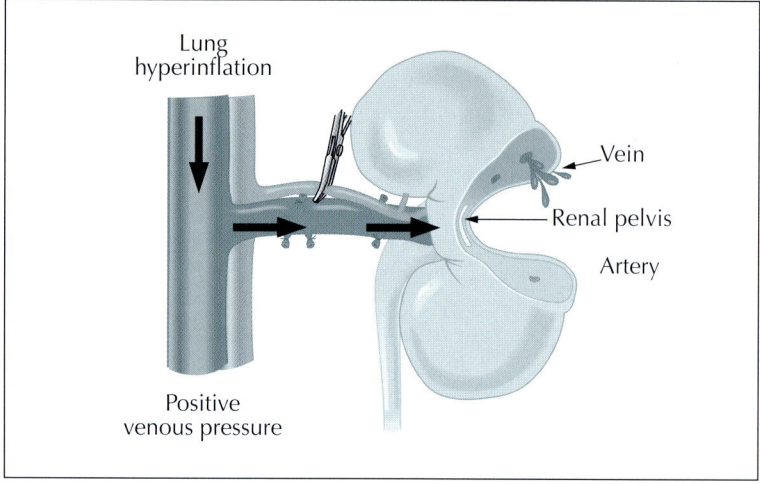

Lung
hyperinflation

Vein

Renal pelvis

Artery

Positive
venous pressure

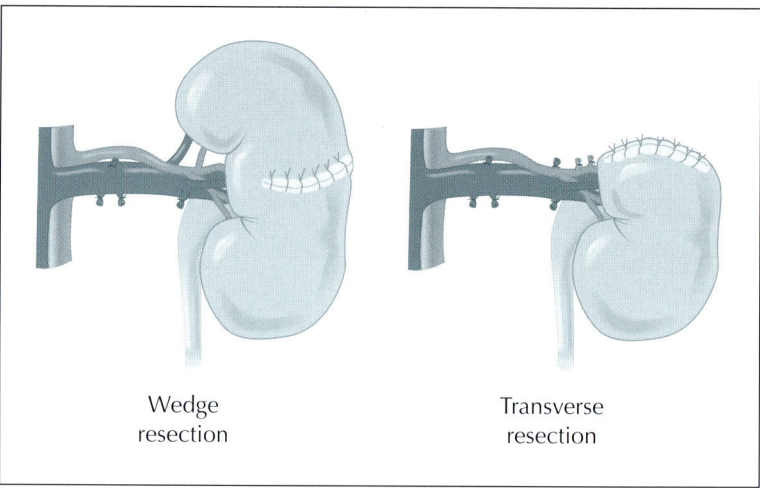

Wedge
resection

Transverse
resection

▶ FIGURE 4-15. Hyperinflation of the lungs. After excision of the tumor, the remaining transected blood vessels on the renal surface are secured with figure eight 4.0 chromic sutures. Bleeding at this point is usually minimal, and the operative field can be kept satisfactorily clear by gentle suction during placement of hemostatic sutures. Residual collecting system defects are similarly closed with interrupted or continuous 4.0 chromic sutures. With the renal artery still clamped but with the renal vein open, the anesthesiologist is asked to hyperinflate the lungs and thereby raise the central and renal venous pressure. This forces blood out through residual unsecured transected veins on the renal surface and thereby facilitates their detection. Once identified, these veins are secured with interrupted figure eight 4.0 chromic sutures. The argon beam coagulator is a useful adjunct for achieving hemostasis on the transected peripheral renal surface.

▶ FIGURE 4-16. Closure of the kidney after tumor excision. In most cases, after securing the renal vasculature and collecting system, the kidney is closed upon itself by approximating the transected cortical margins with simple interrupted 3.0 chromic sutures after placing a small piece of oxidized cellulose at the base of the defect. This is an important additional hemostatic measure. When this is done, there must be no tension on the suture line and no significant angulation or kinking of blood vessels supplying the kidney. After closure of the renal defect, the renal artery is unclamped and circulation to the kidney is restored.

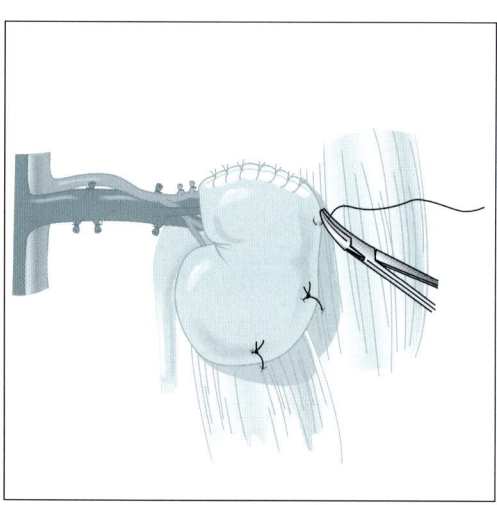

▶ FIGURE 4-17. Nephropexy of the remnant kidney. When the remnant kidney resides within a large retroperitoneal fossa, the kidney is fixed to the posterior musculature with interrupted 3.0 chromic sutures to prevent postoperative movement or rotation of the kidney. Kidney movement or rotation may compromise the blood supply. A retroperitoneal drain is always left in place for at least 7 days, and an intraoperative ureteral stent is placed only when major reconstruction of the intrarenal collecting system has been performed.

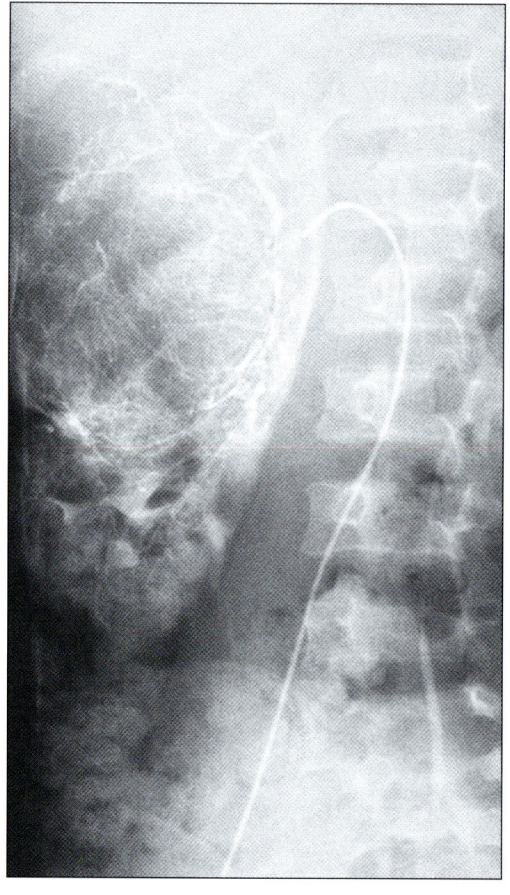

▶ FIGURE 4-18. Arteriogram depicting a large vascular centrally located tumor involving the upper two thirds of the right kidney. Extracorporeal partial nephrectomy with renal autotransplantation is rarely necessary, and even large centrally located tumors can be satisfactorily managed in situ. The function of the left kidney in this patient is impaired and, therefore, nephron-sparing tumor excision is indicated.

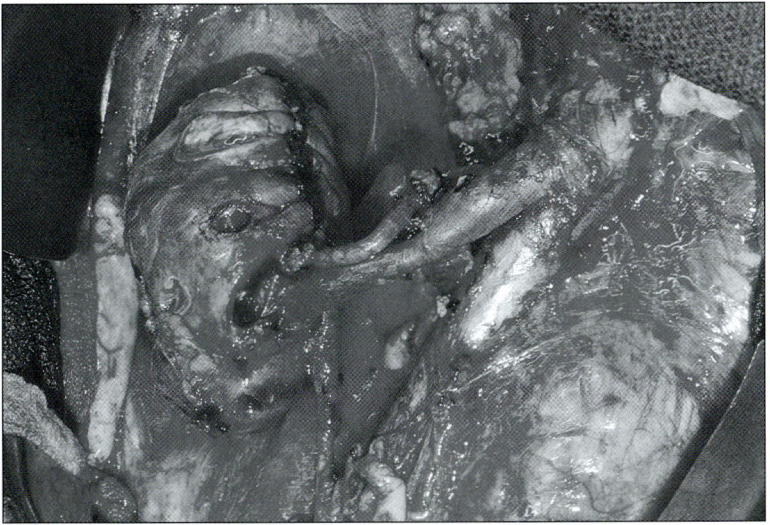

▶ **FIGURE 4-19.** (*See* Color Plate) Operative photograph depicting the repaired remnant lower third of the right kidney following nephron-sparing tumor excision in the same patient as in Figure 4-18. The remnant kidney is well-perfused via segmental branches of the renal artery and vein.

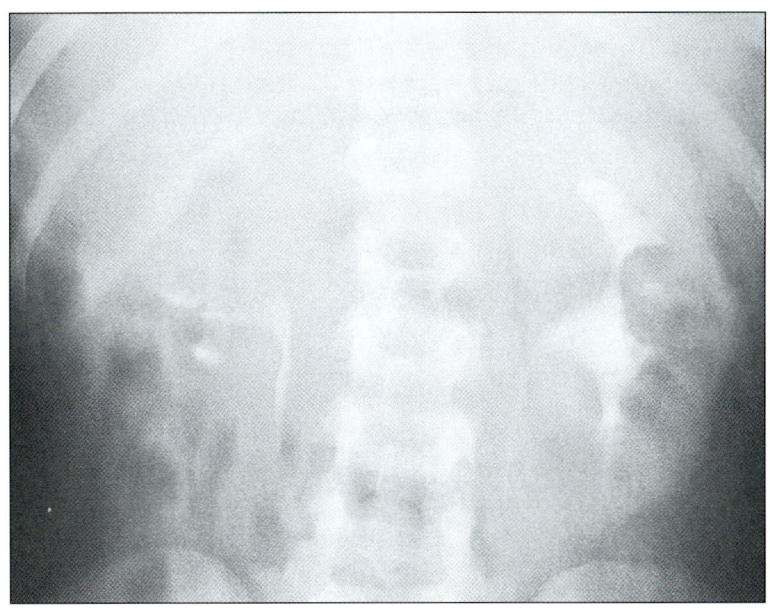

▶ **FIGURE 4-20.** Postoperative intravenous pyelogram of the same patient described in Figures 4-18 and 4-19. This radiograph reveals excellent function of the remaining lower portion of the right kidney, as well as of the left kidney.

COMPLICATIONS OF SURGERY

Complications of Nephron-Sparing Surgery for Renal Tumors*

Type	Incidence
Urinary fistula	45
Acute renal failure	33
Wound infection	11
Other	11

* Data from 259 nephron-sparing operations (1956 to 1992). After 78 operations 100 complications occurred (30.1%).

▶ **FIGURE 4-21.** Complications of nephron-sparing surgery for renal tumors. A recent study detailed the incidence and clinical outcome of technical or renal-related complications occurring after 259 nephron-sparing operations for renal tumors at The Cleveland Clinic [3]. In the overall series, local or renal-related complications occurred after 78 operations (30.1%). The incidence of complications was significantly less for operations performed after 1988 and also significantly less for incidentally detected versus suspected tumors. The most common complications were urinary fistula formation and acute renal failure, with the remainder composed of wound infections or other general complications. Overall, only eight complications (3.1%) required repeat open surgery for treatment, whereas all other complications resolved with noninterventive or endourologic management. Surgical complications contributed to an adverse clinical outcome in only seven patients (2.9%).

Development of Urinary Fistulas After Nephron-Sparing Surgery for Renal Tumors*

Risk Factors	
Central location	$P=0.001$
Size >4.0 cm	$P=0.001$
Major repair	$P=0.001$
Ex vivo	$P=0.001$
Outcome	
Spontaneous resolution	30
Endoscopic management	14
Repeat open surgery	1

* Of 259 surgeries, 45 (17%) patients developed urinary fistulas.

▶ **FIGURE 4-22.** Development of urinary fistulas after nephron-sparing surgery for renal tumors. A urinary fistula occurred after 45 of 259 operations (17%). Significant predisposing factors for a urinary fistula included central tumor location, tumor size greater than 4 cm, the need for major reconstruction of the collecting system, and ex vivo surgery. Only one urinary fistula required open operative repair, whereas the remainder resolved either spontaneously (*n* = 30) or with endoscopic management (*n* = 14).

Acute Renal Failure After Nephron-Sparing Surgery for Renal Tumors*

Risk factors	
Size > 7.0 cm	$P = 0.008$
> 50% Excision	$P = 0.001$
Ex vivo	$P = 0.0001$
Spontaneous resolution	16
Temporary dialysis	9 (7.8%)
Permanent dialysis	5 (4.3%)

Of 115 patients, 30 (26%) experienced acute renal failure in solitary kidneys after nephron-sparing surgery for renal tumors.

▶ **FIGURE 4-23.** Acute renal failure after nephron-sparing surgery for renal tumors. Acute renal failure occurred after 30 of 115 operations (26%) performed on a solitary kidney. Significant predisposing factors for acute renal failure were a tumor size greater than 7 cm, more than 50% parenchymal excision, more than 60 minutes ischemia time, and ex vivo surgery. Acute renal failure resolved completely in 25 patients, of whom nine (8%) required temporary dialysis; five patients (4%) required permanent dialysis. Patients undergoing nephron-sparing surgery for malignancy in a solitary kidney should be apprised of the small risk of temporary or permanent dialysis postoperatively.

POSTOPERATIVE RESULTS AND SURVIVAL RATES

Results of Nephron-Sparing Surgery for Renal Cell Carcinoma

Study	Patients, n	Local tumor recurrence, n (%)	5-Year cancer-specific survival rate, %
Morgan and Zincke [4]	104	6 (5.8)	89
Steinbach et al. [5]	121	5 (4.1)	90
Licht et al. [6]	216	9 (4.2)	87

▶ **FIGURE 4-24.** Results of nephron-sparing surgery for renal cell carcinoma. The technical success rate with nephron-sparing surgery for renal cell carcinoma is excellent, and large studies have reported 5-year cancer-specific survival rates of 87% to 90% in such patients [4–6]. These survival rates are comparable to those obtained after radical nephrectomy, particularly for low-stage renal cell carcinoma. The major disadvantage of nephron-sparing surgery for renal cell carcinoma is the risk of postoperative local tumor recurrence in the operated kidney, which has occurred in 4% to 6% of patients. These local recurrences are most likely a manifestation of undetected microscopic multifocal renal cell carcinoma in the remnant kidney. The risk of local tumor recurrence after radical nephrectomy has not been studied, but it is presumably very low.

Tumor Characteristics and Survival Rate of Patients With Renal Cell Carcinoma

Tumor characteristics	Radical nephrectomy (n=42)	Nephron-sparing surgery (n=46)
Mean tumor size	2.7 cm ± 0.8 cm	2.5 cm ± 0.8 cm
Pathologic stage		
T1	9 (21%)	13 (28%)
T2	28 (67%)	28 (61%)
T3a	5 (12%)	5 (11%)
Tumor location within kidney		
Upper kidney	16 (38%)	16 (36%)
Mid kidney	12 (29%)	15 (32%)
Lower kidney	14 (33%)	15 (32%)
5-Year cancer-specific survival rate	97%	100%

▶ **FIGURE 4-25.** Tumor characteristics and survival rate of patients with renal cell carcinoma. These patients underwent radical nephrectomies or nephron-sparing surgery. Recent data have suggested that nephron-sparing surgery may be an acceptable therapeutic approach in patients who have a single, small (less than 4 cm) renal cell carcinoma and a normal contralateral kidney [7,8]. To test this hypothesis, we conducted a study wherein the outcome following radical nephrectomy versus nephron-sparing surgery was evaluated in 88 patients with a single, small (< 4 cm), localized, unilateral, sporadic, renal cell carcinoma. The radical (n = 42) and nephron-sparing (n = 46) surgical groups were well-matched for patient age, gender, renal function, diabetes, hypertension, tumor size, tumor location, and tumor stage. All patients in both groups had low pathologic stage renal cell carcinoma. Tumor location within the kidney was similar for patients in the radical and nephron-sparing surgical groups. A single patient in each group developed recurrent malignancy postoperatively. The cancer-specific 5-year survival rate for patients in the radical and nephron-sparing surgical groups was 97% and 100%, respectively. The results of this study demonstrated that radical nephrectomy and nephron-sparing surgery each provide safe and effective curative treatment for patients with a single, small, unilateral, localized renal cell carcinoma.

Effect of Tumor Location in Small, Solitary, and Unilateral Renal Cell Carcinoma

Tumor characteristics and outcomes	Central location (n=35)	Peripheral location (n=110)
Tumor size	2.5 cm	2.65 cm
Tumor stage		
T1	18	38
T2	15	53
T3a	1	17
T3b	1	2
Tumor grade		
I	4	18
II	24	67
III	7	22
IV	0	3
5-Year survival rate	100%	97%
Recurrent RCC	2 (5.7%)	5 (4.5%)

FIGURE 4-26. Effect of tumor location in small, solitary, and unilateral renal cell carcinoma. An issue related to the role of nephron-sparing surgery in patients with a normal opposite kidney is whether the location of the tumor in the involved kidney is a significant factor affecting treatment outcome in the setting of a single, small, unilateral, localized, sporadic renal cell carcinoma (RCC). To address this issue, another study was conducted in which tumor characteristics and cancer-free survival were compared in patients with centrally versus peripherally located renal cell carcinomas fulfilling the above criteria [9]. This study comprised 145 patients treated with either radical nephrectomy or nephron-sparing surgery, and the mean postoperative follow-up was 4.3 years. Pathologic tumor stage was T1 to 2 in 94% and 82% of central versus peripheral RCCs, respectively. Grade I to II RCC was present in 80% and 77% of central versus peripheral RCCs, respectively. Postoperatively, when comparing patients with central versus peripheral RCCs, there was no difference in 5-year cancer-specific survival (100% vs 97%) or tumor recurrence (5.7% vs 4.5%). These parameters were also equivalent in patients treated with nephron-sparing surgery versus radical nephrectomy both overall and within the central versus peripheral RCC subgroups. The results of this study indicate that there are no significant biologic differences between centrally versus peripherally located small, solitary, unilateral renal cell carcinomas. Treatment with nephron-sparing surgery or radical nephrectomy is equally effective regardless of tumor location in these patients.

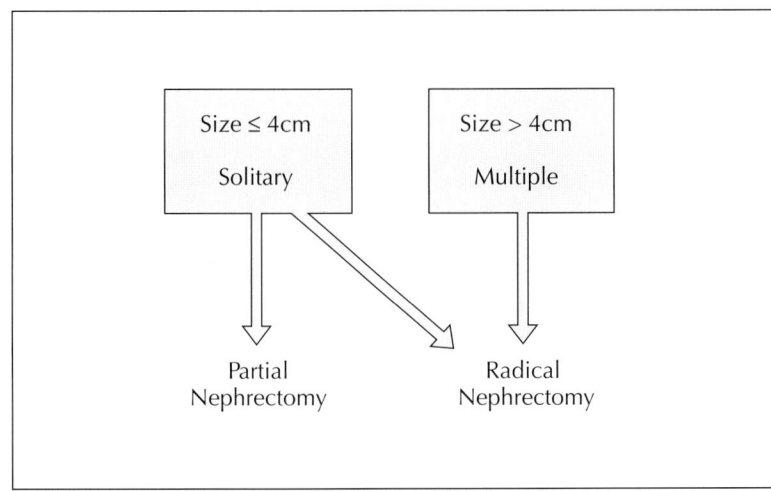

FIGURE 4-27. Algorithm of renal cell carcinoma with a normal contralateral kidney. Recent studies have clarified the role of nephron-sparing surgery in patients with localized, unilateral renal cell carcinoma and a normal contralateral kidney. These data indicate that radical nephrectomy and nephron-sparing surgery provide equally effective curative treatment for patients who present with a single, small (less than 4 cm), and clearly localized renal cell carcinoma. The results of nephron-sparing surgery are less satisfactory in patients with larger (greater than 4 cm) or multiple localized renal cell carcinomas, and radical nephrectomy remains the treatment of choice in such cases when the opposite kidney is normal. The long-term renal functional advantage of nephron-sparing surgery with a normal opposite kidney requires further study.

Tumor Recurrence After Nephron-Sparing Surgery According to Pathologic Tumor Stage

Tumor stage	Patients, n	Local recurrence		Metastatic recurrence	
		n, (%)	MTR, mo	n, (%)	MTR, mo
T1	68	0 (0)	—	3 (4.4)	44.8
T2	151	3 (2.0)	62.0	8 (5.3)	40.0
T3a	61	5 (8.2)	36.4	7 (11.5)	5.0
T3b	47	5 (10.6)	30.4	7 (14.9)	28.6

FIGURE 4-28. Tumor recurrence after nephron-sparing surgery according to pathologic tumor stage. A detailed analysis of tumor recurrence patterns after nephron-sparing surgery for sporadic localized renal cell carcinoma (RCC) in 327 patients was recently completed at The Cleveland Clinic [10]. The purpose of this study was to develop appropriate guidelines for long-term surveillance after nephron-sparing surgery for RCC. Recurrent RCC occurred postoperatively in 38 patients (11.6%), including 13 patients (4.0%) who developed local tumor recurrence (LTR) and 25 patients (7.6%) who developed metastatic disease (MD). MTR—mean time to recurrence.

Recommended Postoperative Surveillance After Nephron-Sparing Surgery for Sporadic Localized Renal Cell Carcinoma

Pathologic tumor stage	History, examination, blood tests*	Chest radiograph	Abdominal CT scan
T1	Yearly	—	—
T2	Yearly	Yearly	Every 2 y
T3	Yearly	Yearly	Every 6 mo for 2 y, then every 2 y

* Medical history, physical examination, and measurement of serum calcium, alkaline phosphatase, liver function, and renal function.

▶ **FIGURE 4-29.** Recommended postoperative surveillance after nephron-sparing surgery for sporadic localized renal cell carcinoma (RCC). The above data indicate that surveillance for recurrent malignancy after nephron-sparing surgery for RCC can be tailored according to the initial pathologic tumor stage. All patients should be evaluated with a medical history, physical examination, and selected blood studies on a yearly basis. Patients who undergo nephron-sparing surgery for T1 RCC do not require any radiographic imaging postoperatively in view of the very low risk of recurrent malignancy. In patients who undergo nephron-sparing surgery for T2 RCC, a yearly chest radiograph is recommended because the lung is the most common site of postoperative metastasis. However, follow-up abdominal CT scanning is only occasionally needed (< every 2 years) due to the low risk of abdominal or retroperitoneal tumor recurrence in this group. Patients with T3 RCC have a higher risk of developing local recurrence during the first 2 years after nephron-sparing surgery; in these patients, follow-up abdominal CT scanning is recommended every 6 months for 2 years and every 2 years thereafter. This tailored approach for surveillance after nephron-sparing surgery for RCC is similar to that which has been described following radical nephrectomy for RCC [11].

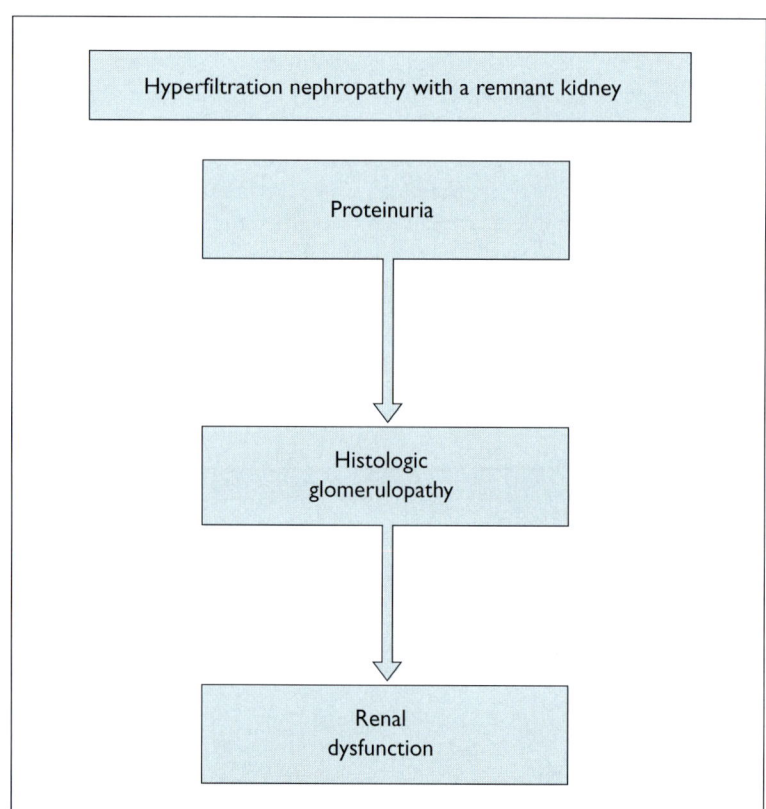

▶ **FIGURE 4-30.** Hyperfiltration nephropathy with a remnant kidney. Another important issue relevant to postoperative follow-up is the potential development of hyperfiltration nephropathy in patients with a remnant kidney. Recent data suggest that patients with a greater than 50% reduction in overall renal mass are at increased risk for developing proteinuria, glomerulopathy, and progressive renal failure [12]. Structural or functional renal damage in such cases is usually antedated by the appearance of proteinuria. Therefore, the follow-up of patients after nephron-sparing surgery should include a 24-hour urinary protein determination in addition to a serum creatinine level and glomerular filtration rate. Patients who have proteinuria may be treated with a low protein diet and a converting enzyme inhibitor agent. Both methods of treatment appear to be beneficial in preventing glomerulopathy caused by reduced renal mass.

REFERENCES

1. Licht MR, Novick AC, Goormastic M: Nephron-sparing surgery for renal cell carcinoma. *J Urol* 1994, 149:1–7.

2 Campbell SC, Fichtner J, Novick AC, *et al.*: Intraoperative evaluation of renal cell carcinoma: prospective study of the role of ultrasonography and histopathological frozen sections. *J Urol* 1996, 155:1191–1195.

3 Campbell SC, Novick AC, Streem SB, *et al.*: Complications of nephron-sparing surgery for renal tumors. *Urology* 1994, 151:1177–1180.

4. Morgan WR, Zincke H: Progression and survival after renal-conserving surgery for renal cell carcinoma: experience in 104 patients and extended follow-up. *J Urol* 1990, 144:852–857.

5. Steinbach F, Stockle M, Muller SC, *et al.*: Conservative surgery of renal cell tumors in 140 patients: 21 years of experience. *J Urol* 1992, 148:24–29.

6. Licht MR, Novick AC, Goormastic M: Nephron-sparing surgery in incidental versus suspected renal cell carcinoma. *J Urol* 1994, 152:39–42.

7. Butler B, Novick AC, Miller D, *et al.*: Management of small unilateral renal cell carcinomas: radical versus nephron-sparing surgery. *Urology* 1995, 45:34–41.

8. Lerner SE, Hawkins CA, Blute ML, *et al.*: Disease outcome in patients with low-stage renal cell carcinoma treated with nephron-sparing or radical surgery. *J Urol* 1996, 155:1868–1873.

9. Hafez KS, Novick AC, Butler B: Management of small, solitary, unilateral renal cell carcinomas: impact of central versus peripheral tumor location. *J Urol* 1998, 159:1156–1160.

10. Hafez KS, Novick AC, Campbell SC: Patterns of tumor recurrence and guidelines for follow-up after nephron-sparing surgery for sporadic renal cell carcinoma. *J Urol* 1997, 157:2067–2070.

11. Sandock DS, Seftell AD, Resnick MI: A new protocol for the followup of renal cell carcinoma based on pathological stage. *J Urol* 1995, 154:28–31.

12. Novick AC, Gephardt G, Guz B, *et al.*: Long-term follow-up after partial removal of a solitary kidney. *N Engl J Med* 1991, 325:1058–1062.

Renal Cell Carcinoma With Vena Caval Involvement

Thomas J. Polascik and Fray F. Marshall

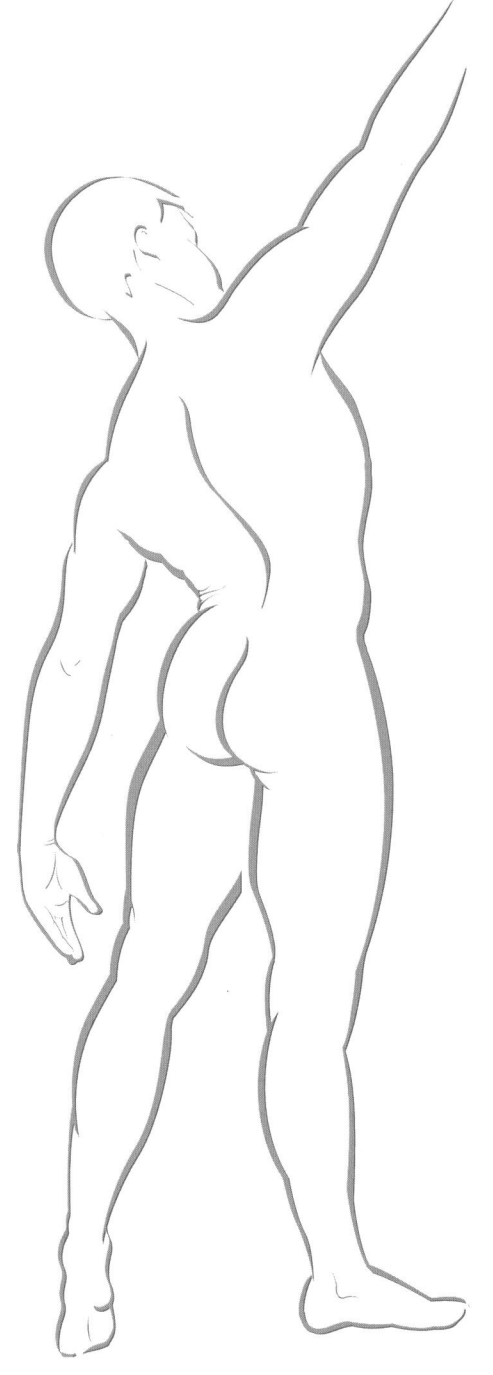

Renal cell carcinoma has an intriguing ability to extend directly into the renal vein and vena cava, often in the absence of known metastases or further local extension. In 1970, Marshall *et al.* [1] reported that 4% to 10% of patients with renal cell carcinoma have neoplastic extension of tumor into the ipsilateral renal vein and inferior vena cava. The extent of intracaval tumor may vary, although focal extension of tumor into the renal vein is more common than intracaval extension to the heart. Early attempts at radical nephrectomy and caval thrombectomy were limited by unacceptably high rates of morbidity and mortality. With improvements in surgical technique, intraoperative monitoring, and postoperative care, these extensive surgical procedures are now considered technically feasible and reasonably safe. Use of cardiopulmonary bypass, hypothermia, and circulatory arrest have greatly improved our clinical ability to resect caval tumors extending above the diaphragm [2–4]. Because chemotherapy and radiotherapy offer little efficacy, radical surgery remains the primary treatment for these tumors.

The principal indication for radical nephrectomy and venacavotomy is a renal mass with intracaval tumor extension in the absence of metastatic disease. The patient should be otherwise healthy with a good performance status and be medically able to tolerate an extensive surgical procedure. Preoperative evaluation may include cardiac stress testing, echocardiography, or coronary angiography if the patient has a significant risk of cardiovascular disease. Radical nephrectomy and venacavotomy can be rarely performed for palliative purposes in patients with metastatic disease who are symptomatic or have imminent risk of catastrophic death. In these extenuating circumstances, surgery will not increase life and can actually shorten it. At present, therapeutic alternatives to surgery for these large tumors with vascular extension and metastatic disease are lacking. Expectant therapy or systemic protocols may be applicable if the patient is a candidate.

CLINICAL PRESENTATION

A. Clinical Presentation

Abdominal mass
Abdominal pain
Hematuria
Weight loss
Fever

B. Signs and Symptoms Related to Caval Occlusion

Bilateral lower extremity edema
Varicocele
Proteinuria
Hepatic dysfunction with hepatomegaly
Dilated abdominal wall veins
Pulmonary embolus

▶ **FIGURE 5-1.** Clinical presentation and signs and symptoms related to caval occlusion. **A,** Clinical presentation. Because these tumors are often relatively large, patients frequently present with typical signs or symptoms such as an abdominal mass (25% to 55%), flank or abdominal pain (23% to 33%), or hematuria (42% to 58%) [5,6]. Approximately one third of patients experience weight loss and a significant percentage have fever [5]. **B,** Signs and symptoms related to caval occlusion. Approximately 25% to 50% of patients with significant tumor involvement of the vena cava have signs and symptoms related to complete or partial caval occlusion [5,7]. Development of adequate venous collaterals diminishes the clinical manifestations of caval occlusion.

In addition to palpating for an abdominal mass, the physical examination should focus on detecting signs associated with caval occlusion, such as a varicocele that does not collapse in the supine position, dilated superficial abdominal wall veins, or hepatomegaly. In one report, bilateral lower extremity edema was identified in 16% of 48 patients presenting with vena caval tumor involvement [8]. In addition, the supraclavicular nodes should be examined for evidence of enlargement.

Laboratory analysis should include hematology, chemistry, and coagulation studies. Anemia is common and has been demonstrated in nearly 60% of patients with caval tumor involvement [9]. A serum chemistry panel is helpful to detect abnormalities in liver function, which are often found when the intracaval tumor hinders hepatic venous drainage into the inferior vena cava. An elevated alkaline phosphatase level can provide an indication of bone metastasis. A baseline serum creatinine level should be determined to evaluate renal function. In addition to detecting hematuria, urinalysis often identifies proteinuria that can accompany this disease process.

RADIOLOGIC EVALUATION

A. Goals of Radiologic Staging

Determine the local extent of the cancer
Define the inferior and superior limits of the caval tumor extension
Exclude metastatic disease

B. Preoperative Radiologic Evaluation

Intravenous pyelography
Transabdominal sonography
Transthoracic echocardiography
CT of abdomen and chest
Magnetic resonance imaging

▶ **FIGURE 5-2.** Radiologic evaluation. **A,** The goals of radiologic staging when considering imaging options. Defining the superior extent of the caval tumor is necessary to plan the surgical approach and determine the need for cardiac bypass. Surgical outcome is significantly improved in the absence of metastatic disease. **B,** Options for preoperative radiologic evaluation.

In the past, many of these tumors were diagnosed by intravenous pyelography (IVP). Vena caval involvement is suspected in the presence of a renal mass associated with a nonfunctioning or hypofunctioning kidney. Today, no indication exists for IVP to stage these tumors unless suspicion suggests that the renal mass may represent a transitional cell carcinoma. With encroachment of tumor into the renal vein or caval lumen, the ability of IVP to image the renal mass is diminished by obstruction of the venous outflow.

Often, transabdominal sonography is the first imaging modality to detect a renal mass because of this technique's widespread clinical use and relatively low cost. Renal masses detected by transabdominal ultrasound are typically further studied with CT. Transabdominal sonography is of less value for staging large renal cell cancers with vena caval involvement. The sensitivity of transabdominal ultrasound for detecting caval thrombi approaches 50% to 70% at best, with one fourth of the studies deemed indeterminate because of the inability to visualize the renal vein and the subhepatic vena cava [10]. Intraoperative ultrasound and transesophageal echocardiography (sonography), however, are valuable adjuncts for real-time intraoperative imaging. Alternatively, transthoracic echocardiography can preoperatively be used to verify the presence of tumor in the right atrium.

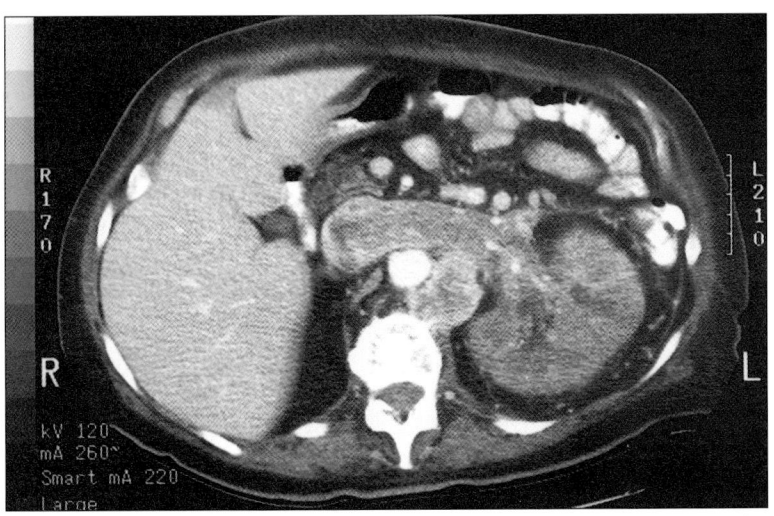

▶ **FIGURE 5-3.** Abdominal CT scan reveals tumor filling the left renal vein and extending into the inferior vena cava. Most patients presenting with a renal mass and intracaval tumor extension today are diagnosed by CT, which is obtained primarily to diagnose metastatic disease and determine patency of the ipsilateral renal vein. CT usually provides the initial suggestion that the renal tumor is extending into the lumen of the renal vein or vena cava. The sensitivity of CT for detecting caval tumors is less than 80% [10]. Spiral CT can provide additional information about the dynamic vascular function of the involved kidney when compared with conventional CT [11]. Although a standard chest roentgenogram is usually obtained, CT evaluation of the chest is recommended because it provides superior information regarding subtle pulmonary lesions and mediastinal lymphadenopathy. (*Courtesy of* SJ Savader, MD.)

•• MAGNETIC RESONANCE IMAGING ••

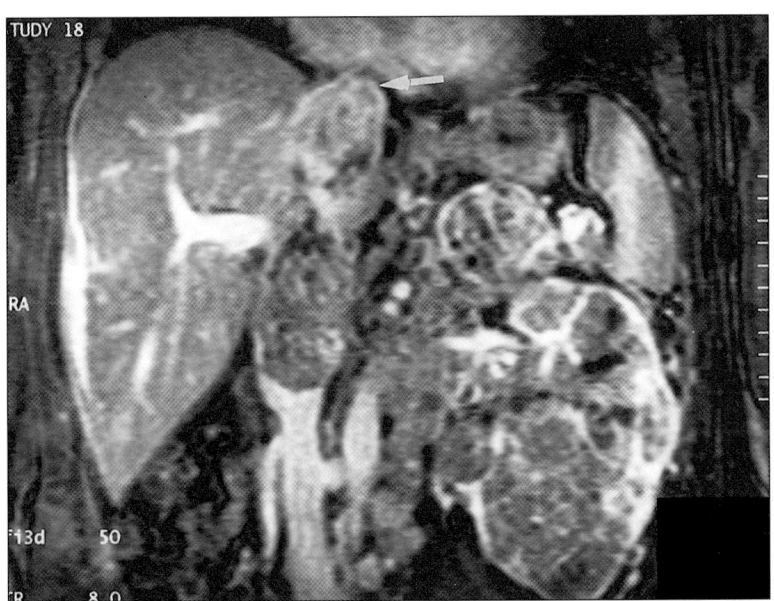

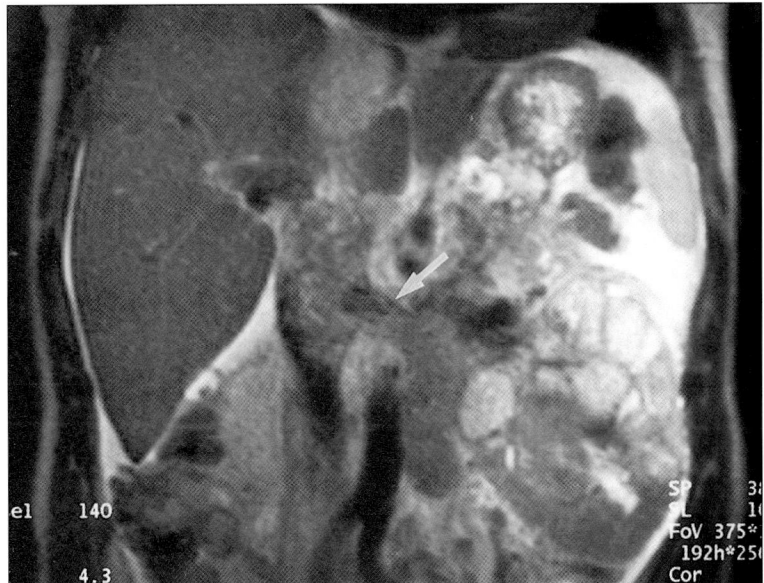

▶ **FIGURE 5-4.** Coronal T_1-weighted gadolinium-enhanced three-dimensional gradient echo magnetic resonance image (repetition time, 8.0; echo time, 2.7; FA, 45°) of a patient with a large left-sided renal neoplasm extending into the vena cava. The superior extent of the tumor (*arrow*) can be seen at the level of the diaphragm. The tumor does not appear to enter the heart (superior to the arrow) on magnetic resonance imaging, which was confirmed at surgery. (*Courtesy of* JP Earls, MD.)

▶ **FIGURE 5-5.** Coronal T_2-weighted HASTE (Half Fourier Acquisition Turbo Spin-Echo) (repetition time, ω; echo-time, 60) magnetic resonance imaging of the same patient as in Figure 5-4 showing the tumor filling the renal vein (*arrow*) and extending into the inferior vena cava. (*Courtesy of* JP Earls, MD.)

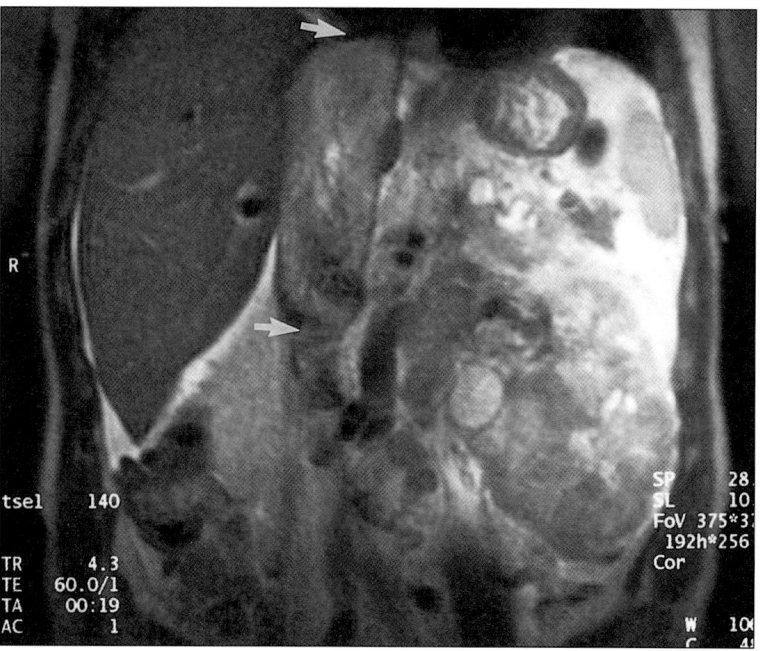

FIGURE 5-6. Coronal T_2-weighted image delineating the inferior and superior extent of the caval tumor (*arrows*). The tumor does not appear to enter the heart. After demonstrating caval tumor involvement, usually by CT, the proximal and distal limits of the caval tumor should be determined. Magnetic resonance imaging (MRI) has become the preferred modality to document and delineate the extent of a caval tumor because of its accuracy and noninvasive nature. The superior limit of the caval thrombus can usually be identified using MRI unless the thrombus is mobile. In such cases, artifact registration diminishes the accuracy for delineating the superior extent of the intracaval tumor. MRI is also effective for defining the extent of caval tumor involvement in cases in which the lumen of the vena cava is completely occluded. For complete identification of the extent of a large caval tumor, MRI combined with intraoperative transesophageal echocardiography provide the best results [12]. These noninvasive imaging modalities avoid the risk of tumor embolism that can occur with venacavography. (*Courtesy of* JP Earls, MD.)

•• INFERIOR VENACAVOGRAPHY ••

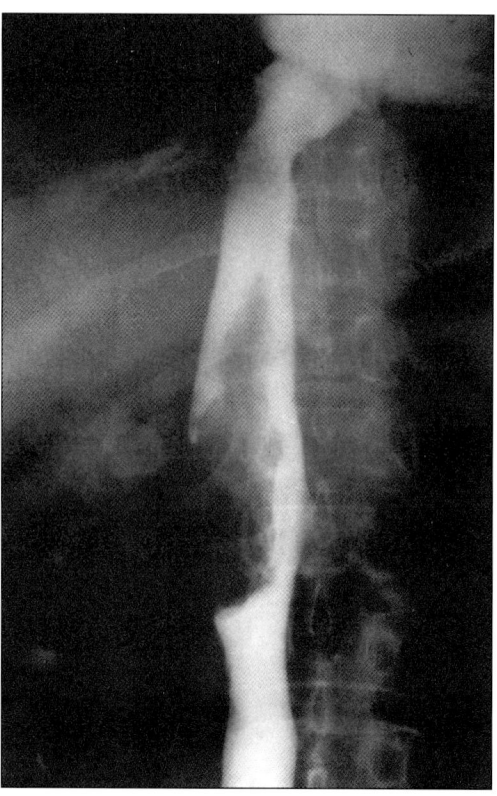

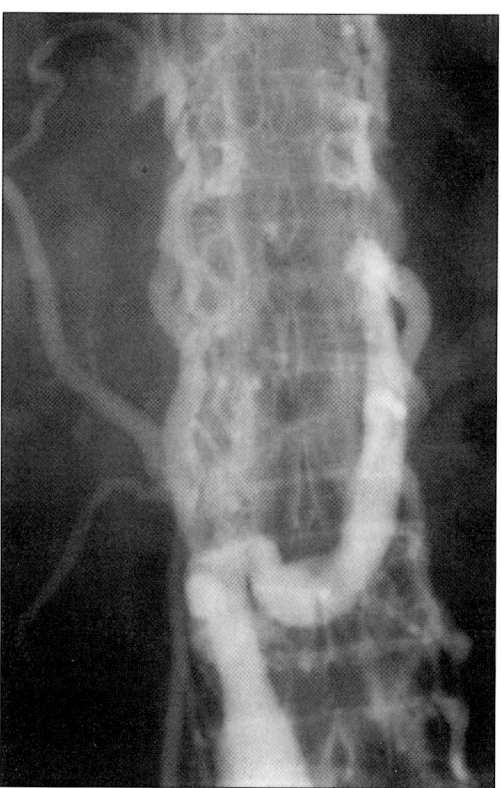

FIGURE 5-7. Inferior venacavogram of a renal cell carcinoma partially obstructing the vena cava. The superior and inferior extent of the caval tumor (seen as a filling defect) is well delineated; flow is demonstrated around the tumor. For many years, inferior venacavography was the definitive diagnostic study to evaluate the presence and extent of caval tumor involvement. If the vena cava is completely occluded, combined inferior and superior venacavography can be performed.

FIGURE 5-8. Inferior venacavogram of a renal neoplasm with tumor extension completely occluding the inferior vena cava. Abundant collateral vessels can be identified in this image.

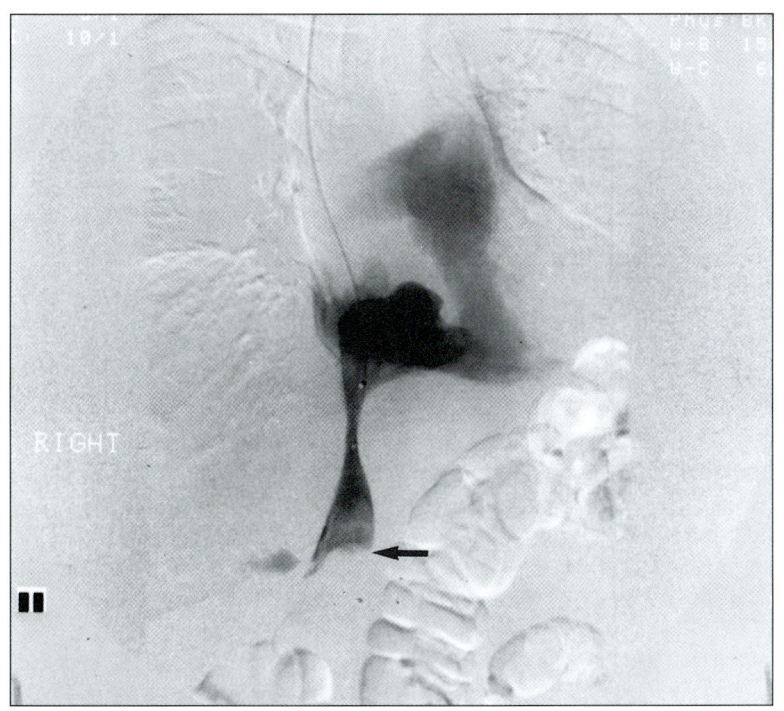

▶ **FIGURE 5-9.** Digital subtraction superior venacavogram showing the superior extent of a caval tumor (*arrow*, same patient as Fig. 5-3). Evaluation of the superior vena cava is commonly approached through the brachial vein. However, magnetic resonance imaging generally delineates the caval tumor accurately in this setting and is less invasive. In a study comparing venacavography and MRI for detecting vena caval tumors, the sensitivity and specificity for both modalities approached 100% and 85%, respectively [10]. When the ability to predict the extent of caval tumor was studied, the diagnostic accuracy of MRI was 90% and venacavography 75% [13]. With respect to the level of intracaval tumor extension, preoperative radiographic staging primarily using MRI was accurate in 94% of patients [14].

Transesophageal echocardiography can improve the diagnostic accuracy of either MRI or venacavography when determining the superior level of caval involvement [12,13]. Although venacavography can be used to define a caval tumor, its invasive nature, false-positive and false-negative results, and decreased ability to define the superior extent of the tumor all combine to limit its use. Today, venacavography is more often used as an alternative to MRI when MRI is contraindicated or nondiagnostic. Venacavography or MRI combined with intraoperative transesophageal echocardiography have been used to fully delineate the superior extent of the tumor when undergoing cardiopulmonary bypass [12]. A preoperative transesophageal echocardiography is not recommended because it necessitates a separate procedure and it can easily be performed at the time of operation. (*Courtesy of SJ Savader, MD.*)

OPERATIVE TECHNIQUE

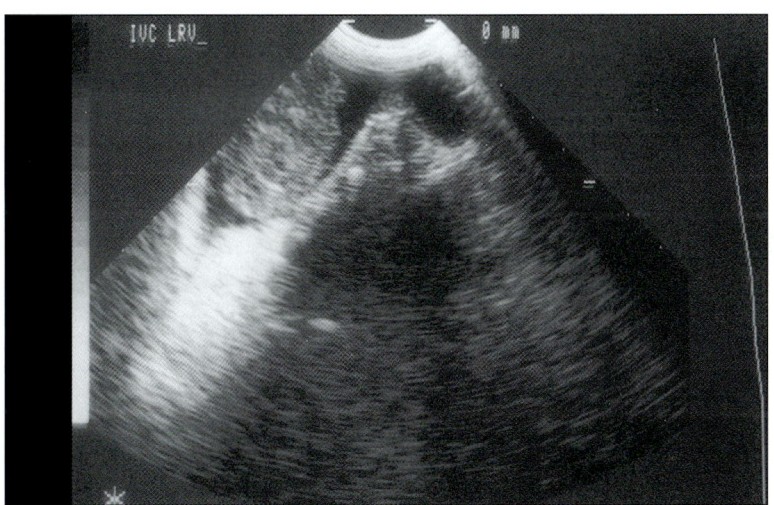

▶ **FIGURE 5-10.** Transesophageal echocardiogram of an intracaval renal tumor in the inferior vena cava just superior to the liver. Transesophageal echocardiography should be routinely used for all intrahepatic and supradiaphragmatic intracaval tumors. This modality can identify and confirm the superior extent of the caval tumor, thus enabling the surgeon to select the location of the incision and the need for cardiopulmonary bypass. It may also detect adherence of the tumor to the caval wall for which cardiac bypass would be advisable [15]. Moreover, it has also proven beneficial for visualization of correct placement of the superior vena caval lines to monitor cardiac function intraoperatively and to verify complete extraction of the caval tumor.

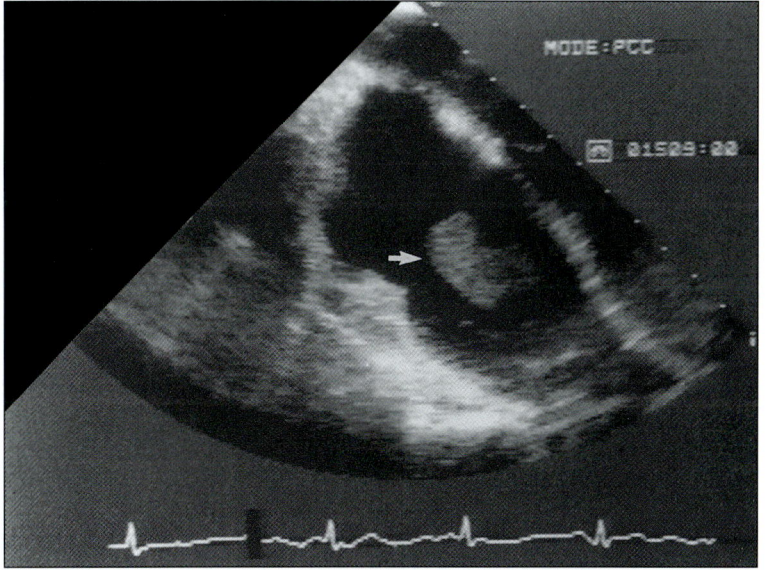

▶ **FIGURE 5-11.** Transesophageal echocardiogram depicting the tumor thrombus (*arrow*) within the right atrium. Several other techniques and devices for intraoperative monitoring deserve comment. Standard intraoperative monitoring includes central venous pressure, arterial pressure tracings, electrocardiography, and urinary output. For extensive vena caval tumors, additional monitoring would include a Swan-Ganz catheter, esophageal and rectal temperature probes, transesophageal sonography, and measurement of oxygen and carbon dioxide levels. Body temperature is maintained by use of a hypothermic blanket. To prevent lower extremity venous stasis, elastic stockings and sequential compression devices are used. A thoracic epidural can be used as an adjunct to general anesthesia because the epidural can effectively control postoperative pain with most flank incisions.

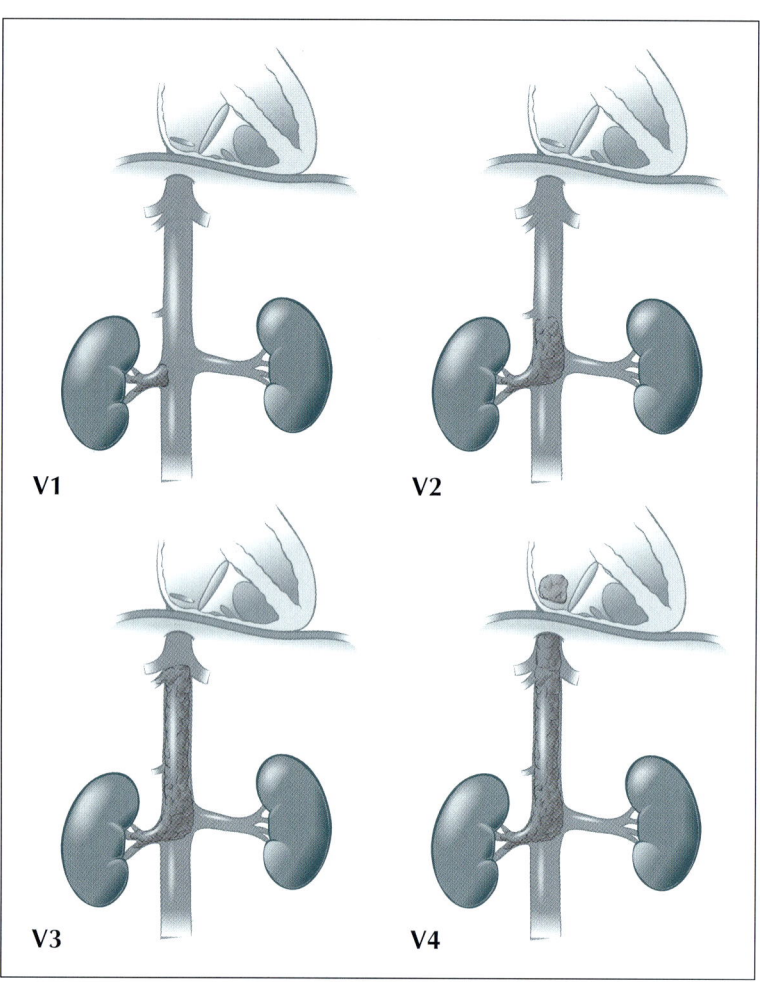

▶ **FIGURE 5-12.** Clinical and histopathologic classification of the venous (V) stages (levels of intracaval neoplastic extension of renal cell carcinoma). A V1 tumor extends into the renal vein and can include the renal vein ostium, V2 involvement includes tumor extension into the lumen of the vena cava but inferior to the first hepatic vein tributary, V3 includes neoplastic extension into the intrahepatic vena cava inferior to the diaphragm, and V4 refers to intracaval tumor extension superior to the diaphragm. These various levels of caval tumor involvement are important when considering the surgical approach.

Various incisions can be used to approach the renal primary tumor with intracaval tumor extension. In general, the extent of the tumor and body habitus of the patient should determine the surgical approach. For left- or right-sided renal tumors with involvement solely of the renal vein or with minimal involvement of the inferior vena cava, a thoracoabdominal approach at the level of the 11th rib or above is ideal, especially in obese patients.

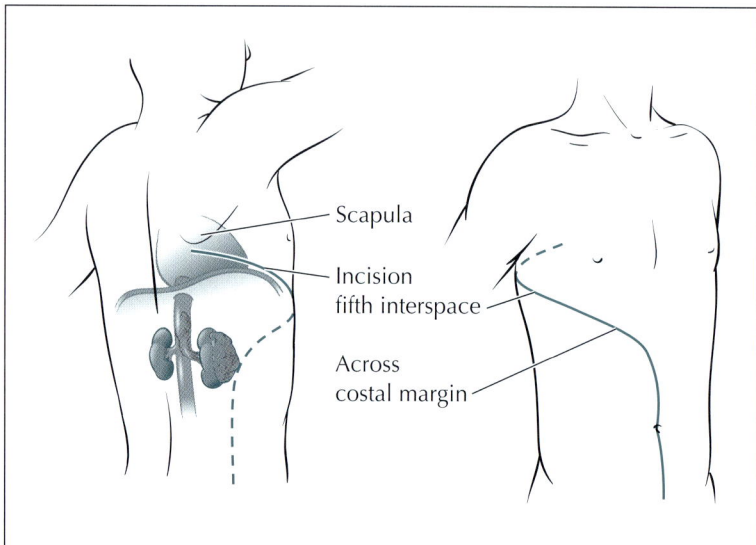

▶ **FIGURE 5-13.** For right-sided renal tumors with significant tumor extension into the vena cava (*ie*, V3 to V4), a thoracoabdominal incision (5th intercostal space) can be used. The extended thoracoabdominal incision extends from the inferior angle of the scapula, across the costal margin to the midline halfway between the xyphoid process and the umbilicus. The midline incision can be extended inferiorly beyond the umbilicus to the lower abdomen.

The best exposure for this incision is achieved by rotating the patient's shoulder while maintaining the pelvis in the supine position. The advantage of this approach is that it provides good exposure of the renal primary and the vena cava. Although it is possible to use this incision for caval tumors extending into the heart, this exposure is more difficult for the cardiac surgeon, especially for cannulation of the aortic arch for cardiopulmonary bypass. (*Adapted from* Marshall [16].)

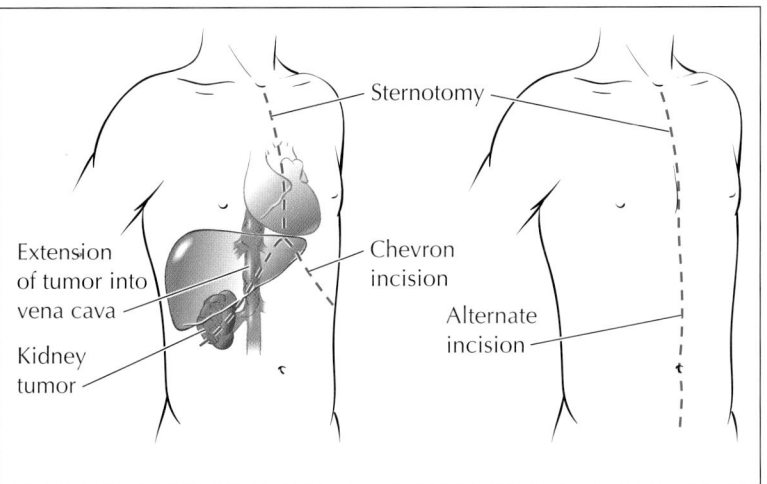

FIGURE 5-14. Anterior incisions. Anterior incisions provide good exposure for more extensive caval tumors (*ie*, V3 to V4) and left-sided tumors. When the intracaval neoplasm extends into or beyond the liver and cardiopulmonary bypass is considered, a median sternotomy extending into either a midline abdominal (for thin patients) or a chevron incision (for patients with a wide abdominal girth) is recommended. The entire length of the incision is made from commencement of the operation because it facilitates exposure and dissection. The advantage of this approach is that it provides better access to the heart for cardiopulmonary bypass and less musculature is divided compared with the extended thoracoabdominal incision. Although the excellent exposure obtained with these extensive incisions allows for additional operations to be performed including coronary artery bypass grafting, we recommend limiting the procedure to nephrectomy and caval thrombectomy whenever possible. (*Adapted from* Marshall [16].)

ISOLATION OF VENA CAVA WITH
•• INTRACAVAL NEOPLASTIC EXTENSION ••
AT THE LEVEL OF THE RENAL VEIN

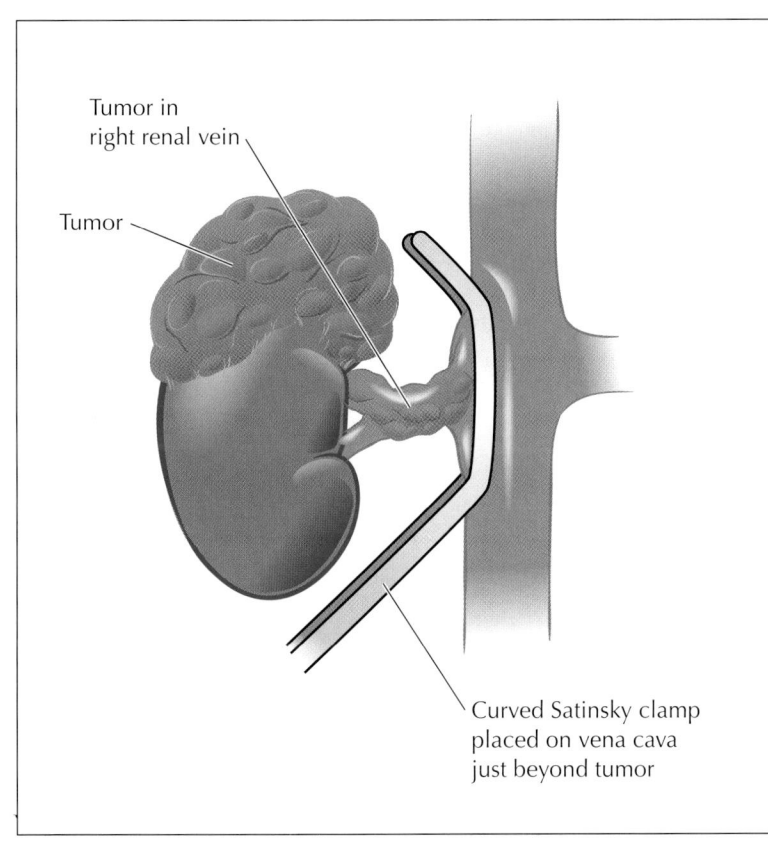

FIGURE 5-15. Use of the Satinsky clamp to isolate a renal cell carcinoma with V1 tumor extension. For caval tumors extending slightly (< 2 cm) beyond the ostium of the renal vein into the vena cava, a Satinsky vascular clamp is placed on the sidewall of the vena cava beyond the tumor. This segment of caval wall is excised en bloc with the renal neoplasm, and the cava is then oversewn with 4-0 or 5-0 polypropylene cardiovascular suture. A flank or low thoracoabdominal incision is used to approach a right renal tumor involving only the renal vein or with minimal neoplastic extension into the vena cava. The retroperitoneum and abdomen are grossly inspected to exclude metastatic disease. The OmniTract (Minnesota Scientific Inc., Minneapolis, MN) retractor provides excellent superficial and deep exposure of the surgical field. The kidney is first approached posterolaterally by developing the plane between the quadratus and psoas muscles and Gerota's fascia. Anteriorly, the mesocolon is reflected medially from the anterior surface of Gerota's fascia to the vena cava. Kocher's maneuver provides additional medial exposure along the vena cava. After the entire kidney is mobilized within Gerota's fascia, the renal artery is ligated, preferably from the posterior approach. The adrenal vein is ligated and divided followed by dissection of the adrenal superiorly. The gonadal vein and ureter are sequentially ligated, completing the inferior dissection. The entire kidney should now only be attached to the vena cava via the renal vein. Isolation of the vena cava should be in proportion to the extent of the intracaval tumor for right-sided renal tumors. The involved renal vein and vena cava should be judiciously dissected to prevent potential dislodgment of caval tumor.

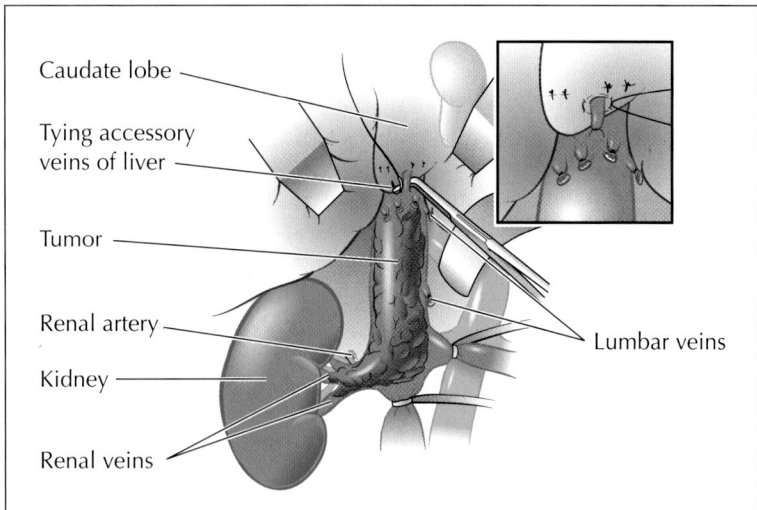

◗ FIGURE 5-16. Vena caval isolation and ligation of individual hepatic tributaries. With a more extensive intrahepatic intracaval tumor (V3), a midline transperitoneal approach is recommended. After incising the line of Toldt from the cecum to the ligament of Treitz, the ascending colon is reflected medially to expose the right kidney. The small intestine can be placed in a bowel bag for additional exposure. The entire right kidney is dissected within Gerota's fascia as previously mentioned, leaving only its renal vein attached to the vena cava. Control of the vena cava must be obtained below both renal veins. Ligation of several posterior lumbar veins entering the involved segment of vena cava is usually necessary to prevent unexpected bleeding. Lumbar veins drain into the vena cava posterolaterally and should be handled delicately, because these often are the cause of troublesome intraoperative hemorrhage. The left renal vein is partially mobilized and a Rummel's tourniquet is placed loosely should vascular control become

required. If necessary, superior exposure to the vena cava can be achieved through division of the triangular ligament and rotation of the liver medially. With extension of the tumor into the liver (V3), several venous branches draining the caudate lobe of the liver may require ligation and division. This maneuver can expose an additional 2 to 3 cm of vena cava superiorly. Suture ligatures placed into the liver parenchyma can control these veins draining the caudate lobe if they are short. Cardiopulmonary bypass can be avoided if a vascular clamp or a Rummel's tourniquet can be placed across the cava above the superior extent of the tumor.

After the vena cava is sufficiently mobilized, Satinsky clamps or Rummel's tourniquets are placed on the vena cava just beyond the superior and inferior limits of the intracaval tumor. The vena cava is first clamped inferiorly, followed by the contralateral renal vein and the vena caval vein superiorly above the tumor. An elliptical incision circumscribing the ostium of the involved renal vein is made. It is good practice to excise the renal vein ostium in that this is a common area of tumor adherence seen with V3 to V4 caval tumors. After the caval tumor has been removed, the vascular clamp located on the superior extent of the vena cava can be removed concurrently with a positive pressure ventilation delivered by the anesthesiologist. This will flush out any residual fragments of tumor superiorly. Following cavotomy, the interior of the cava is irrigated with saline. After closing the venacavotomy, the inferior vascular clamp is first released, followed by the clamp on the contralateral renal vein. Before securing the knot on the cavotomy closure, all air within the cava is removed and the superior vascular clamp is released.

On occasion, adherence of the tumor to the vascular wall is found. Bypass is recommended if intrahepatic caval extension with tumor adherent to the caval wall is present because it provides superior exposure and adequate time for "endarterectomy" or caval resection and reconstruction. (*Adapted from* Marshall *et al.* [3].)

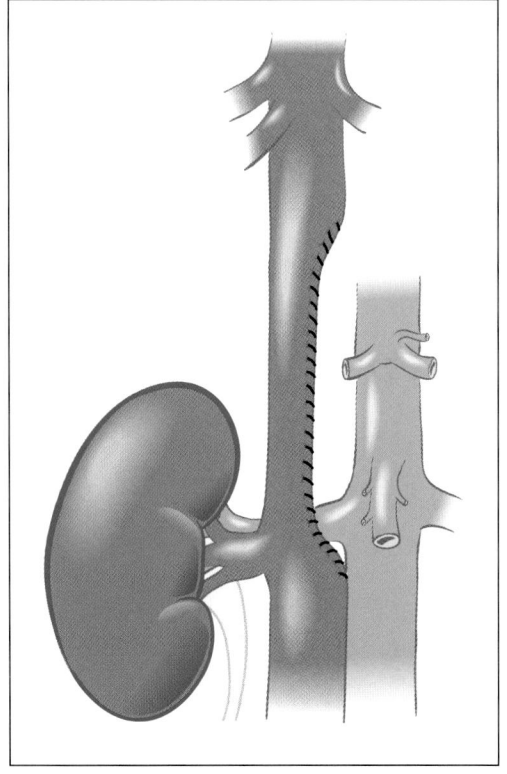

◗ FIGURE 5-17. Reduction of caval lumen by 50%, with reconstruction. In this figure, a segment of the caval wall is resected and the cavotomy closed leaving the caval diameter at 50% of its original caliber. If preexisting collaterals are not apparent or if excision of the caval wall reduces the vascular diameter by greater than 50%, the vena cava should be reconstructed. If collateral circulation is not present, resection and ligation of the inferior vena cava can create marked lower extremity edema that usually improves after several months.

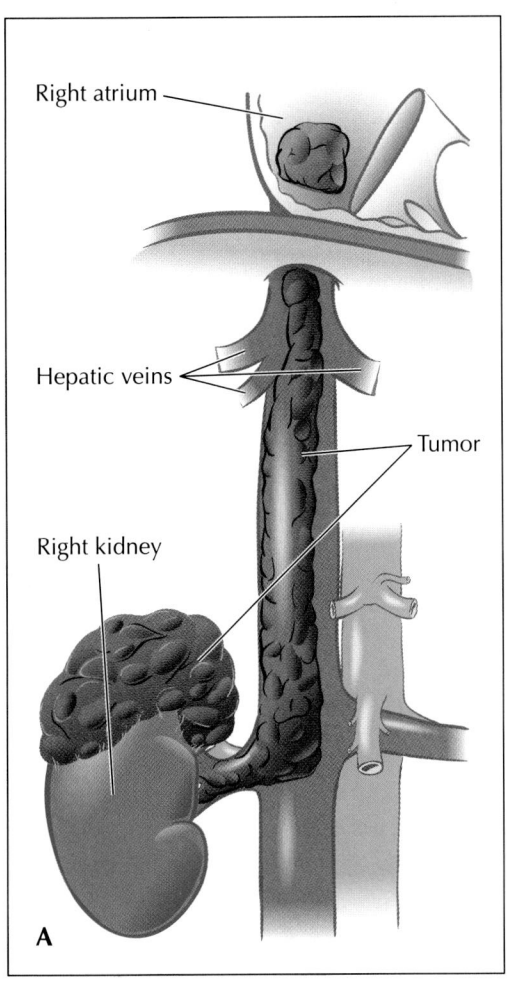

Right atrium

Hepatic veins

Right kidney

Tumor

A

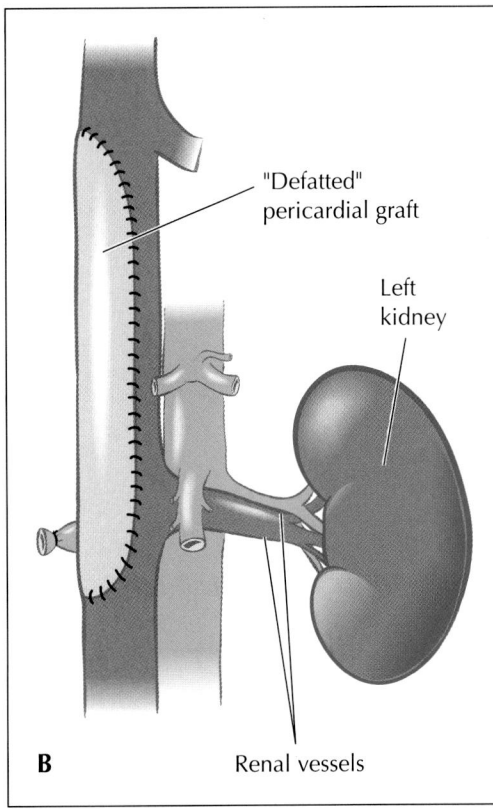

"Defatted" pericardial graft

Left kidney

Renal vessels

B

▶ **FIGURE 5-18.** Excision and reconstruction of the vena cava. Following excision of a right renal tumor with supradiaphragmatic caval tumor extension (**A**) requiring partial resection of the caval wall, a defatted pericardial graft is used for vena caval reconstruction (**B**). An adequate caliber caval lumen is necessary to ensure venous drainage of the lower extremities and contralateral kidney. To reconstruct the caval wall, we prefer using autologous material, such as pericardium, because it is less thrombogenic, although prosthetic grafts of a material such as Gore-Tex (WL Gore and Associates, Inc., Flagstaff, AZ) can be used [16]. (*Adapted from* Marshall and Reitz [17].)

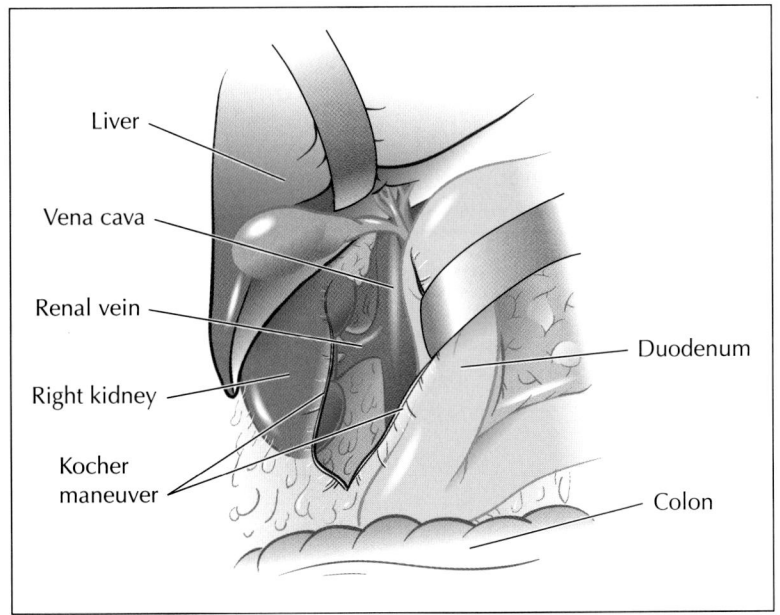

Liver

Vena cava

Renal vein

Right kidney

Kocher maneuver

Duodenum

Colon

▶ **FIGURE 5-19.** Intraoperatic exposure of a left renal cell carcinoma with vena caval tumor extension. The surgical approach to a left-sided renal neoplasm with caval tumor extension requires special consideration. These procedures are often more difficult than those for a right-sided lesion because both sides of the abdomen must be dissected to access the vena cava and the left kidney. This precludes an extended thoracoabdominal approach. Depending on the superior extent of the caval tumor, an anterior incision provides adequate exposure. After incising the line of Toldt, the descending colon is reflected medially. In a dissection similar to a right-sided tumor, the entire kidney within Gerota's fascia is mobilized until only the left renal vein remains attached to the vena cava. The ascending colon is then reflected medially and the duodenum is mobilized by the Kocher maneuver. After the vena cava has been adequately exposed, the remainder of the procedure is as previously described. (*Adapted from* Marshall and Reitz [18].)

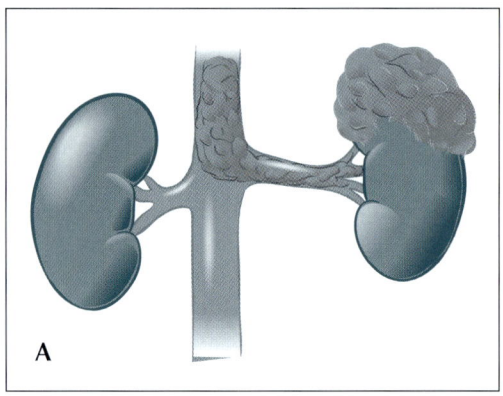

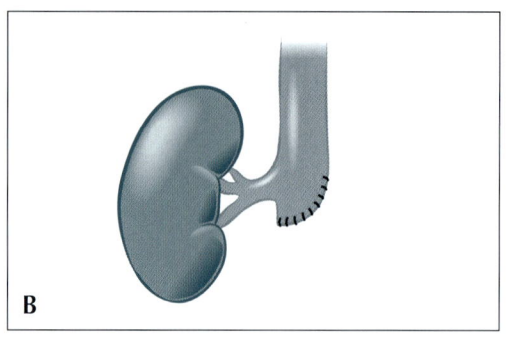

▶ **FIGURE 5-20.** Reconstruction of vena cava following resection of left-sided renal cell carcinoma. Preservation of venous drainage of the uninvolved right kidney is paramount to prevent venous infarction resulting from a lack of collateral vessels. When reconstructing the vena cava following extraction of a left-sided renal primary with caval tumor (**A**), a segment of vena cava around the ostium of the right renal vein must be preserved to ensure adequate venous drainage (**B**). If it is necessary to resect the suprarenal vena cava and the cava cannot be reconstructed to provide drainage of the right kidney, the surgeon should be prepared to use an interposition graft or consider using the splenic vein.

CARDIOPULMONARY BYPASS, HYPOTHERMIA, AND TEMPORARY CARDIAC ARREST

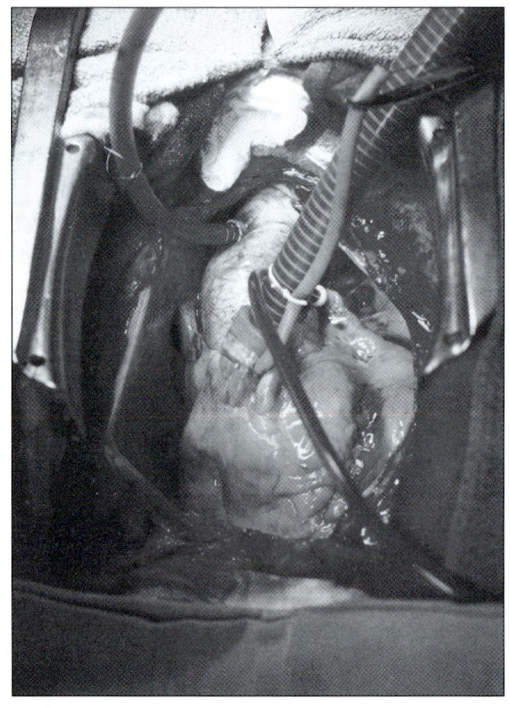

▶ **FIGURE 5-21.** (*See* Color Plate) Intraoperative view of cardiopulmonary bypass. The resection of a suprahepatic caval thrombus (V4) is immensely facilitated by the use of cardiopulmonary bypass, hypothermia, and temporary cardiac arrest [2–4]. We have also used bypass and cardiac arrest for extraction of intrahepatic tumors (V3), because the alternative approach using temporary occlusion of the thoracic vena cava, the porta hepatis (Pringle's maneuver), and the superior and inferior mesenteric arteries (to maintain intravascular volume) entails significant risk of hepatic venous congestion and problematic venous backbleeding. In addition, the alternative approach as described allows the porta hepatitis to be occluded for approximately 20 minutes versus the occlusion time for cardiopulmonary bypass, which can last for as long as 1 hour. To keep the duration of cardiac bypass as short as possible, the kidney and the vena cava should first be fully dissected. After the renal tumor has been isolated, the pericardium is opened and retracted with stay sutures. We usually cannulate the right atrial appendage with a 32-F venous cannula and the aortic arch with a 22-F Bardic cannula.

Hemostasis should be confirmed before intravenously administering heparin to maintain an activated clotting time longer than 450 seconds. The patient is placed on bypass with flow rates maintained between 2.5 and 3.5 L/min. Maintaining an 8° to 10°C gradient between the patient's core temperature and the perfusion, a core temperature of 18° to 20°C is achieved within 30 minutes. When a rectal temperature of 20°C is reached and the heart is in ventricular fibrillation, the aorta is cross-clamped and 500 mL of cooled cardioplegic solution is infused. After cardiac arrest has been achieved, bypass is terminated and the patient is temporarily exsanguinated into an oxygen reservoir. The brain is protected with ice bags around the head. At this point, no anesthesia or ventilatory or circulatory support is provided. Circulatory arrest time should be limited to 45 minutes to reduce the incidence of complications.

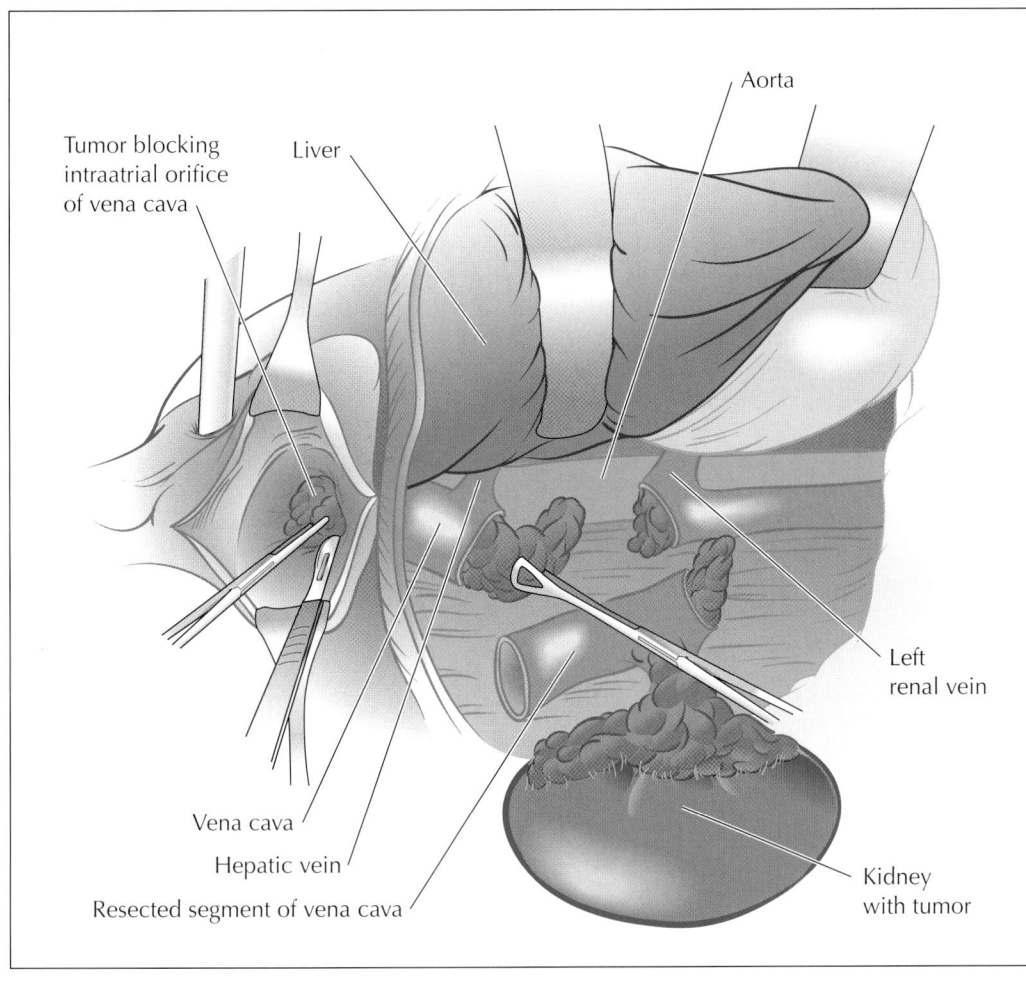

▶ FIGURE 5-22. Excision of a segment of infra-hepatic vena cava and extraction of intracaval and intra-atrial tumor through a right thoracoabdominal incision. Note that thrombus in the vena cava inferior to the renal veins is typically a blood thrombus without neoplastic cells. When the tumor is inseparable from the caval endothelium superior to the renal veins, excising the involved segment of cava is recommended. It is usually only necessary to perform segmental caval resection rather than circumferential resection. If the vena cava had been completely occluded with tumor preoperatively and sufficient venous collaterals had formed, little risk exists in oversewing the vena cava. Additionally, if significant concern arises regarding postoperative embolism, the vena cava can be oversewn inferiorly. If the vena cava is ligated, venous drainage of the uninvolved left kidney must be preserved by sparing the adrenal and gonadal veins. However, it is still preferable to attempt to restore continuity of the left renal vein and the vena cava. (*Adapted from* Marshall *et al.* [2].)

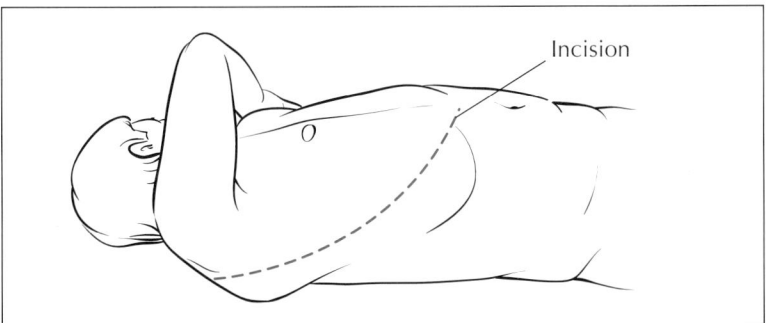

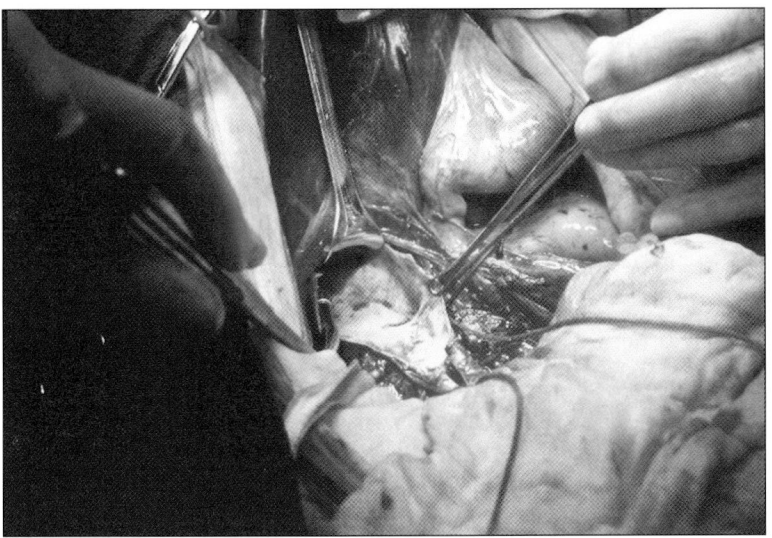

▶ FIGURE 5-23. (*See* Color Plate) Intraoperative view of the interior of the vena cava while the patient is on cardiopulmonary bypass with deep hypothermic circulatory arrest. Occasionally, a Fogarty or Foley catheter may be used to extract the tumor from difficult to reach segments of the cava. We have used a dental mirror or a flexible cystoscope to inspect difficult-to-visualize caval segments (*ie*, the hepatic veins) during bypass and circulatory arrest. Transesophageal or direct sonography can be used intraoperatively to determine whether the superior extent of the thrombus has been completely removed. The intracaval tumor is removed and the interior of the vena cava and heart can be inspected under direct vision in a bloodless field using cardiopulmonary bypass and deep hypothermic circulatory arrest. It is not uncommon to find some degree of adherence of the tumor to the caval endothelium in which case the tumor thrombus can be "endarterectomized" from the interior of the vena cava or atrium.

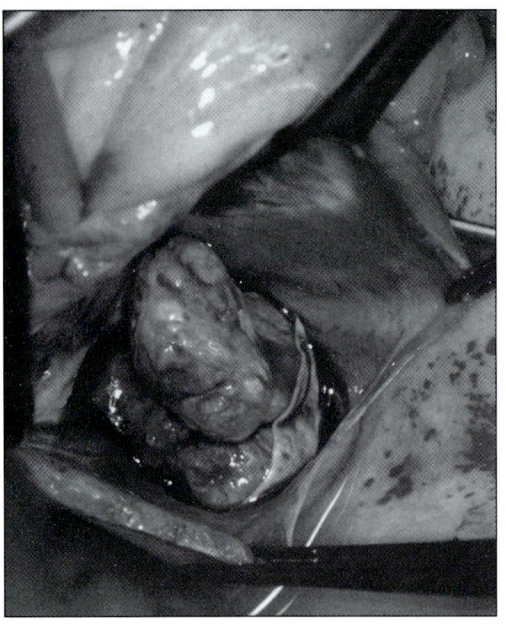

FIGURE 5-24. (*See* Color Plate) Tumor thrombus is extracted from the right atrium. For tumors extending into the right atrium, the atrial wall is opened to facilitate tumor extraction and inspection of the interior of the heart. After removing the intracaval tumor, the vena cava is irrigated and reconstructed as previously mentioned. Following closure of the venacavotomy, cardiopulmonary bypass is initiated. Using a 10°C gradient between the patient and the bypass machine, the patient is slowly warmed with a heating blanket. The warming process can sometimes take as long as 1 hour. When the core temperature reaches 25°C, 12.5 g of mannitol and 1 g of CaCl are intravenously administered. Following the rewarming process, the heart is electrically defibrillated if spontaneous beating has not resumed. After cardiac activity commences, the patient's blood is returned from the oxygen reservoir and cardiopulmonary bypass is terminated. The bypass cannulas are removed and the anticoagulant effect of heparin is neutralized with protamine. Mediastinal chest tubes are placed; however, the retroperitoneum is usually not drained. The patient is returned to the cardiac intensive care unit on ventilatory support.

RESULTS OF SURGERY

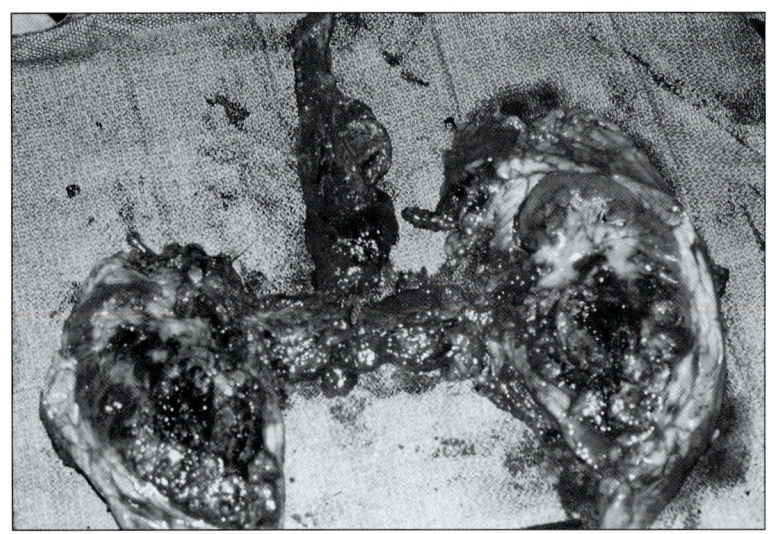

FIGURE 5-25. (*See* Color Plate) A bivalved kidney with renal cell carcinoma and intracaval extension of tumor. Although renal cell carcinoma with vena caval neoplastic extension is usually associated with more advanced disease (pathologic T3 to T4), many patients are potentially curable by radical nephrectomy and caval thrombectomy in the absence of metastases. The 5-year survival rates in most reported large series range from 14% to 68% following complete surgical removal of the renal primary and caval tumor extension [6,7,14,19,20]. The predominant factor affecting cancer-specific survival is the presence of metastatic disease.

Most authorities agree that the presence of metastasis portends a poor prognosis despite an otherwise technically successful surgery [5,7,8,14,15,19]. A significant proportion of patients presenting with renal cell carcinoma and intracaval tumor have metastatic disease. Owing to limitations in resolution using contemporary radiologic imaging, some metastases escape preoperative radiographic detection only to be subsequently identified intraoperatively. Preoperative or intraoperative metastases have been demonstrated in 27% to 57% of patients with a renal primary and caval tumor extension [7,8,14,15]. In addition, many patients develop metastases postoperatively, accounting for the most common cause of death after surgery [8,14,19].

Disease-specific survival varies significantly between those patients with and without metastatic disease. Following surgery, the cancer-specific survival curves separate into two groups. For those patients developing metastasis, median survival of 13 to 14 months [7,15] and a mean survival of 18.8 months have been reported [19]. In patients without metastatic disease, the 5-year survival rates following complete surgical removal of the primary renal tumor and the accompanying caval extension range from 47% to 68% [6,7,15,19,20].

Local (perinephric) extension of primary tumor
Presence of lymphatic or visceral metastases
Level of caval tumor extension
Invasion into the vascular wall

▶ **FIGURE 5-26.** It is common for patients with renal neoplasms extending into the vena cava to have perinephric extension of the renal primary. Polascik *et al.* [14] identified perinephric extension in 67% of 34 patients with V3 to V4 tumors, whereas Glazer and Novick [19]found perinephric extension in eight of 18 patients (44%) with V4 tumors. Whether perinephric extension of tumor affects survival has been debated in the literature. When evaluating survival, some authors demonstrated poorer outcomes with perinephric extension of tumor [5,6,19,21], whereas others reported no difference in survival [7] when compared with tumors locally confined to the renal capsule.

The relationship between the cephalad extent of the caval tumor and survival following radical nephrectomy and caval thrombectomy has also been controversial. Some authors suggest that survival correlates with the level of intracaval tumor [5,6], whereas others do not [4,7,19,21]. Several investigators found that adverse prognostic factors, such as perinephric extension of tumor or lymph node metastases, might be more prevalent with higher level caval tumors [5,6]. Novick *et al.* [4] found no difference in lymph node involvement or distant metastases when comparing renal tumors having atrial extension with tumors having lesser degrees of intracaval involvement. In three large series of patients undergoing radical nephrectomy with caval thrombectomy, no difference in survival was demonstrated between supradiaphragmatic (V4) and intrahepatic (V3) caval tumors [7,14], and in patients with tumors extending into the right atrium [19].

Another factor that may adversely affect survival is invasion of tumor into the venous wall. Fortunately, these tumors infrequently invade the vascular endothelium [20]. Some tumors have been noted to be more adherent at the renal vein ostium [6]. Adherence or invasion of the renal vein ostium was common with large, intracaval neoplastic extension in our experience. Invasion into the inferior vena caval wall by tumor suggests a poor prognosis [21]. Further studies are needed to prospectively evaluate this issue.

COMPLICATIONS AND POSTOPERATIVE MANAGEMENT

Potential Surgical Complications

Intraoperative

Excessive hemorrhage
Coagulopathy
Prolonged renal ischemia
Tumor embolism

Postoperative

Caval thrombosis
Deep venous thrombosis
Pulmonary embolus
Bleeding or hematoma
Cirrhotic hemorrhage from esophageal varices
Sepsis
Bowel obstruction
Adrenal insufficiency
Pneumonia
Atelectasis
Renal insufficiency
Hepatic dysfunction
Pancreatitis

▶ **FIGURE 5-27.** Potential intraoperative and postoperative complications. Because of the magnitude of the surgical procedure, a spectrum of medical and surgical complications can occur both during or after surgery. The use of cardiopulmonary bypass, hypothermia, and temporary circulatory arrest has greatly improved the efficacy of removing intracaval tumors with intrahepatic (V3) and supradiaphragmatic (V4) extension into the vena cava. Similarly, this technique has largely reduced the incidence of major hemorrhage and allows extraction of these large intracaval tumors in a bloodless field.

Although coagulopathy can occur secondary to extensive blood loss, coagulopathy is also common with prolonged cardiopulmonary bypass and cardiac arrest. Several of these potential complications can be prevented intraoperatively. For example, erythrocytes, platelets, fresh frozen plasma, and calcium chloride are routinely administered intraoperatively when using cardiopulmonary bypass to preclude coagulopathy. To prevent renal ischemia, we attempt to minimize the cross-clamp time of the contralateral renal vein and reconstruct the vena cava to ensure adequate venous drainage of the remaining kidney. Furosemide (alone or combined with mannitol) is administered if the intraoperative urine output remains low. Transient hypotension can occur when clamping the vena cava, especially in cases involving partial caval occlusion without the development of adequate venous collaterals. This hypotension can be managed with volume expansion. Finally, great care should be taken when handling the vena cava to prevent tumor embolism, a potentially lethal intraoperative complication.

Significant morbidity ranges from 15% to 30% [6,7,15]. The perioperative mortality rate is approximately 3.5% to 7.3% [6,7,9,14]. Early postoperative deaths have been attributed to air embolus, myocardial infarction, renal and hepatic failure with sepsis, and multisystem organ failure.

REFERENCES

1. Marshall VF, Middleton RG, Holswade GR, *et al.*Surgery for renal cell carcinoma in the vena cava. *J Urol* 1970, 103:414–420.

2. Marshall FF, Reitz BA, Diamond DA: A new technique for management of renal cell carcinoma involving the right atrium: hypothermia and cardiac arrest. *J Urol* 1984, 131:103–107.

3. Marshall FF, Dietrick DD, Baumgartner WM, *et al.*: Surgical management of renal cell carcinoma with intracaval neoplastic extension above the hepatic veins. *J Urol* 1988, 139:1166–1172.

4. Novick AC, Kaye MC, Cosgrove DM, *et al.*: Experience with cardiopulmonary bypass and deep hypothermic circulatory arrest in the management of retroperitoneal tumors with large vena caval thrombi. *Ann Surg* 1990, 212: 472–477.

5. Sosa RE, Muecke EC, Vaughan Jr ED, *et al.*: Renal cell carcinoma extending into the inferior vena cava: the prognostic significance of the level of vena caval involvement. *J Urol* 1984, 132:1097–1100.

6. Suggs WD, Smith RB III, Dodson TF, *et al.*: Renal cell carcinoma with inferior vena caval involvement. *J Vasc Surg* 1991, 14:413–418.

7. Libertino JA, Zinman L, Watkins E, Jr: Long-term results of resection of renal cell cancer with extension into inferior vena cava. *J Urol* 1987, 137:21–24.

8. Montie JE, Pontes JE, Novick AC, *et al.*: Resection of inferior vena cava tumor thrombi from renal cell carcinoma. *Am Surg* 1991, 57:56–61.

9. Montie JE, Ammar R, Pontes JE, *et al.*: Renal cell carcinoma with inferior vena cava tumor thrombi. *Surg Gynecol Obstet* 1991, 173:107–115.

10. Kallman DA, King BF, Hattery RR, *et al.*: Renal vein and inferior vena cava tumor thrombus in renal cell carcinoma: CT, US, MRI, and venacavography. *J Comput Assist Tomogr* 1992, 16:240–247.

11. Smith PA, Marshall FF, Fishman EK: Spiral computed tomography evaluation of the kidneys: state of the art. *Urology* 1998, 51:3–11.

12. Treiger BFC, Humphrey LS, Peterson JCV, *et al.*: Transesophageal echocardiography in renal cell carcinoma: an accurate diagnostic technique for intracaval neoplastic extension. *J Urol* 1991, 145:1138–1140.

13. Glazer A, Novick AC: Preoperative transesophageal echocardiography for assessment of vena caval tumor thrombi: a comparative study with venacavography and magnetic resonance imaging. *Urology* 1997, 49:32–34.

14. Polascik TJ, Partin AW, Pound CR, *et al.*: Frequent occurrence of metastatic disease in patients with renal cell carcinoma and intrahepatic or supradiaphragmatic intracaval extension treated with surgery: an outcome analysis. *Urology*, 1998, 52:995–999.

15. Reissigl A, Janetschek G, Eberle J, *et al.*: Renal cell carcinoma extending into the vena cava: surgical approach, technique and results. *Br J Urol* 1995, 75:138–142.

16. Marshall FF (ed.): *Operative Urology*. Philadelphia: WB Saunders; 1996:265.

17. Marshall FF, Reitz BA: Supradiaphragmatic renal cell carcinoma tumor thrombus: indications for vena caval reconstruction with pericardium. *J Urol* 1985, 133:266–268.

18. Marshall FF, Reitz BA: Technique for removal of renal cell carcinoma with suprahepatic vena caval tumor thrombus. *Urol Clin North Am* 1986, 13:551–557.

19. Glazer AA, Novick AC: Long-term follow-up after surgical treatment for renal cell carcinoma extending into the right atrium. *J Urol* 1996, 155:448–450.

20. Skinner DG, Pfeister RF, Colvin R: Extension of renal cell carcinoma into the vena cava: the rationale for aggressive surgical management. *J Urol* 1972, 107:711–716.

21. Hatcher PA, Anderson EE, Paulson DF, *et al.*: Surgical management and prognosis of renal cell carcinoma invading the vena cava. *J Urol* 1991, 145:20–23.

Combined-modality Treatment of Renal Cell Carcinoma

Ronald M. Bukowski

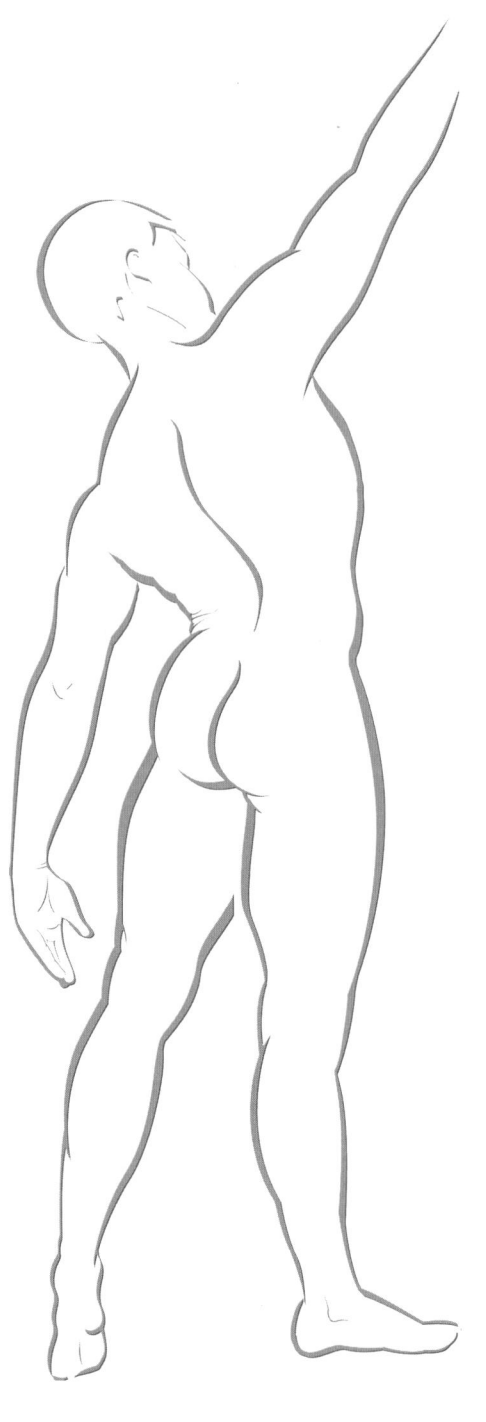

Adenocarcinoma is the most common neoplasm arising in the kidney, representing more than 85% of these tumors [1]. Of patients with renal cancer, 30% present with metastatic disease, and ultimately another 40% develop dissemination of the tumor [2]. Therapy depends on tumor stage, with surgery being the major modality used in early and locally advanced disease. Despite new surgical approaches, the outcome for these patients has not changed appreciably over the past 20 years.

The demonstration of an active immune response in patients with renal cell carcinoma (RCC) [3,4], the reports of spontaneous regression [5], and the results of immunotherapy support the combined-modality approach to patients with this neoplasm. Cytokines such as interferon-alfa and interleukin-2 are now commonly used, and although response rates are low, selected patients do appear to benefit. Integration of surgery and radiation therapy with treatment using cytokines is now being explored. Combined-modality approaches involving cytoreductive surgery before or after therapy, postoperative adjuvant treatment, and novel immunotherapeutic strategies are under development. These approaches and results illustrate the potential and future directions of combined-modality strategies for the treatment of RCC.

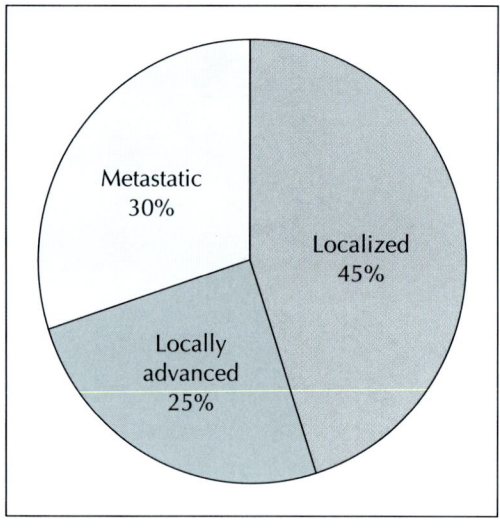

▶ **FIGURE 6-1.** Percentage rates of metastatic renal cell carcinoma. Adenocarcinoma of the kidney, the most common renal neoplasm, is diagnosed in more than 30,600 individuals annually in the United States [6]. As shown in this figure, 30% of patients have distant metastases at the time of diagnosis [2] and 25% have locally advanced disease. In the group of patients who undergo surgery with curative intent, 40% ultimately develop metastatic disease [2].

Staging of Renal Cell Carcinoma

TNM Stage	TNM Categories			Robson stage
III	T1	N1	M0	IIIB
	T2	N1	M0	IIIB
	T3a	N0,1	M0	IIIA or B
	T3b	N0,1	M0	IIIA or B
IV	T4	N (any)	M0	IV
	T4	N (any)	M0	III or IV
	T (any)	N (any)	M1	IV

Tumor characteristics	Lymph node characteristics
T$_1$ ≤ 7.0 cm (limited to kidney)	N0 No regional node metastases
T$_2$ 7.0 cm (limited to kidney)	N1 Single node involved
T$_3$ a, Perinephric invasion	N2 Metastases in more than one regional node
b, Venous (major) invasion below diaphragm	**Metastases**
c, Venous invasion above diaphragm	M0 Absent
T$_4$ Invasion of Gerota's fascia	M1 Present

▶ **FIGURE 6-2.** Staging of renal cell carcinoma (RCC). The clinical or pathologic stage of a patient with RCC is the major factor that determines prognosis. Most clinicians use the Robson modification of the Flocks/Kadesky system [7]. In this system, lymph node involvement, local organ invasion, and distant spread define metastatic disease categories (stages III and IV). The TNM (tumor, node, metastasis) classification may more accurately define the various groups by differentiating the extent of lymph node involvement (N0, N1, or N2). The Robson and the 1997 revision [8] of the TNM staging systems for RCC are illustrated. (*Data from* Robson *et al.* [7] and Guinan *et al.* [8].)

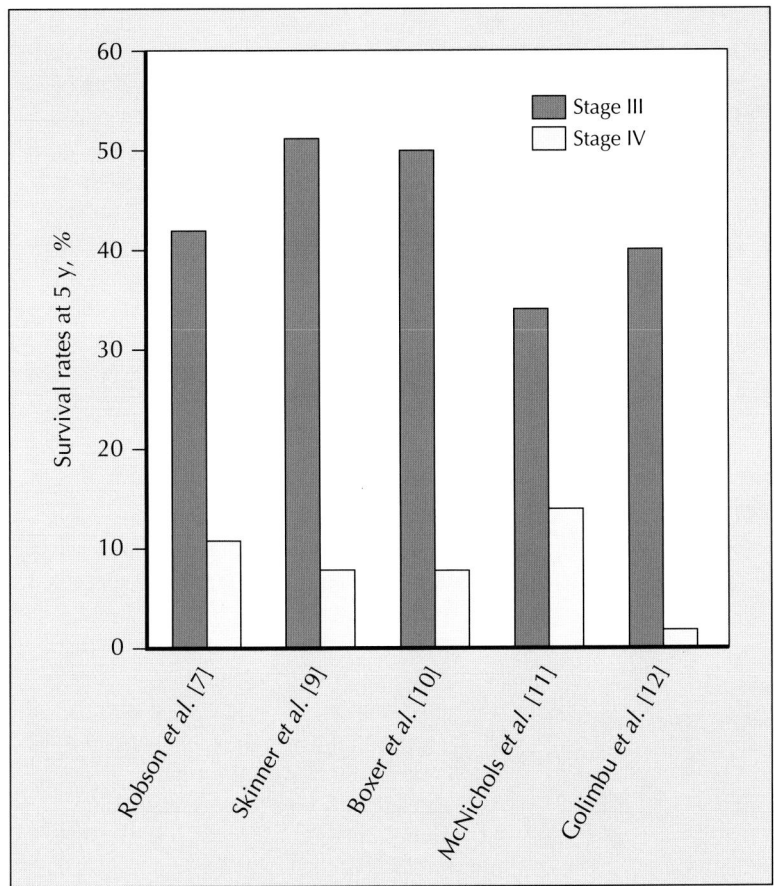

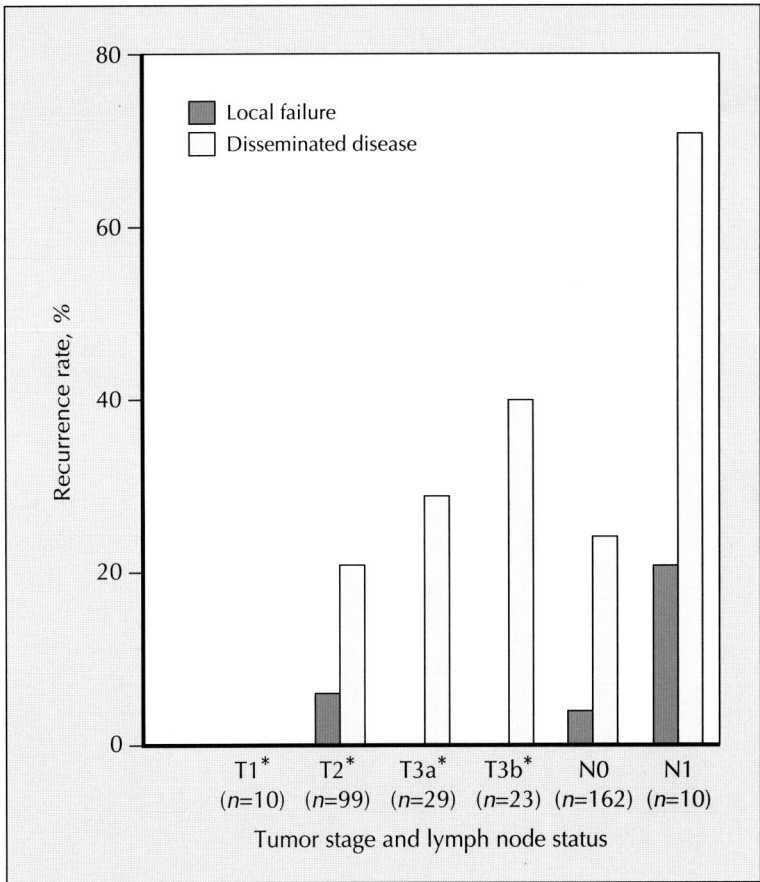

FIGURE 6-3. Prognosis of renal cell carcinoma (RCC). The outcome for patients with metastatic RCC has not changed significantly over the past 25 years. In patients with stage III disease, the 5-year survival rate has been reported to vary from 30% to 50%. In those with stage IV or metastatic (M1) disease, the 5-year survival rate is generally less than 10%. This figure illustrates survival rates for patients with advanced stages of RCC reported by various authors [7,9,12]. Subsets of patients appear to have improved survival rates, including patients with solitary metastases [9], patients developing metastases more than 2 years after nephrectomy [14], and patients who respond completely to cytokine-based therapy [15].

FIGURE 6-4. Patterns of treatment failure in renal cell carcinoma (RCC). This figures shows the actuarial frequency of recurrent RCC following nephrectomy. The outcome for patients with resected RCC is generally reported in terms of survival. The analysis of patterns of failure in these patients is also of interest because it provides information regarding the potential role of adjuvant and combined-modality therapy. In a recent analysis of 172 patients, the frequency of local failure was only 5% [16]. Distant metastases occur much more commonly, and in a regression analysis, lymph node involvement and renal vein involvement were independent risk factors predicting disseminated disease [16]. *Asterisks* indicate no node involvement. N—node; T—tumor. (*Data from* Rabinovitch *et al.* [16].)

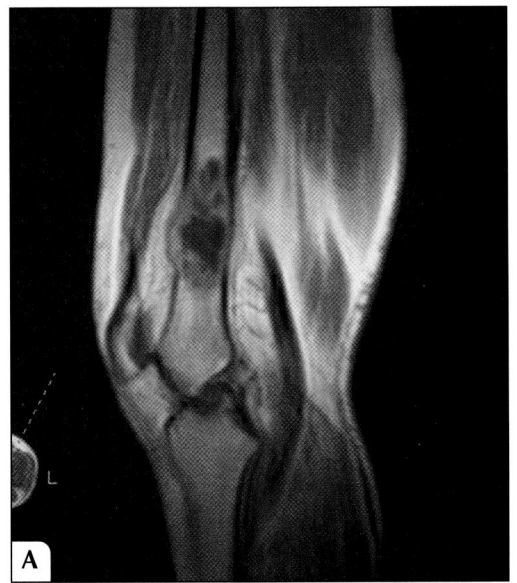

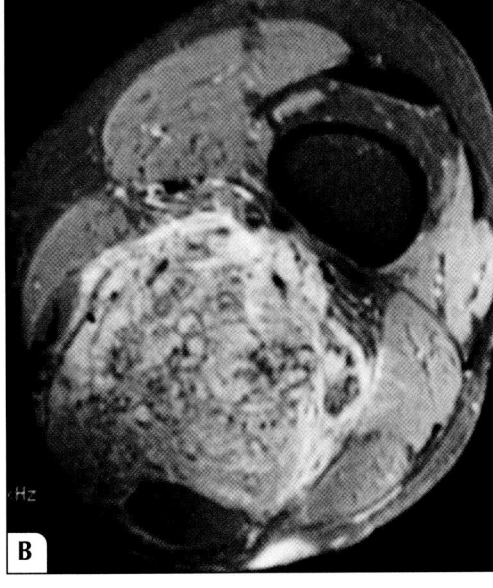

FIGURE 6-5. The major sites of metastatic disease in patients with metastatic renal cell carcinoma (RCC) [17] are the lung (75%), lymph nodes and soft tissue (36%), bone (20%), liver (10%), and central nervous system (< 10%). **A,** Magnetic resonance imaging (MRI) study of a metastatic lesion of the left femur presenting secondary to an RCC. In addition, patients frequently develop metastatic lesions in unusual sites such as the pancreas [18] and thyroid [19]. **B,** MRI study of a metastatic lesion involving the muscles of the posterior thigh.

Factors Predicting Improved Survival in Metastatic Renal Cell Carcinoma

Factors	Study
Performance status, disease-free interval, weight loss, number of metastatic sites, prior chemotherapy	Elson et al. [20]
Prior nephrectomy, lung metastases only	Maldazys and Dekernion et al. [17]
Time from diagnosis to therapy	Palmer et al. [23]
Sedimentation rate	Fossa et al. [24]
Disease-free interval >24 mo	Landonio et al. [25]

FIGURE 6-6. Prognostic factors in metastatic renal cell carcinoma. In patients with metastatic disease, various factors associated with improved survival have been identified. Characteristics such as absence of symptoms, metastases in the lung only, and a previous nephrectomy [17,20,21] are included among these variables. This figure lists a series of findings associated with an improved prognosis. Fyfe et al. [22] recently noted that performance status in patients receiving high-dose recombinant inter-leukin-2 for metastatic disease was the only factor predicting response and a favorable outcome.

Prognostic Factors in Metastatic Renal Cell Carcinoma

Risk factor assessment

ECOG performance status 0, 1, etc.
Time from initial diagnosis to metastatic disease
 < 1 y, 0
 ≥ 1 y, 1
Number of metastatic sites
 0 or 1 site, 0
 ≥ 2 sites, 1
Weight loss in the prior 6 mo
 No, 0
 Yes, 1
Prior chemotherapy
 No, 0
 Yes, 1

Risk grouping

Risk factors, n*	Risk group	Median survival, mo
0,1	1	12.8
2	2	7.7
3	3	5.3
4	4	3.4
≥5	5	2.1

* Equals the sum of ECOG performance status and other variables. If the number of metastatic sites, weight loss, and prior chemotherapy all equal 1, the risk factor number is calculated by subtracting 1.

FIGURE 6-7. Risk assessment in metastatic renal cell carcinoma (RCC). In patients with advanced and metastatic RCC, various models have been devised to predict survival. Because these patients can have indolent disease in some instances, methods to assess outcomes and permit comparisons of various populations are relevant. Elson et al. [20] identified a series of factors associated with survival in patients with metastatic disease. By multivariate analysis, patients were separated into five subgroups according to the number of risk factors present. This model is presented in the figure. ECOG—Eastern Cooperative Oncology Group. (Adapted from Elson et al. [20].)

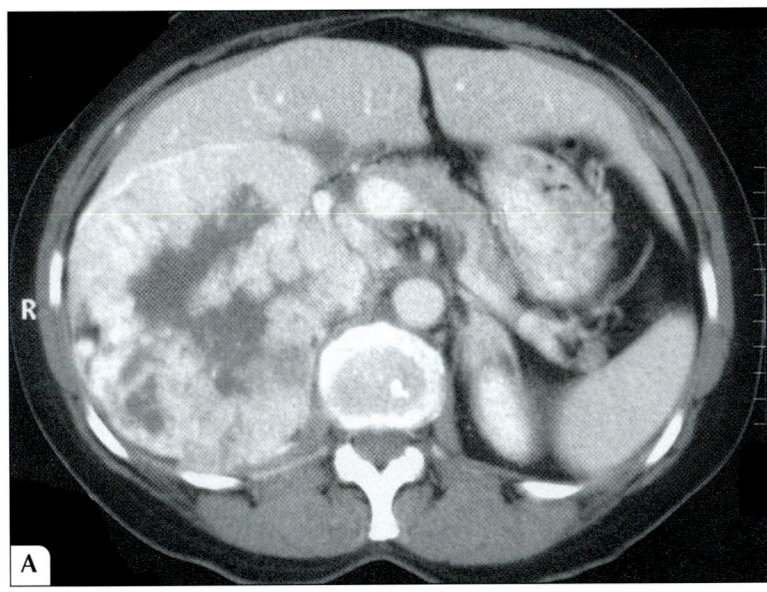

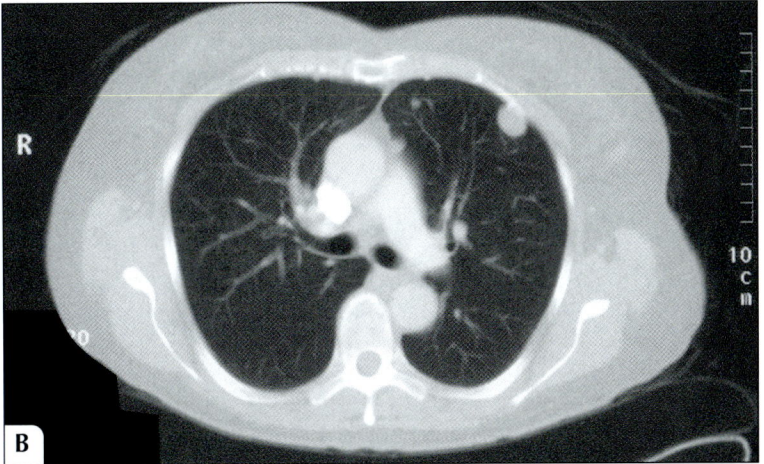

▶ **FIGURE 6-8.** Nephrectomy for metastatic renal cell carcinoma (RCC). The role of nephrectomy in patients who present with metastatic disease is controversial. In the presence of symptoms such as pain, hematuria, hypercalcemia, fatigue, and fever, removal of the primary tumor may have palliative effects and alleviate such symptoms [2]. Spontaneous regression of metastatic lesions has been reported after nephrectomy, but the incidence in a recent review [26] appears to be less than 1%. In addition, adjuvant nephrectomy in these patients does not appear to affect survival [27]. Finally, in patients receiving cytokine therapy for metastatic disease, higher response rates and more favorable outcomes have been reported for individuals who have had prior nephrectomy [21,22]. This finding has not been demonstrated prospectively, but adjuvant nephrectomy in preparation for subsequent systemic therapy is an alternative that is being explored. A primary tumor in place (**A**) and synchronous metastatic disease in the lung (**B**) of the same patient are shown in these magnetic resonance imaging studies.

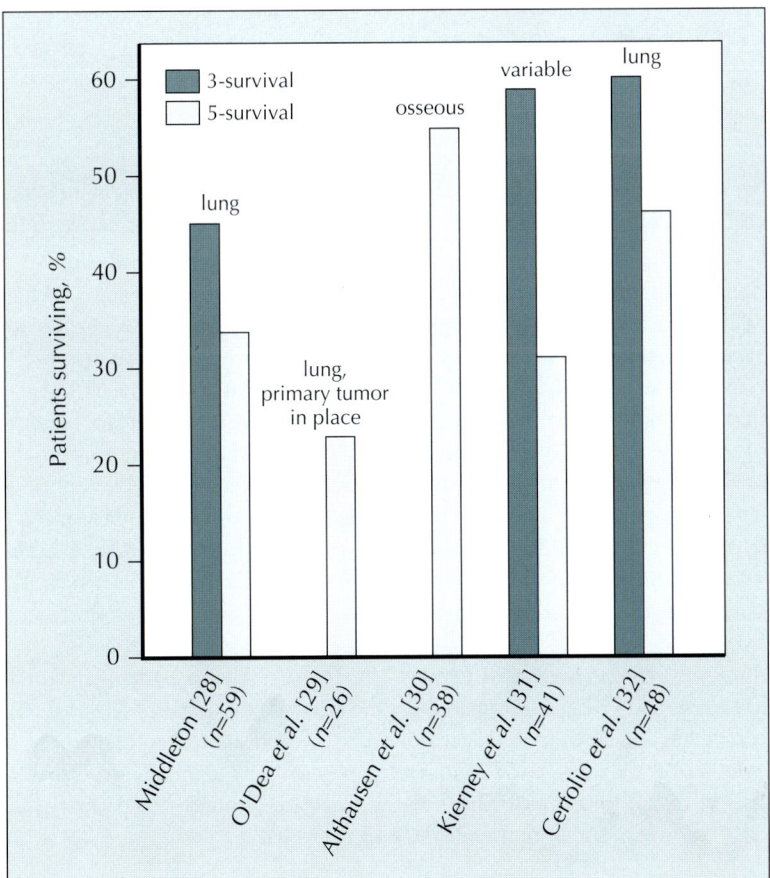

▶ **FIGURE 6-9.** Outcomes in patients undergoing surgery for solitary metastases from renal cell carcinoma. The frequency of isolated or solitary metastases in this tumor is low, with estimates ranging from 1.5% to 3.5% of patients with metastatic disease [9,28]. This subset of patients is managed by surgical resection when possible, even in the setting of synchronous metastatic disease. Survival rates in patients treated by surgical resection, reported by various authors [28–32], are shown. Five-year survival rates for this group appear to range from 30% to 50%. The sites of solitary metastases are given.

Outcomes in Patients With Multiple Pulmonary Metastases Following Surgery				
Study	**Patients, n**	**Patient characteristics**	**Survival rate, %**	
			3 y	**5 y**
Hoffman *et al.* [33]	39	33% with solitary lesions	NS	14
Cerfolio *et al.* [32]	48	Patients with two or more lesions	≈ 45*	27
Tanguay *et al.* [34]	22	Eight patients with two or more lesions	≈ 65	≈ 40

* *Estimated from survival curves.*

▶ **FIGURE 6-10.** Outcomes in patients with multiple pulmonary metastases following surgery. Patients with multiple metastatic sites are also frequently considered candidates for surgical resection. Pulmonary metastases are often multiple despite preoperative staging that suggests a solitary lesion. The outcome for these patients is related to the number of metastatic lesions and the length of the disease-free interval from the time of initial diagnosis [33]. The overall survival in these patients is limited, but clearly in selected instances, resection can be associated with prolonged survival [32–34], as shown in the figure. NS—not stated.

IMMUNOTHERAPY FOR RENAL CELL CARCINOMA

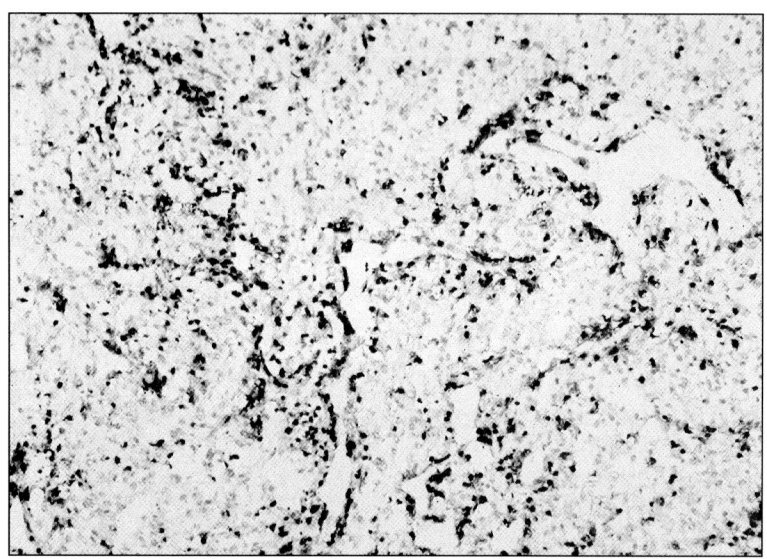

▶ **FIGURE 6-11.** (*See* Color Plate) Microscopic section of a renal tumor. Therapeutic approaches to patients with metastatic renal cell carcinoma (RCC) involve manipulation of the immune response. The rationale for this manipulation is based on observations of spontaneous regression of metastatic lesions [5] and tumor regressions that occur during therapy with various biologic agents such as cytokines. The immunobiologic features of this neoplasm also provide evidence of an existing immune response. The existence of specific cytotoxic T lymphocytes [3], the presence of antigens on tumor cells recognized by T cells in an HLA-restricted fashion [35], and the significant T-cell infiltrate seen in renal tumors [4] are recent observations demonstrating the existence of an active immune response in these patients with metastatic RCC. This section of tumor was stained immunohistologically with conjugated monoclonal antibodies against the CD3 complex on T lymphocytes. The T-cell infiltrate is clearly demonstrated.

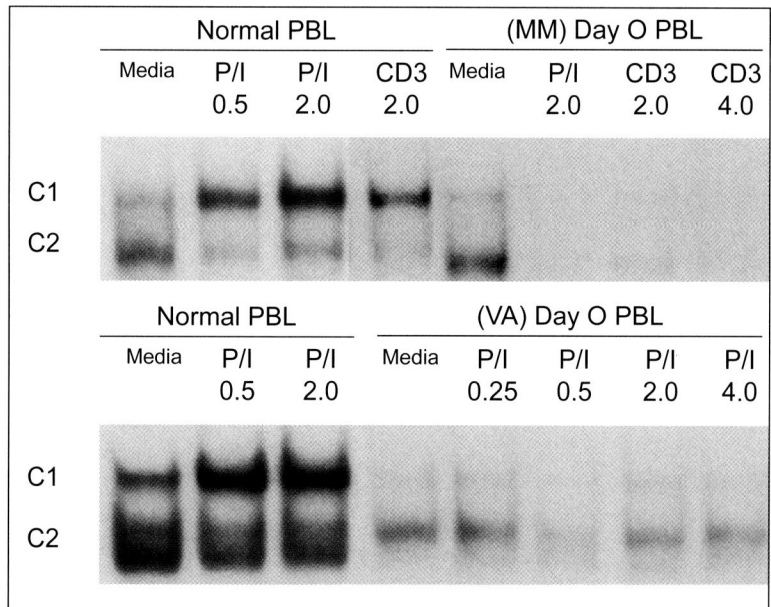

▶ **FIGURE 6-12.** Acquired immune dysregulation in renal cell carcinoma. Impairment of various cellular immune responses in patients with advanced tumors has been noted for several decades [36]. The clinical relevance and effects on the efficacy of immunotherapy are not clear, but the possibility exists that this impairment may diminish the effectiveness of immunotherapy. Recent investigations have demonstrated that the causes of immune dysregulation may be multifactorial, including tumor-associated suppressive factors [37], enhanced apoptosis of activated T lymphocytes [38], and production of immunosuppressive cytokines such as interleukin-10 [39]. In addition, T cells from patients with renal cancer exhibit various abnormalities of the T-cell antigen receptor, such as decreases in T-cell receptor chain and impaired translocation of nuclear transcription factors such as NFκB [41]. In the electrophoretic mobility shift assay shown, T lymphocytes from two patients (MM, VA) and normal control T lymphocytes (PBL) are compared. In the normal lymphocytes, C1 and C2 complexes appear in the nuclear isolates at 0.5 and 2.0 hours following stimulation with PMA and ionomycin P/I, or CD3 (monoclonal antibody against the CD3 complex). In contrast, these are absent in the patient's cells following stimulation with the same mitogens.

Cytokines and Cytokine Regimens Used in Renal Cell Carcinoma

Interferon-alfa
Interleukin-2
Interferon-alfa + interleukin-2
Interferon-alfa + vinblastine
Interferon-alfa + *cis*-retinoic acid
Interferon-alfa + interleukin-2 + 5-fluorouracil

▶ **FIGURE 6-13.** Cytokines and cytokine regimens used in metastatic renal cell carcinoma (RCC). Cytokine therapy of metastatic RCC has been investigated since the early 1980s. A variety of agents have been used, with recombinant interleukin-2 and interferon-alfa producing tumor regression in 10% to 15% of patients in a reproducible fashion. Combinations of these agents as well as the addition of various chemotherapeutic agents, such as fluorouracil or vinblastine, to these cytokines are also used therapeutically.

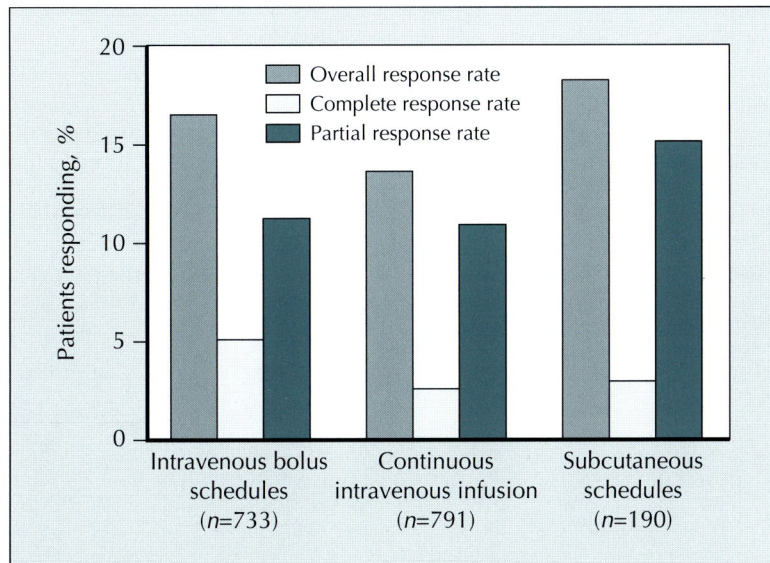

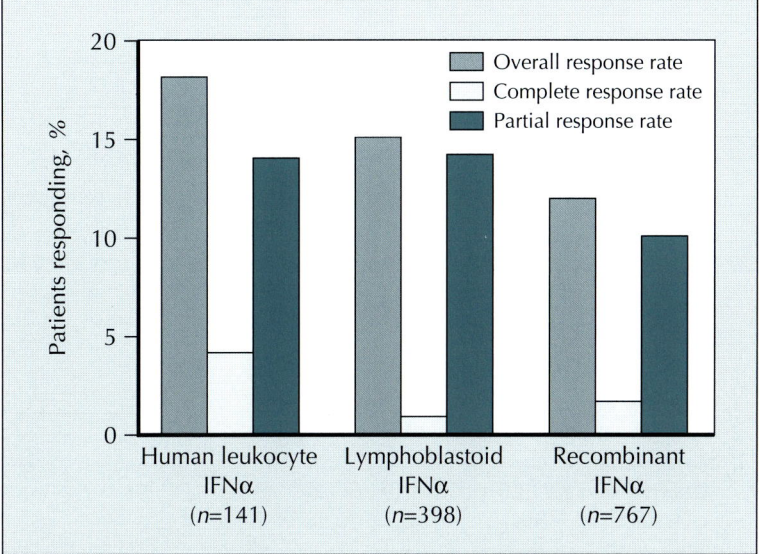

▶ **FIGURE 6-14.** Results of immunotherapy with recombinant interleukin-2 (rIL-2). Interleukin-2 is a 15-kD glycoprotein produced by CD4+ T lymphocytes that supports proliferation and activation of T cells [42]. A recombinant form was approved by the Food and Drug Administration in 1992 for treatment of metastatic renal cell carcinoma. Various schedules and dose levels have been used, and clinical results are shown in the figure. These data represent a review of more than 1700 patients who have received rIL-2 [43]. Complete and durable responses occur and have been reported most frequently with the high-dose bolus schedule [22]. Overall, response rates associated with rIL-2 administration are 15%, with complete responses occurring in 3% to 5% of patients [43]. (*Adapted from* Bukowski [43].)

▶ **FIGURE 6-15.** Results of immunotherapy with interferon-alfa. The first cytokine investigated in patients with advanced renal cell carcinoma was interferon-alfa [44]. This cytokine includes a family of glycoproteins produced in response to various stimuli and having antiproliferative and immune-modulating activities [45]. Various interferon-alfa preparations have been used, including natural and recombinant ones, and a recent overview [46] of more than 1300 patients suggests that response rates vary from 12% to more than 18% (see figure). Various dosing schedules, such as subcutaneous daily or orally three times weekly, and dose levels from 1.0 to 50 MU/m^2 have been used. Optimal results appear to be associated with doses from 5 to 10 MU/m^2 [46]. (*Adapted from* Bukowski and Novick [46].)

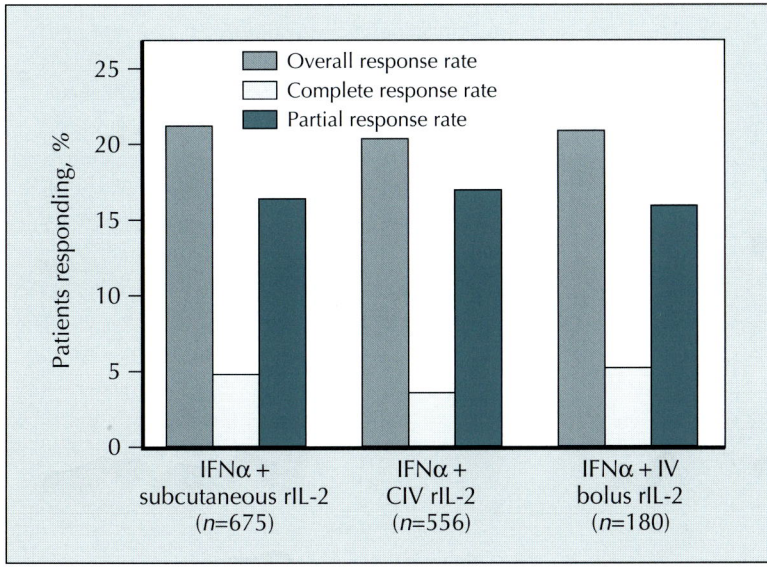

▶ **FIGURE 6-16.** Immunotherapy with combination cytokine regimens. The single-agent activities of recombinant interleukin-2 (rIL-2) and interferon-alfa as well as the synergistic activity of the combination observed in murine tumor models [47] stimulated development of clinical regimens using this combination. This overview of published results suggests an overall response rate of 20% [43]. Preliminary results from a recent randomized trial conducted in France indicate that the combination of continuous-infusion (CIV) rIL-2 and subcutaneous interferon-alfa produced a response rate of 18.6% compared with 6.5% and 7.5%, respectively, for either cytokine alone [48]. Patients receiving the combination also had an improved event-free survival at 1 year. These findings suggest that the combination of rIL-2 and interferon-alfa may result in a slightly higher rate of tumor regression than either cytokine used as a single agent. IV—intravenous. (*Adapted from* Bukowski [43].)

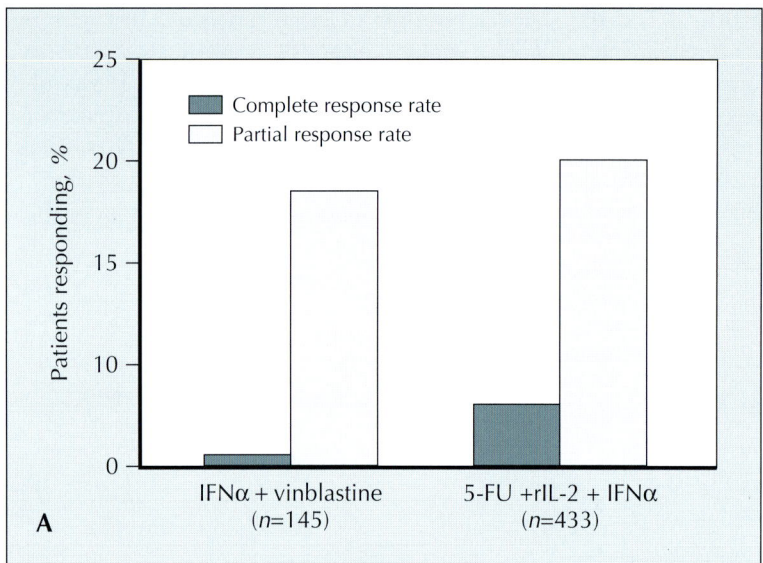

A

▶ **FIGURE 6-17.** Immunotherapy with cytokines and chemotherapy. Metastatic renal cell carcinoma is a chemotherapy-resistant tumor; a review of more than 3000 patients found an overall response rate of less than 5% [49] in patients treated with this modality. The agents vinblastine and the fluoropyrimidines are reported to have modest effects, with regression rates from 2% to 10% for vinblastine [50,51] and 8% to 20% for continuous-infusion floxuridine [52,53]. Alone, these agents are of limited value but they have been combined with cytokines in a variety of chemoimmunotherapy regimens. The combination of vinblastine and interferon-alfa was not superior to interferon-alfa alone [54], but improved response rates and survival compared with vinblastine alone have been reported [52]. The results of this study are consistent with an effect of interferon-alfa on overall patient survival. Phase II studies suggest that regimens containing 5-fluroruracil, recombinant interleukin-2 (rIL-2), and interferon-alfa may have response rates higher than 25% [43]. Confirmation in randomized trials is now required. In a preliminary report comparing rIL-2 and interferon-alfa with and without 5-fluorouracil [55], however, no differences were noted. The results of these chemoimmunotherapy regimens are presented in overview form (**A**) and broken down by study (**B**).

B. Summary of Results With Chemoimmunotherapy in Metastatic Renal Cell Carcinoma

Regimen and study	Patients, n	Complete response, %	Partial response, %
Vinblastine + interferon-alfa			
Fossa *et al.* [54]	66	2	23
Pyrohönen *et al.* [50]	79	—	16
5-Fluorouracil + rIL-2 + interferon-alfa			
Hänninen *et al.* [56]	120	11	28
Hofmockel *et al.* [57]	25	9	29
Dutcher *et al.* [58]	50	4	12
Sella *et al.* [59]	19	16	31
Olencki *et al.* [60]	39	—	8
Jaffe *et al.* [61]	55	—	16
Aztpodien *et al.* [62]	41	17	22
Gitilitz *et al.* [63]	23	—	22
Negrier *et al.* [55]	61	—	8

A. Outpatient Regimen of Recombinant Interleukin-2 Interferon-alfa in Renal Carcinoma*

Regimen	Weeks 1 and 4					Weeks 2, 3, 5, and 6				
	Day					Day				
	1	2	3	4	5	1	2	3	4	5
rIL-2										
20 MIU/m², SC	—	—	+	+	+	—	—	—	—	—
5 MIU/m², SC	—	—	—	—	—	+	—	+	—	+
rIFN-alfa2										
6 MIU/m², SC	+	—	—	—	—	+	—	+	—	+

* Cycles repeated every 8 weeks as tolerated.

▶ **FIGURE 6-18.** Immunotherapy with the recombinant interleukin-2 (rIL-2) and interferon-alfa regimen and example of results. Various schedules and doses of rIL-2 and interferon-alfa have been used in this combination; however, a frequently used outpatient regimen in which both cytokines are subcutaneously administered is illustrated in **A**. The *plus signs* indicate day of treatment. The toxicity of this regimen is moderate, however, and will vary depending on patient selection and comorbid factors. Responses in parenchymal organs are unusual when cytokines are used; however, they do occur, and one such partial response in a patient receiving continuous-infusion rIL-2 and subcutaneous (SC) interferon-alfa is illustrated in **B** and **C**.

(Continued on next page)

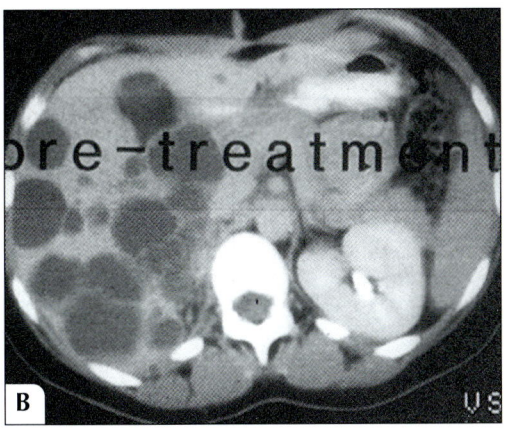

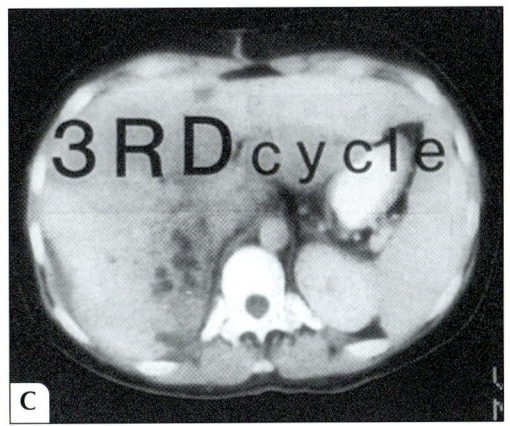

▶ **FIGURE 6-18.** (*Continued*) *Panel B*, Hepatic metastases on a CT scan prior to treatment. *Panel C*, Partial regression of these lesions after three cycles of treatment. This response lasted more than 6 months. (Part A *adapted from Atzpodien et al.* [64].)

Comparative Toxicity of Cytokine Regimens

Type of Toxicity	High-dose rIL-2 (≥ grade 3), %*‡	Subcutaneous rIL-2†	Subcutaneous rIL-2 and interferon-alfa†	Chemoimmunotherapy with 5-Fluorouracil, rIL-2, and Interferon-alfa†
Nausea or vomiting	32	34%	75% (4% ≥ grade 3)	64% (≤ grade 2)
Diarrhea	17	—	25% (≤ grade 2)	29% (1% grade 3)
Creatinine	2§	Mild	—	—
Oliguria (<80 mL/8 h)	21	—	—	—
Hypotension	54	52% (11%)¶	28% (≤ grade 2)	19% (≤ grade 2)
Central nervous system toxicity	12	—	9% (grade 1)	—
Hyperbilirubinemia	6	4% (grade 1)	—	—
Arrhythmia	4	—	2% (grade 1)	2% (grade 1)
Thrombopenia	9	—	—	—
Anemia	NS§	NS	34% (≤ grade 2)	—
Pulmonary abnormalities	4	—	47% (7% ≥ grade 3)	23% (1% grade 3)

* National Cancer Institute common toxicity criteria.
† World Health Organization toxicity criteria.
‡ Percentage of patients reported with toxicity.
§ Creatinine ≥ 8 mg/dL.
¶ Value in parentheses indicates the percentage of patients with blood pressure <90 mm Hg.

▶ **FIGURE 6-19.** Cytokine toxicity in immunotherapy. The side effects of cytokines depend on the agent, dose, route of administration, and patient comorbid factors. Acute toxicity may be dramatic, with chills, fever, hypotension, and renal abnormalities. Chronic side effects may include neuropathy, depression, hematologic abnormalities, and dermatologic findings. The figure illustrates the kinds of toxicity reported with four regimens including high-dose bolus recombinant interleukin (rIL-2) [65], rIL-2 subcutaneously administered on an outpatient basis with [64] or without interferon-alfa [66], and the chemoimmunotherapy regimen of 5-fluorouracil (5-FU), rIL-2, and interferon-alfa [56]. The choice of treatment regimen is guided by patient status, comorbid factors, and the degree and severity of side effects that are acceptable. NS—not stated.

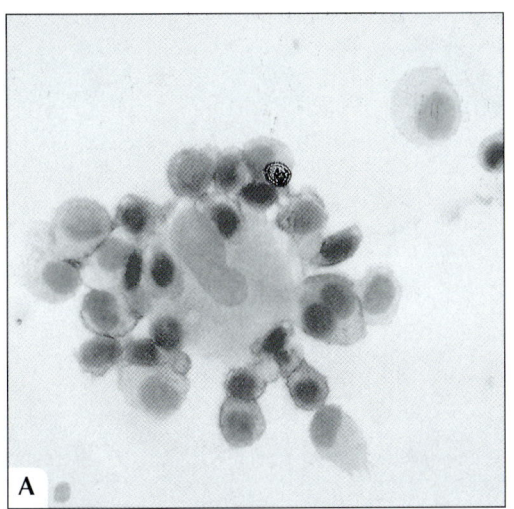

▶ **FIGURE 6-20.** (*See* Color Plate) Adoptive immunotherapy. The transfer of immune or activated lymphocytes to enhance cellular immunity has been actively investigated in patients with renal cell carcinoma. Lymphokine-activated killer (LAK) cells, tumor-infiltrating lymphocytes (TIL), autolymphocyte therapy (ALT), and tumor-sensitized T cells are approaches that have been reported [43,67–69]. The sources of these cells include peripheral blood (LAK, ALT), tumor specimens (TIL), and regional lymph nodes (sensitized T cells). Various culture methods, media, concentrations of recombinant interleukin-2 (rIL-2), and absence or presence of other stimuli such as anti-CD3 monoclonal antibodies have been used. The optimal cell population is unclear, but in view of the role of T lymphocytes in tumor rejection, it probably includes subpopulations of these cells. **A**, Photomicrograph of activated T lymphocytes surrounding a tumor cell. Clinical results and outcomes with adoptive immunotherapy (AIT) have been variable and have often been accompanied by coadministration of rIL-2, making interpretation of results difficult.

(*Continued on next page*)

B. Clinical Results With Adoptive Immunotherapy in Renal Cell Carcinoma

Approach	Patients, n	Response rate, %
LAK cells + rIL-2 [43]	461	21
TIL ± rIL-2 [67,70,71]	92	24
ALT [68]	45	18
Tumor-sensitized T lymphocytes [69]	12	33

COMBINED-MODALITY APPROACHES

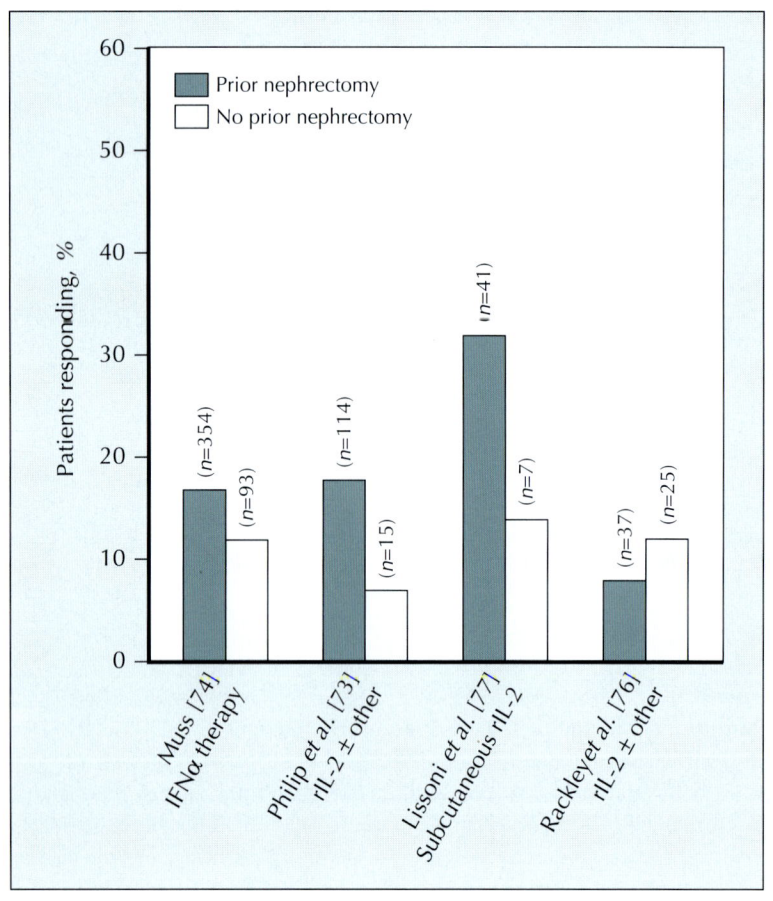

◗ **FIGURE 6-21.** Clinical responses in patients receiving cytokine therapy: influence of previous nephrectomy. The possibility that immunotherapy may be more effective in low-volume disease [72] has resulted in the use of debulking adjunctive nephrectomy prior to systemic administration of cytokines. Reports on the use of recombinant interleukin-2 (rIL-2) [22,73] and interferon-alfa [74] have noted that prior nephrectomy is associated with a higher likelihood of response and survival. It is probable that the performance of a nephrectomy introduces bias because patients with high-risk disease are frequently not considered surgical candidates and variable percentages (20% to 30%) of patients do not survive long enough to receive therapy [67,70,75]. The impact of adjuvant nephrectomy was also investigated by Rackley *et al.* [76] in a group of 62 patients receiving rIL-2–based therapy. No differences in response rates in sites outside the primary tumor were found whether nephrectomy was performed prior to therapy or delayed until response was determined. The figure shows results reported in patients undergoing adjunctive nephrectomy prior to cytokine treatment. Analysis of data generally suggests higher response rates in previously nephrectomized patients. An ongoing study of interferon-alfa with and without adjunctive nephrectomy will provide important prospective data to assess this approach.

Results of Immunotherapy Followed by Cytoreductive Surgery

Study	Patients, n	Type of immunotherapy	Sites resected	Median survival, mo
Krishnamurthy *et al.* [83]	3	NS	Kidney, partial nephrectomy	6+, 7.0, 20.0*
Sherry *et al.* [80]	16	rIL-2 based	Lung, kidney, brain	11.0
Tanguay *et al.* [34]	29	Interferon-alfa, -gamma, tumor necrosis factor-α + rIL-2	Lung, liver, lymph nodes	>48.0 (5/29 remain DF)
Fleischman *et al.* [81]	2	rIL-2 + LAK cells	Kidney, soft tissue	9+, 18.0
Rackley *et al.* [76]	3	rIL-2 based	Kidney, lymph nodes	14+, 18+ (2/3 remain DF)

* Survival time of three patients.

▶ **FIGURE 6-22.** Cytokine therapy and cytoreductive surgery in responding patients. In patients who respond incompletely to immunotherapy, surgical resection of areas of residual disease is being explored as part of a combined-modality approach. Preliminary evidence suggests that this approach may be of value in selected patients who have been treated with either interferon-alfa [78] or recombinant interleukin-2 (rIL-2)–based regimens [79]. Resection of residual pulmonary [34], hepatic [80], and retroperitoneal lesions [81] has been reported, and no evidence of increased surgical morbidity in this highly selected group of patients has been found [34]. Patients with synchronous metastatic disease whose primary tumors do not respond have also been treated in this fashion [76,81,82]. This figure summarizes reports on cytokine therapy followed by cytoreductive surgery. Randomized trials demonstrating the benefit of this approach have not been performed, but selected patients appear to benefit when a combination of modalities is used in a sequential fashion. DF—disease free; LAK—lymphokine-activated killer; NS—not stated.

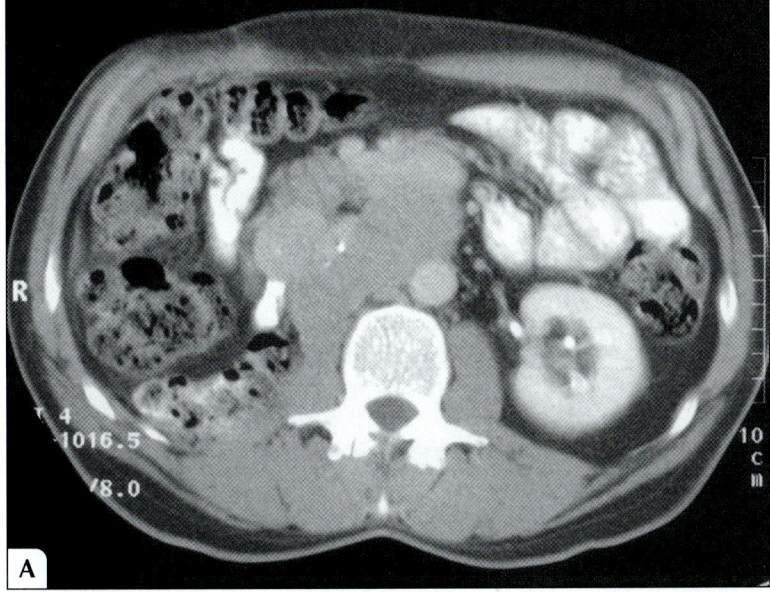

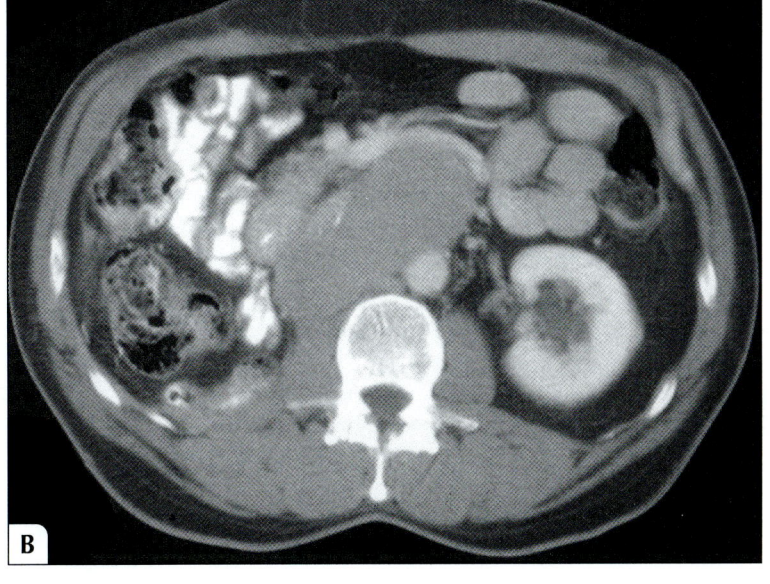

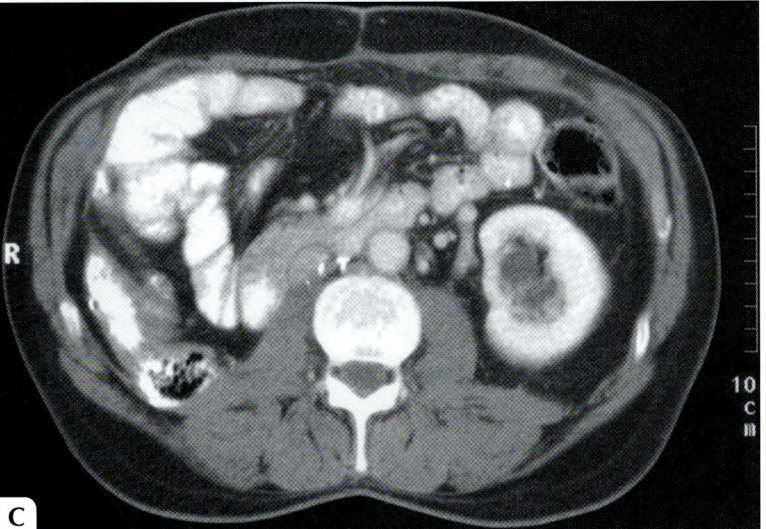

▶ **FIGURE 6-23.** Cytoreductive surgery following cytokine therapy. The findings noted in Figure 6-13 suggest that in selected responding and stable patients who have been treated with cytokine-based regimens, resection of areas of residual disease is possible. These CT scans show a patient with recurrent clear-cell carcinoma who was treated with 5-fluorouracil (5-FU), recombinant interleukin (rIL-2), and interferon-alfa [60]. The pretreatment scan (**A**) demonstrates significant retroperitoneal adenopathy. Following three cycles of 5-FU, rIL-2, and interferon-alfa, a minimal decrease in the size of the lymph nodes areas can be seen (**B**). Resection of residual retroperitoneal disease were resected (**C**), and the patient remained disease free for more than 8 months.

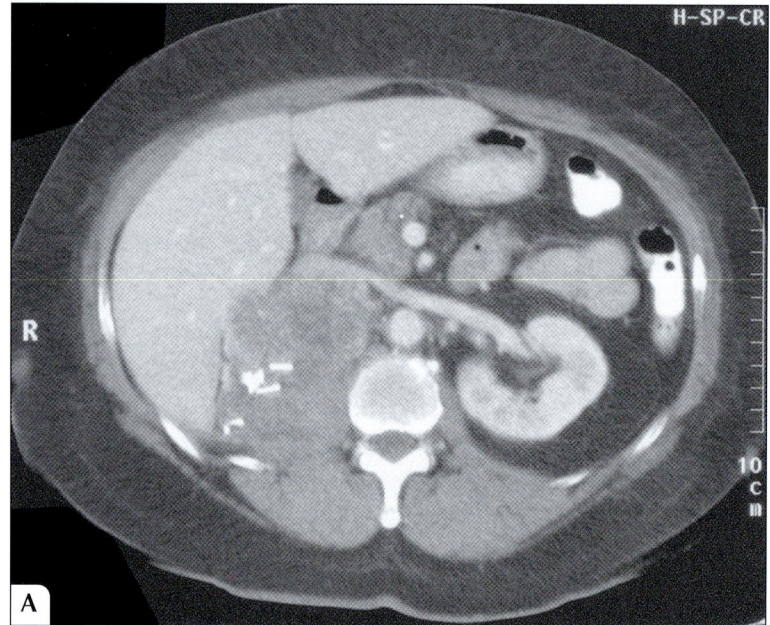

A

B

Preoperative external-beam radiation therapy (4500–5040 cGy) → Cytoreductive surgery + Intraoperative external-beam radiation therapy (1000–2500 cGy)

• Eight patients
• Sites of disease: renal fossa (6), primary tumor (2)
• 6/8 patients alive at 10.5 mo
• Four patients remain free of disease

▶ **FIGURE 6-24.** Radiation therapy and cytoreductive surgery. **A,** Resection of recurrent lesions in the renal fossa of patients with previously resected renal cell carcinoma (RCC) has been reported to be associated with extended survival [84]. The addition of preoperative external irradiation (4500 to 5040 cGy) and intraoperative external-beam radiation therapy (1000 to 2500 cGy) has been investigated in this group of individuals [85].

Eight patients with RCC and either recurrent disease in the renal fossa (six patients) or locally advanced primary tumors (two patients) were treated in this fashion. **B,** Summary of results. Previous reports investigating preoperative radiation therapy (3000 cGy) followed by nephrectomy, however, have not demonstrated any advantages over surgery alone [86].

—•• ADJUVANT THERAPY ••—

Adjuvant Therapy for Renal Cell Carcinoma

Radiation therapy: preoperative, postoperative
Cytokines: interferon-alfa; recombinant interleukin
Autologous tumor cell vaccines

▶ **FIGURE 6-25.** Adjuvant therapy for renal cell carcinoma. Patients in advanced stages of disease, including venous involvement (T3b, T3c), involvement of the perinephric fat (T3a), lymph node metastases (N+) or invasion of Gerota's fascia (T4) are candidates for adjuvant therapy. The outcome for these individuals has not changed over the past several decades. Adjuvant therapy approaches that have been investigated are listed.

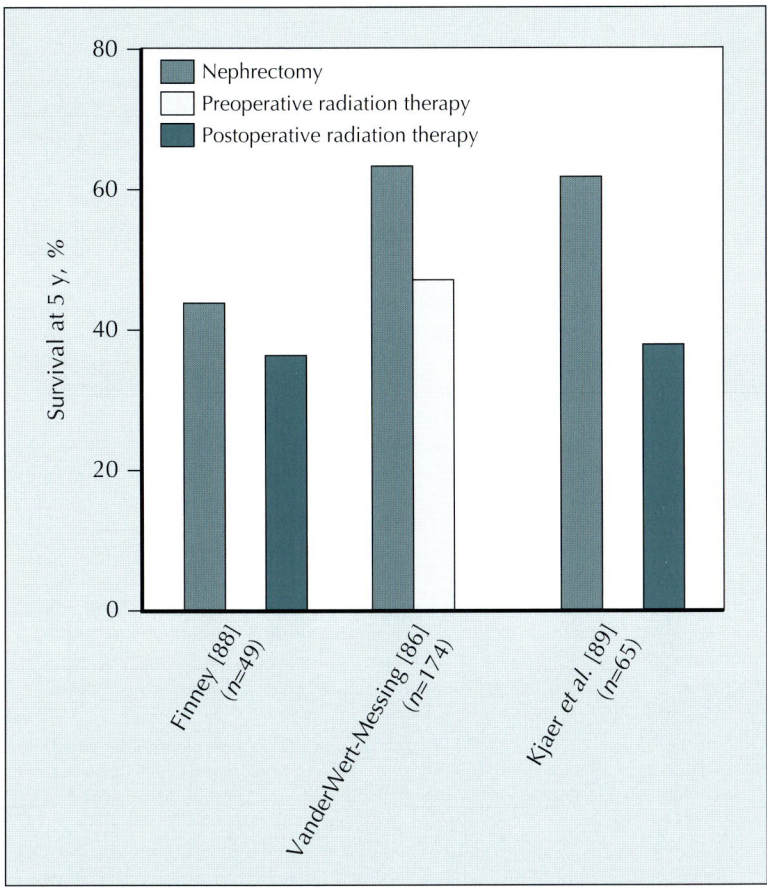

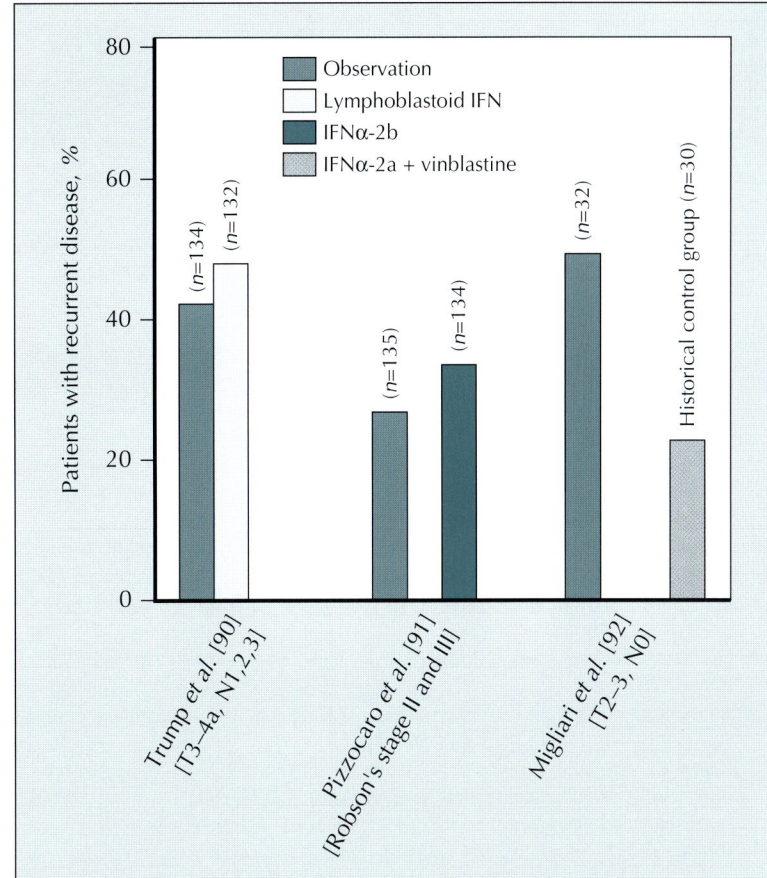

▶ **FIGURE 6-26.** Radiation therapy results. Adjuvant radiation therapy has been studied in a series of randomized trials in high-risk patients with renal cancer following nephrectomy, and improved outcomes have not been demonstrated. Two studies have investigated preoperative radiation therapy (3000 to 3600 cGy) followed by nephrectomy [86,87], and two trials have focused on the sequence of nephrectomy followed by postoperative radiation therapy (3600 to 5000 cGy) [88,89]. These reports yielded negative results; however, patients with T1 and T2 tumor were included, making demonstration of any benefit difficult.

▶ **FIGURE 6-27.** Results of adjuvant interferon-alfa in patients with renal cell carcinoma following nephrectomy. Interferon-alpha has been used following nephrectomy in several randomized and nonrandomized trials to investigate its ability to decrease recurrence rates and enhance survival in patients with high-risk stages of RCC. Entry criteria for these studies have varied, and preliminary results from the two largest trials [90,91] have been reported as negative. As shown in the figure, the randomized trials illustrate no benefit in terms of recurrence rates in patients receiving various interferon-alfa preparations. Studies using various schedules of recombinant interleukin-2 are now in progress, but results are not available. Therefore, data obtained so far do not support the routine use of postoperative adjuvant cytokine therapy in RCC patients. N—node; T—tumor.

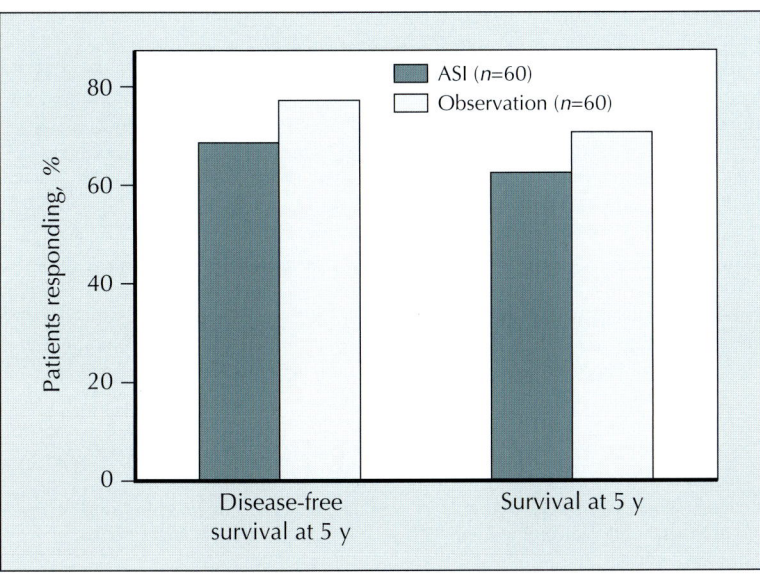

▶ **FIGURE 6-28.** Results of active specific immunotherapy with autologous tumor cells plus bacillus Calmette-Guérin (BCG). Active specific immunotherapy (ASI) generally uses vaccine preparations including either tumor cells or tumor-associated antigens with an adjuvant such as BCG to enhance the specific antitumor immune response. Studies in patients with metastatic disease [92] have been reported, with occasional responses noted. Galligioni *et al.* [93] conducted a randomized trial of adjuvant therapy consisting of autologous irradiated tumor cells mixed with BCG. Patients in stages I, II, and III of disease were included, with 97% in stage II or III. Results are summarized in the figure. In treated patients, 70% developed delayed hypersensitivity to autologous tumor cells. Clinical results do not suggest that ASI is of benefit.

1. McDougal WS, Garnick M: Clinical signs and symptoms of renal cell carcinoma. In *Comprehensive Textbook of Genitourinary Oncology*. Edited by Vogelzang NJ, Scardino PT, Shipley WV, Coffey DS. Baltimore: Williams & Wilkins; 1996:154–159.

2. Linehan WM, Shipley W, Parkinson D: Cancer of the kidney and ureter. In *Cancer Principles and Practice of Oncology*. Edited by Divita VT, Hellman S, Rosenberg SA. Philadelphia: JB Lippincott; 1993:1023–1051.

3. Finke JH, Rayman P, Hart L, *et al.*: Characterization of TIL subsets from human renal carcinoma: specific reactivity defined by cytotoxicity, IFN*alpha* secretion, and proliferation. *J Immunother* 1994, 15:91–104.

4. Finke JH, Tubbs R, Connelly B, *et al.*: Tumor-infiltrating lymphocytes in patients with RCC. *Ann N Y Acad Sci* 1988, 532:387–394.

5. Oliver RTD, Mehta A, Barnett MJ: A phase 2 study of surveillance in patients with metastatic renal cell carcinoma and assessment of response of such patients to therapy on progression. *Mol Biother* 1988, 1:14–20.

6. American Cancer Society: Cancer Facts & Figures: 1996. Atlanta: American Cancer Society; 1996.

7. Robson CJ, Churchill BM, Anderson W: The results of radical nephrectomy for RCC. *J Urol* 1969, 101:297–301.

8. Guinan P, Sobin LH, Algaba F, *et al.*: TNM staging of renal cell carcinoma. 1997, 80:992–993.

9. Skinner DG, Calvin RB, Vermillion CD, *et al.*: Diagnosis and management of renal cell carcinoma. *Cancer* 1971, 28:1165–1177.

10. Boxer RJ, Waisman J, Leiber MM, *et al.*: Renal carcinoma: computer analysis of 96 patients treated by nephrectomy. *J Urol* 1979, 122:598–601.

11. McNichols DW, Segrura JW, DeWeerd JH: Renal cell carcinoma: long-term survival and late recurrence. *J Urol* 1901, 126.17–23.

12. Golimbu M, Joshi P, Sperber A, *et al.*: Renal cell carcinoma: survival and prognostic factors. *Urology* 1986, 27:291–301.

13. Tolia BM, Whitmore WF: Solitary metastasis from renal cell carcinoma. *J Urol* 1975, 114:836–840.

14. Stenzl A, DeKernion JB: Pathology, biology, and clinical staging of renal cell carcinoma. *Semin Oncol* 1989, 16(suppl 1):3–11.

15. Jones M, Phillip T, Palmer P, *et al.*: The impact of interleukin-2 on survival in renal cancer: a multivariate analysis. *Cancer Biother* 1993, 8:275–288.

16. Rabinovitch RA, Zelefsky MJ, Gaynor JJ, Fuks Z: Patterns of failure following surgical resection of renal cell carcinoma: implications for adjuvant local and systemic therapy. *J Clin Oncol* 1994, 12:206–212.

17. Maldazys JD, DeKernion JB: Prognostic factors in metastatic renal carcinoma. *J Urol* 1986, 136:376–379.

18. Zhao B, Kimura W, Futakawa N, *et al.*: Renal cell carcinoma of the spindle cell type with metastasis to the pancreas: a case report. *Jpn J Clin Oncol* 1997, 27:58–61.

19. Nakhjavani MK, Gharib H, Goellner JR, van Heerelen JA: Metastases to the thyroid gland: a report of 43 cases. *Cancer* 1997, 79:574–578.

20. Elson PJ, Witte RS, Trump DL: Prognostic factors for survival in patients with recurrent or metastatic renal cell carcinoma. *Cancer Res* 1988, 48:7310–7313.

21. Minisian LM, Motzer RJ, Gluck L, *et al.*: Interferon alpha 2-a in advanced renal cell carcinoma: treatment results and survival in 159 patients with long-term follow-up. *J Clin Oncol* 1993, 11:1368–1375.

22. Fyfe G, Fisher RI, Rosenberg SA, *et al.*: Results of treatment of 255 patients with metastatic renal cell carcinoma who receive high dose recombinant interleukin-2 therapy. *J Clin Oncol* 1995, 13:688–696.

23. Palmer PA, Finke J, Phillip T, *et al.*: Prognostic factors for survival in patients with advanced renal cell carcinoma treated with recombinant interleukin-2. *Ann Oncol* 1992, 3:475–480.

24. Fossa SD, Kramar A, Droz JP: Prognostic factors and survival in patients with metastatic renal cell carcinoma treated with chemotherapy or interferon-alpha. *Eur J Cancer* 1994, 30A:1310–1314.

25. Landonio G, Baiocchi C, Cattaneo D, *et al.*: Retrospective analysis of 156 cases of metastatic renal cell carcinoma: evaluation of prognostic factors and response to different treatments. *Tumori* 1994, 80:468–472.

26. Montie JE, Steward BH, Straffon RA, *et al.*: The role of adjunctive nephrectomy in patients with metastatic renal cell carcinoma. *J Urol* 1977, 117:272–277.

27. DeKernion JB, Ramming KP, Smith RB: The natural history of metastatic renal cell carcinoma: a computer analysis. *J Urol* 1978, 120:148–158.

28. Middleton RG: Surgery for metastatic renal cell carcinoma. *J Urol* 1967, 97:973–977.

29. O'Dea MJ, Zincke H, Utz D, Bernatz PE: The treatment of renal cell carcinoma with solitary metastasis. *J Urol* 1978, 120:540–542.

30. Althausen P, Althausen A, Jennings LC, Mankin HJ: Prognostic factors and surgical treatment of osseous metastases secondary to renal cell carcinoma. *Cancer* 1977, 80:1103–1109.

31. Kierney PC, van Heerden JA, Segura JW, Weaver AL: Surgeon's role in the management of solitary renal cell carcinoma metastases occurring subsequent to initial curative nephrectomy: an institutional review. *Ann Surg Oncol* 1994, 1:345–352.

32. Cerfolio RJ, Allen MS, Deschamps C, *et al.*: Pulmonary resection of metastatic renal cell carcinoma. *Ann Thorac Surg* 1994, 57:339–344.

33. Hofmann HS, Neek H, Zerkowski HR: Results and prognostic factors after surgical treatment of lung metastases in renal cell carcinoma [abstract]. *Eur J Cancer* 1997, 33:540.

34. Tanguay S, Swanson DA, Putmam JB: Renal cell carcinoma metastatic to the lung: potential benefit in the combination of biological therapy and surgery. *J Urol* 1996, 156:1586–1589.

35. Gaugler B, Browvenstijn N, Vantomme V, *et al.*: A new gene coding for an antigen recognized by autologous cytolytic T-lymphocytes on a human renal carcinoma. *Immunogenetics* 1996, 44:323–330.

36. Broder S, Waldmann TA: The suppressor-cell network in cancer. *N Engl J Med* 1978, 299:1281–1284.

37. Kolenko V, Wang Q, Riedy MC, *et al.*: Tumor induced suppression of T-lymphocyte proliferation coincides with inhibition of JAK3 expression and IL-2R signaling: role of soluble products from human renal cell carcinomas. *J Immunol* 1977, 159:3057–3067.

38. O'Mahony AM, O'Sullivan GC, O'Connell J, *et al.*: An immune suppressive factor derived from esophageal squamous cell carcinoma induces apoptosis in normal and transformed cells of lymphoid lineage. *J Immunol* 1993, 151:4847–4856.

39. Wang Q, Redovan C, Tubbs R, *et al.*: Selective cytokine gene expression in RCC tumor cells and tumor infiltrating lymphocytes. *Int J Cancer* 1995, 61:1–6.

40. Finke JH, Zea A, Stanley J, *et al.*: Loss of T-cell receptor zeta chain and p56[1ck] in T-cells infiltrating human RCC. *Cancer Res* 1993, 53:5613–5616.

41. Li X, Liu J, Park JK, *et al.*: T cells from renal cell carcinoma patients exhibit an abnormal pattern of kappa B–specific DNA-binding activity: a preliminary report. *Cancer Res* 1994, 54:5424–5429.

42. Gillis S, Union NA, Baker PF, *et al.*: The in vitro generation and sustained culture of nude mouse cytolytic T-lymphocytes. *J Exp Med* 1979, 149:1460–1476.

43. Bukowski RM: Natural history and therapy of metastatic renal cell carcinoma: role of interleukin 2. *Cancer* 1997, 80:1198–1220.

44. Quesada JR, Swanson DA, Trindale A, *et al.*: Renal cell carcinoma: antitumor effects of leukocyte interferon. *Cancer Res* 1983, 43:940–947.

45. Dorr RT: Interferon-alpha in malignant and viral diseases: a review. *Drugs* 1993, 45:177–211.

46. Bukowski RM, Novick AC: Clinical practice guidelines: renal cell carcinoma. *Cleve Clin J Med* 1997, 64(suppl 1):1–48.

47. Chikkala NF, Lewis I, Ulchaker J, *et al.*: Interactive effects of alpha-interferon A/D and interleukin-2 on murine lymphokine-activated killer activity: analysis at the effector and precursor level. *Cancer Res* 1990, 50:1176–1182.

48. Negrier S, Escudier B, Lasset C, *et al.*: The FNCLCC Crecy trial: interleukin-2 (IL2) + interferon (IFN) is the optimal treatment to induce responses in metastatic renal cell carcinoma (MRCC) [abstract]. *Proc Am Soc Clin Oncol* 1996, 15:248.

49. Yagoda A, Abi-Rached B, Petrylak D: Chemotherapy for advanced renal-cell carcinoma: 1983–1993. *Semin Oncol* 1995, 22:42–60.

50. Pyrohönen S, Salminen E, Lehtonem T, *et al.*: Recombinant interferon alpha-2a with vinblastine vs. vinblastine alone in advanced renal cell carcinoma: a phase III study [abstract]. *Proc Am Soc Clin Oncol* 1996, 15:244.

51. Crivellari D, Tumolo S, Fustaci S, *et al.*: Phase II study of five-day continuous infusion of vinblastine in patients with metastatic renal-cell carcinoma. *Am J Clin Oncol* 1987, 10:231–233.

52. Von Roemeling, Hrushesky WJM: Circadian patterning of continuous floxuridine infusion reduces toxicity and allows higher dose intensity in patients with widespread cancer. *J Clin Oncol* 1989, 7:1710–1719.

53. Sampaio C, Olencki T, Murthy G, *et al.*: Phase II trial of circadian infusion of the antimetabolite floxuridine in patients with metastatic RCC. *J Infus Chemother* 1994, 4:100–103.

54. Fossa SD, Martinelli G, Otto U, *et al.*: Recombinant interferon alfa-2a with or without vinblastine in metastatic renal cell carcinoma: results of a European multi-center phase III study. *Ann Oncol* 1992, 3:301–305.

55. Negrier S, Escudier B, Dovillard JY, *et al.*: Randomized study of interleukin-2 (IL2) and interferon (IFN) with or without 5-FU (FUCY study) in metastatic renal cell carcinoma (MRCC) [abstract]. *Proc Am Soc Clin Oncol* 1997, 16:326a.

56. Hänninen EL, Kirchner H, Atzpodien J: Interleukin-2 based home therapy of metastatic renal cell carcinoma: risks and benefits in 215 consecutive single institution patients. *J Urol* 1996, 155:19–25.

57. Hoffmockel G, Langer W, Theiss M, *et al.*: Immunochemotherapy for metastatic renal cell carcinoma using a regimen of interleukin-2, interferon-alpha and 5-fluorouracil. *J Urol* 1996, 156:18–21.

58. Dutcher J, Logan T, Gordon M, *et al.*: 5U + subcutaneous (sc) interleukin-2 (IL2) plus sc Intron (IFN) in metastatic renal cell cancer (RCC) patients (PTS). A CWG study [abstract]. *Proc Am Soc Clin Oncol* 1996, 15:272.

59. Sella A, Zukiwiki A, Robinson E, *et al.*: Interleukin-2 (IL-2) with interferon-alpha and 5-fluorouracil in patients with metastatic renal cell cancer (RCC) [abstract]. *Proc am Soc Clin Oncol* 1994, 13:237.

60. Olencki T, Bukowski RM, Budd GT, *et al.*: Phase I/II trial of simultaneously administered rIL-2/rHuIFNalpha2a and 5-FU in patients (PTS) with metastatic renal cell carcinoma (RCC) [abstract]. *Proc Am Soc Clin Oncol* 1997, 16:339.

61. Jaffe JK, Banks RE, Forbes MA, *et al.*: A phase II study of interferon-alpha, interleukin-2 and 5-fluorouracil in advanced renal carcinoma: clinical data and laboratory evidence of protease activation. *Br J Urol* 1996, 77:638–649.

62. Atzpodien J, Kirchner H, Franzke A, *et al.*: Results of a randomized clinical trial comparing SC interleukin-2, SC alpha-2a-interferon, and IV bolus 5-fluorouracil against oral tamoxifen in progressive metastatic renal cell carcinoma patients [abstract]. *Proc Am Soc Clin Oncol* 1997, 16:326.

63. Gitilitz B, Dolan N, Pierce W: Fluoropyrimidines plus interleukin-2 and interferon-alpha in the treatment of metastatic renal cell carcinoma: the UCLA kidney cancer program [abstract]. *Proc Am Soc Clin Oncol* 1996, 15:248.

64. Atzpodien J, Lopez-Hänninen E, Kirchner H, *et al.*: Multiinstitutional home-therapy trial of recombinant human interleukin-2 and interferon alfa-2 in progressive metastatic RCC. *J Clin Oncol* 1995, 13:497–501.

65. Yang JC, Topalian SI, Parkinson D, *et al.*: Randomized comparison of high-dose and low-dose intravenous interleukin-2 for the therapy of metastatic RCC: an interim report. *J Clin Oncol* 1994, 12:1572–1576.

66. Sleijfer DTH, Janssen FJ, deVries EGE, *et al.*: Phase II study of subcutaneous interleukin-2 in unselected patients with advanced renal cell cancer on an outpatient basis. *J Clin Oncol* 1992, 10:1119–1123.

67. Bukowski RM, Sharfman W, Murthy S, *et al.*: Clinical results and characterization of tumor-infiltrating lymphocytes with or without recombinant interleukin-2 in human metastatic renal cell carcinoma. *Cancer Res* 1991, 51:4199–4205.

68. Graham S, Babayan RK, Lamm DL, *et al.*: The use of ex vivo–activated memory T cells (autolymphocyte therapy) in the treatment of metastatic renal cell carcinoma: final results from a randomized, controlled, multisite study. *Semin Urol* 1993, 11:27–34.

69. Chang AE, Aruga A, Cameron MJ, *et al.*: Adoptive immunotherapy with vaccine-primed lymph node cells secondarily activated with anti-CD3 and IL-2. *J Clin Oncol* 1996, 15:796–807.

70. Rayman P, Finke JH, Olencki T, *et al.*: Adoptive immunotherapy utilizing IL-2 and IL-4 for expansion of tumor-infiltrating lymphocytes in renal cell carcinoma. In *Immunotherapy of Cancer with Sensitized T Lymphocytes*. Edited by Chang AE, Shu S. Boca Raton, FL: RG Landers Co; 1994:123–129.

71. Figlin RA, Gitlitz B, Franklin J, *et al.*: Long term survival of patients with metastatic renal cell carcinoma treated with IL-2 based immunotherapy with or without tumor infiltrating lymphocytes: the UCLA kidney cancer program [abstract]. *Proc Am Soc Clin Oncol* 1996, 15:265.

72. Hrouda D, Muir GH, Dalgleish AG: The role of immunotherapy for urologic tumors. *Br J Urol* 1997, 79:307–316.

73. Philip T, Negrier S, Lasset C, *et al.*: Patients with metastatic renal carcinoma candidate for immunotherapy with cytokines: analysis of a single institution study on 181 patients. *Br J Cancer* 1993, 68:1034–1036.

74. Muss HB: Renal cell carcinoma. In *Biologic Therapy of Cancer*. Edited by DeVita VT, Hellman S, Rosenberg SA. Philadelphia: JB Lippincott; 1991:298–310.

75. Walther MM, Alexander R, Weiss GH, *et al.*: Cytoreductive surgery prior to interleukin-2-based therapy in patients with metastatic renal cell carcinoma. *Urology* 1993, 42:250–258.

76. Rackley R, Novick A, Klein E, *et al.*: The impact of adjuvant nephrectomy on multimodality treatment of metastatic renal cell carcinoma. *J Urol* 1994, 152:1399–1403.

77. Lissoni P, Barni S, Ardizoia A, *et al.*: Prognostic factors of the clinical response to subcutaneous immunotherapy with interleukin-2 alone in patients with metastatic renal cell carcinoma. *Oncology* 1994, 51:59–62.

78. Sella A, Swanson DA, Ro JY, *et al.*: Surgery following response to interferon-alpha-based therapy for residual renal cell carcinoma. *J Urol* 1993, 149:19–22.

79. Kim B, Louie AC: Surgical resection following interleukin-2 therapy for metastatic renal cell carcinoma prolongs remission. *Arch Surg* 1992, 127:1343–1349.

80. Sherry RM, Pass HI, Rosenberg SA, Yang JC: Surgical resection of metastatic renal cell carcinoma and melanoma after response to interleukin-2-based immunotherapy. *Cancer* 1992, 69:1850–1855.

81. Fleischman JD, Kim B: Interleukin-2 immunotherapy followed by resection of residual renal cell carcinoma. *J Urol* 1991, 145:938–941.

82. Spencer WF, Linehan WM, Walther MM, *et al.*: Immunotherapy with interleukin-2 and alpha-interferon in patients with metastatic renal cell cancer with in situ primary cancers: a pilot study. *J Urol* 1992, 147:24–30.

83. Krishnamurthy V, Novick AC, Bukowski R: Nephron sparing surgery in patients with metastatic renal cell carcinoma. *J Urol* 1996, 156:36–39.

84. Esrig D, Ahlering TE, Lieskovsky O, Skinner DG: Experience with fossa recurrence of renal cell carcinoma. *J Urol* 1992, 147:1491.

85. Frydenberg M, Gunderson L, Hahn G, *et al.*: Preoperative external beam radiotherapy followed by cytoreductive surgery and intraoperative radiotherapy for locally advanced primary or recurrent renal malignancies. *J Urol* 1994, 152:15–21.

86. Van der Werf-Messing B: Carcinoma of the kidney. *Cancer* 1973, 32:1056–1062.

87. Juusela H, Malmio K, Alfthan D: Preoperative irradiation in the treatment of renal adenocarcinoma. *Scand J Urol Nephrol* 1977, 11:277–283.

88. Finney R: The value of radiotherapy in the treatment of hypernephroma: a clinical trial. *Br J Urol* 1973, 45:258–269.

89. Kjaer M, Frederiksen PL, Engelholm SA. Postoperative radiotherapy in stage II and III renal adenocarcinoma: a randomized trial by the Copenhagen renal cancer study group. *Int J Radiat Oncol Biol Phys* 1987, 13:665–672.

90. Trump DL, Elson P, Propert R, *et al.*: Randomized controlled trial of adjuvant therapy with lymphoblastoid interferon (L-IFN) in resected high-risk renal cell carcinoma [abstract]. *Proc Am Soc Clin Oncol* 1996, 15:253.

91. Pizzocaro G, Piva L, Costa A, Silvestrini R: Adjuvant interferon (IFN) to radical nephrectomy in Robson's stages II and III renal cell carcinoma (RCC), a multi-center randomized study with some biological evaluations [abstract]. *Proc Am Soc Clin Oncol* 1997, 16:318.

92. McCune CS, O'Donnell RW, Marquis DM, Sahasrabudhe DM: Renal cell carcinoma treated by vaccines for active specific immunotherapy: correlation of survival with skin testing by autologous tumor cells. *Cancer Immunol Immunother* 1990, 32:62–66.

93. Galligioni E, Quara M, Merlo A, *et al.*: Adjuvant immunotherapy treatment of renal cell carcinoma patients with autologous tumor cells and bacillus Calmette-Guèrin. *Cancer* 1996, 77:2560–2566.

Evaluation and Management of Benign and Malignant Adrenal Tumors

Robert C. Flanigan
Fernando J. Kim

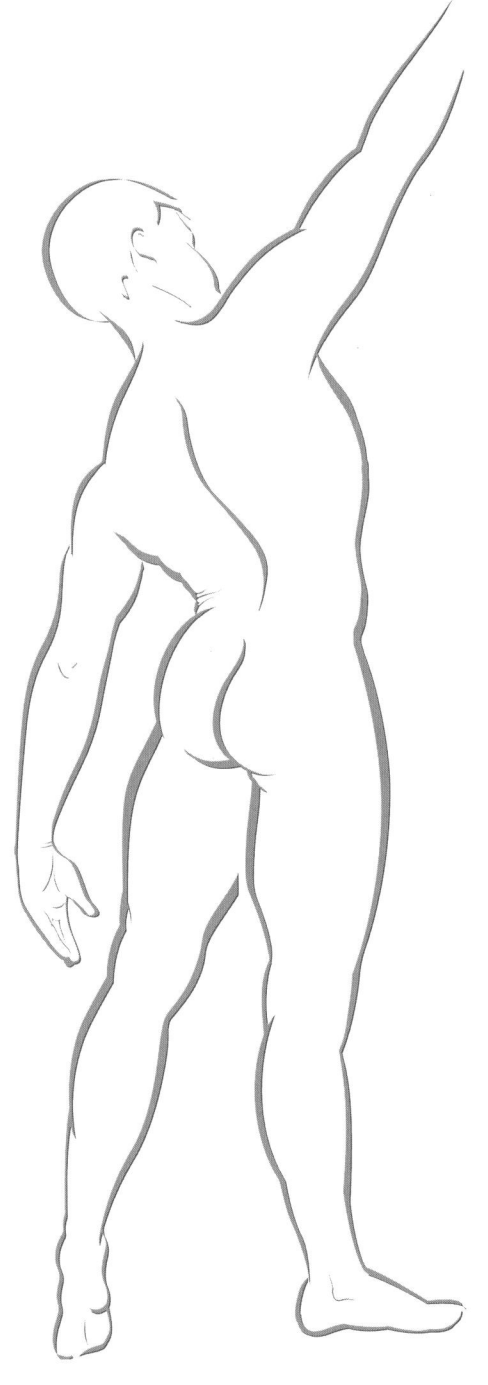

Adrenal tumors are not uncommon [1]. This chapter discusses the major adrenal tumors, which include adrenal cortical adenomas (producing primary hyperaldosteronism) and Cushing's syndrome, adrenal cortical carcinoma, pheochromocytoma, and the incidentally identified adrenal mass. Currently, the diagnosis of adrenal disorders is extremely accurate when using a 1) combination of precise biochemical methods for the measurement of the abnormal secretion of adrenal hormones, and 2) sophisticated radiographic imaging techniques for the localization and characterization of specific adrenal lesions [2].

The treatment of patients with an adrenal disorder is approached on a team basis, including experienced endocrinologists, radiologists, anesthesiologists, and urologists. The management of adrenal tumors requires a clear understanding of the normal physiology of the adrenal medulla and cortex, a three-dimensional concept of the adrenal anatomy as well as adjacent structures, and a knowledge of the various pathologic entities that involve the adrenal glands [3].The operating surgeon must be aware of the different approaches to the diagnosis of the various adrenal entities, the potential intraoperative physiologic changes that are unique to these patients, and the specific postoperative complications that may occur. This chapter reviews the current diagnostic strategies used to identify these diseases as well as their pre- and postoperative management.

Advances in technology provide a better understanding, analysis, and management of different adrenal disorders. The combination of biochemical analysis (to measure the appropriate adrenocortical and medullary hormonal production) with radiologic techniques facilitates the localization of adrenal abnormalities. Following localization, precise surgical techniques are highly successful, resulting in a normalization of both the metabolic abnormalities and their associated clinical manifestations.

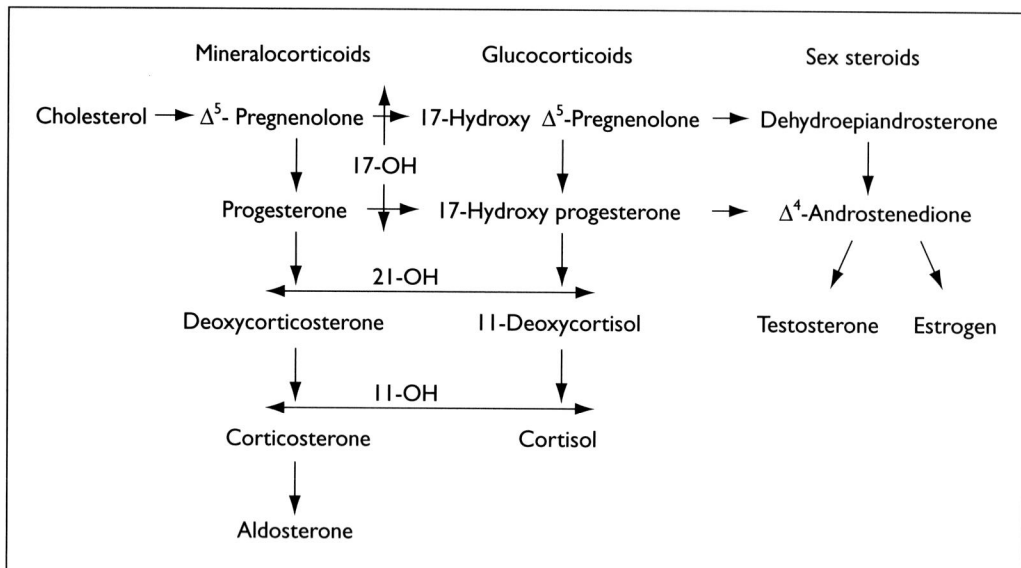

FIGURE 7-1. Routes of hormone synthesis and the enzymes involved. Knowledge of the functional morphology and the regulation of the adrenal gland (especially aldosterone and cortisol production) is pivotal to understanding the meaning of the results of various tests used in the diagnosis of adrenal disease [4–6]. The adrenal glands are paired retroperitoneal organs that lie within perinephric fat at the anterosuperior and medial aspects of the kidneys. Each gland typically weighs 5 g on average, and measures up to 5 cm in length, 3 cm in width, and 1 cm in thickness [3,4].

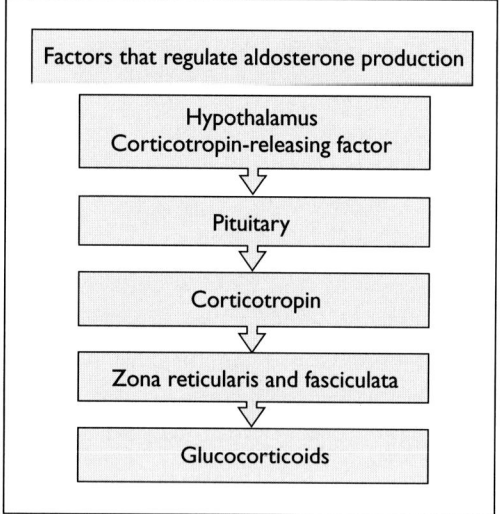

FIGURE 7-2. The interactions among the factors that regulate the production of glucocorticoids. The zona reticularis and zona fasciculata are functionally more versatile than the zona glomerulosa, being the source of cortisol and

adrenal androgens. The structure, growth, and secretory activity of the zona reticularis and the fascicula are regulated entirely by pituitary corticotropin (*see* Fig. 7-3). Among the glucocorticoids, cortisol is the major participant in the feedback mechanism controlling corticotropin secretion. This feedback process can be interrupted by stress, extrapituitary production of corticotropin, or exogenous sources of cortisol. Corticotropin has only a transient effect on aldosterone. Thus, aldosterone production can be sustained at normal levels even in the absence of corticotropin [7].

The adrenal medulla is responsible for the production of adrenal catecholamines. In the brain, nerve fibers from the centers in the medulla, pons, and hypothalamus connect with preganglionic sympathetic neurons in the thoracolumbar spinal cord. These preganglionic fibers leave the cord through the anterior root, proceed into the spinal nerve, pass into the ganglia of the sympathetic chain, and synapse with postganglionic fibers that are distributed to tissues and organs stimulated by the sympathetic nervous system [8]. The neuroanatomy of the adrenal medulla differs in that preganglionic fibers pass from the spinal cord through the sympathetic chains and splanchnic nerves to the adrenal medulla and synapse directly with chromaffin cells, which produce catecholamines. In adults, most chromaffin cells are located in the adrenal medulla, but remnants of chromaffin cell ganglia remain in the sympathetic ganglia and the organs of Zuckerkandl, which may be the site of extra-adrenal pheochromocytomas.

The adrenal medulla and sympathetic nervous system support each other, thus maintaining function when one system is diseased. Adrenal medullary catecholamines reach structures not innervated by sympathetic fibers, and their effects can last five to 10 times longer than direct sympathetic stimulation. Thus, in concert with the sympathetic nervous system, adrenal catecholamines maintain the basal sympathetic tone of the circulation.

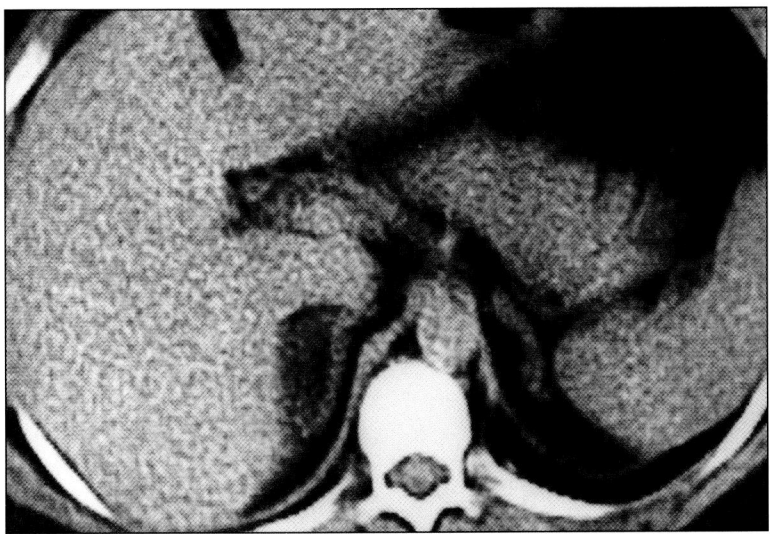

▶ **FIGURE 7-3.** Normal adrenal glands. Currently, the adrenal glands can be readily imaged by CT, sonography, and magnetic resonance imaging (MRI) [9,10]. Hence, invasive procedures such as arteriography, venography, or venous sampling are now seldom required for diagnosis. CT scanning is the most valuable imaging technique [11]. The abundant perinephric fat present in most patients allows the clear display of the

adrenal glands. Tumors as small as 10 mm are routinely identified using contiguous 5-mm collimated slices.

The adenomas of Conn's syndrome (hyperaldosteronism) are the most difficult lesions to detect on CT because they are the smallest lesions, usually measuring less than 2 cm in diameter [12]. Adrenal venous sampling can be helpful in patients with Conn's syndrome because of the small size of the tumor as well as the presence of bilateral disease [13]. In contrast, venous drainage studies are rarely needed in patients with adrenal Cushing's syndrome because of the larger size of the lesions and the abundant retroperitoneal fat. MRI does not provide additional useful information in most patients with Cushing's or Conn's syndrome [14,15].

Sonography may be useful to study the retroperitoneum in children because of the paucity of fat. Although the spatial resolution of MRI is inferior to CT, the intense T_2-weighted signal demonstrated by most pheochromocytomas makes MRI useful in differentiating these tumors from cortical adenomas [16]. Moreover, MRI may help to demonstrate extra-adrenal pheochromocytomas (urinary bladder and paracardiac region) [17]. Although ^{131}I meta-iodobenzyl guanidine (MIBG) scanning seems to be similar in overall accuracy to CT and MR for localization of pheochromocytoma, it is only occasionally used for whole body imaging to detect ectopic tumors or metastatic deposits [18]. Most nonfunctional adrenal masses are incidentally detected on abdominal CT examinations performed for another purpose.

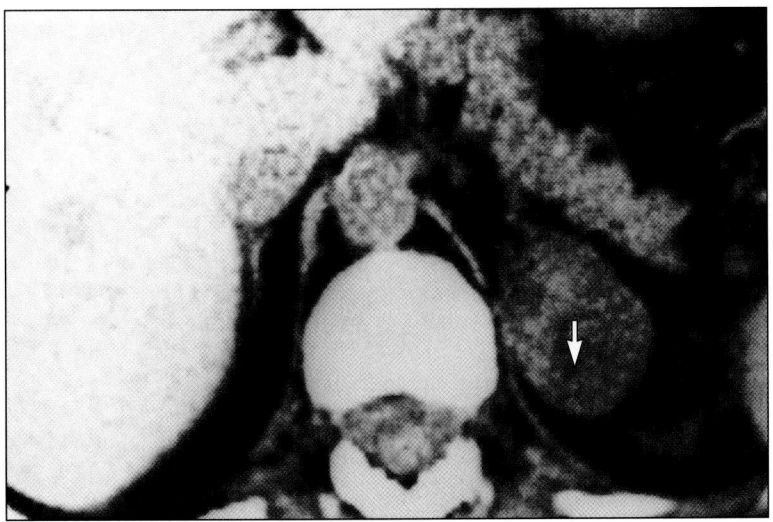

▶ **FIGURE 7-4.** Malignant adrenal tumor (*arrow*). Features indicating such lesions include large size (>6 cm), poorly defined margins, invasion of adjacent structures, nonhomogeneous attenuation, and a thick irregular enhancing rim. Small ovoid lesions with a thin rim and homogenous density are more likely to be benign. However, adrenal carcinomas as small as 1 cm have been reported. The most difficult aspect of CT staging of adrenal carcinoma has been the detection of direct hepatic extension. If no fat plane exists between the tumor and the liver, it is nearly impossible to predict the presence or absence of liver invasion. Magnetic resonance imaging may be useful to detect venous extension of adrenal carcinomas [15].

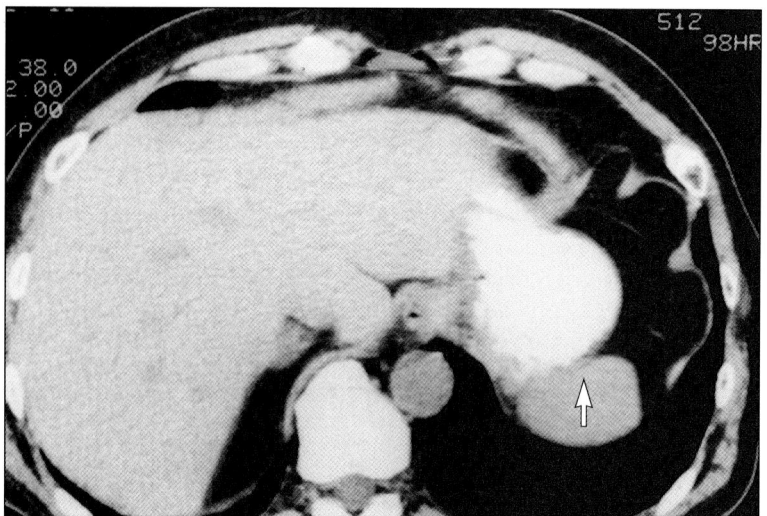

▶ **FIGURE 7-5.** Myelolipoma of the adrenal gland (*arrow*). These nonfunctional masses are usually detected incidentally. A fatty adrenal mass on CT examination is virtually diagnostic of this lesion [19] (*see* Fig. 7-5). Acute adrenal hemorrhage may be identified by its high density on CT. Some areas of adrenal hemorrhage liquefy and persist as an adrenal pseudocyst [20].

used for this purpose and several studies have suggested that there are cutoff points of this ratio below which all lesions are adenomas and above which all lesions are metastases [22]. However, an overlap group exists that contains as many as 31% of the cases. Adrenal cortical scintigraphy using ^{59}Np has also been used to differentiate benign from metastatic adrenal lesions. However, benign lesions such as cysts, hemorrhage, or granulomatous disease do not take up the isotope, thus reducing the accuracy of this study.

Percutaneous aspiration biopsy can be helpful to confirm metastatic adrenal disease [23]. However, patients undergoing percutaneous adrenal aspiration biopsy should first be screened for pheochromocytoma to avoid the risk of precipitating a hypertensive crisis. Obviously, CT evidence of other metastatic lesions supports the diagnosis of adrenal metastasis and lessens the significance of overlooking a primary adrenal malignancy.

Occasionally, "pseudotumors" may be confused with adrenal lesions on CT. Exophytic renal masses may simulate adrenal masses on either side. An adrenal mass on the right side may be mimicked by a hepatic mass, interposition of the colon into the hepatorenal recess, or a dilated inferior vena cava. Adrenal pseudotumors on the left side are more common and include splenic lobulations, accessory spleens, tortuous splenic vessels, splenic artery aneurysms, the tail of the pancreas, the gastric fundus, or a gastric diverticulum. Oral contrast material should distinguish most confusing structures, and bolus intravenous contrast injection should further delineate vascular structures. Repeated CT sections with narrow collimation also may help to establish the true nature of these lesions. If the diagnosis is still in doubt, additional studies such as sonography or MRI may be needed to confirm the diagnosis [19].

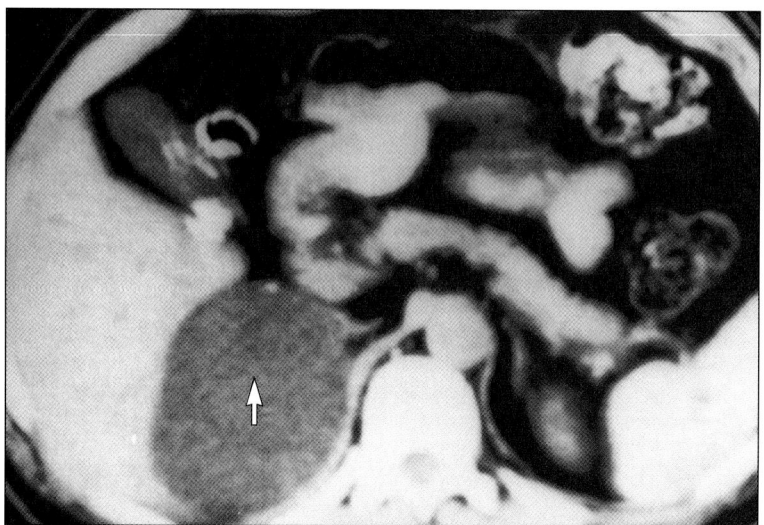

▶ **FIGURE 7-6.** Adrenal cyst (*arrow*). Adrenal cysts may be examined by sonography or CT. In contrast to renal cysts, adrenal cysts may have a thick wall and may have internal septa. Cyst aspiration can be helpful if the fluid is clear and the cytology benign [21].

The adrenal gland is a common site of metastatic disease that cannot be easily distinguished from benign lesions radiographically. Because metastases typically have higher signal intensity on T_2-weighted images, magnetic resonance imaging (MRI) may be useful in this setting. A ratio of the intensity of the adrenal tumor and adjacent liver, muscle, or fat has been

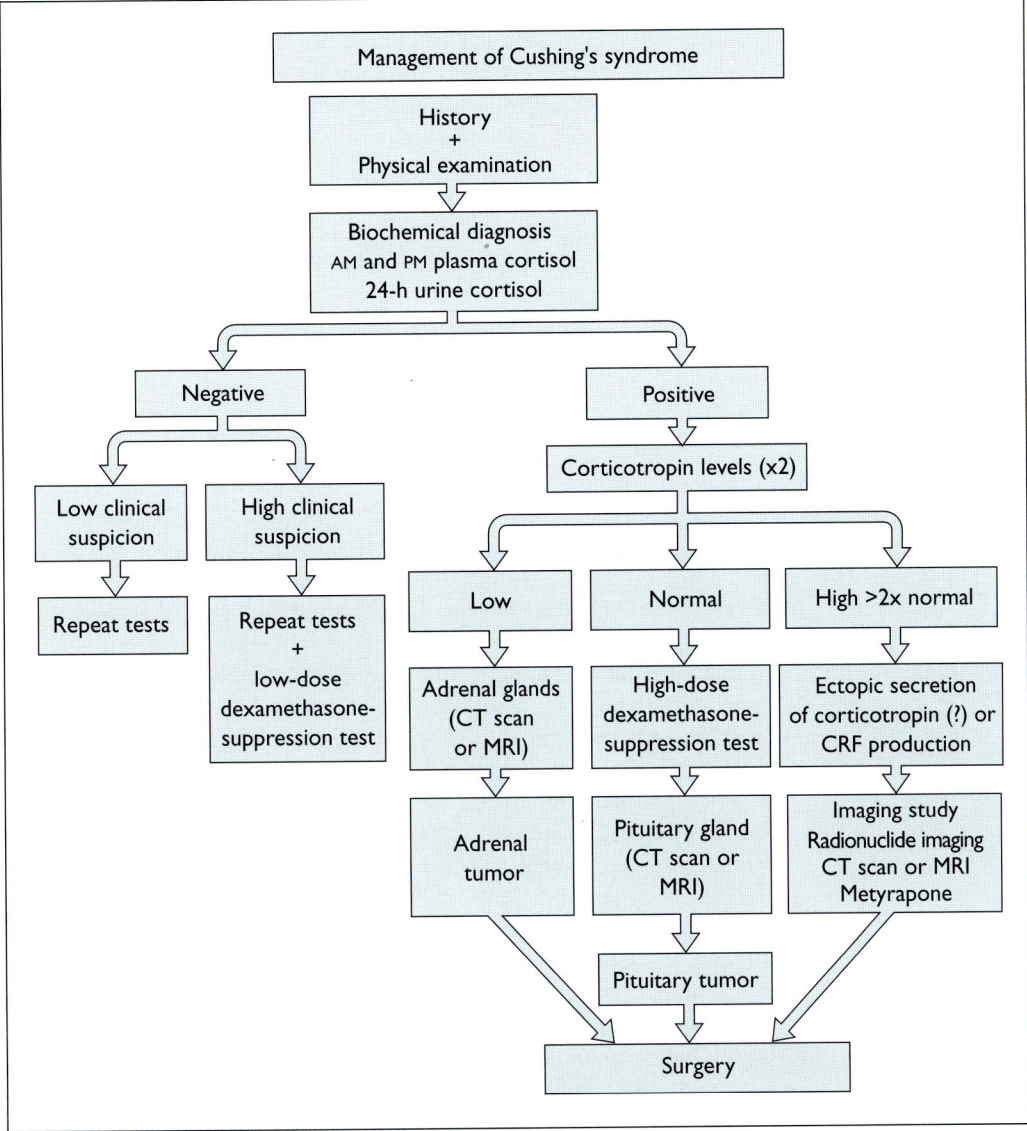

The clinical diagnosis of Cushing's syndrome is confirmed by the demonstration of cortisol hypersecretion [26]. Presently, determination of 24-hour urinary excretion of cortisol is the most direct and reliable index of cortical secretion. It is recommended that urinary cortisol should be measured in two (and preferably three) consecutive 24-hour urine specimens, collected on an outpatient basis. Presently, the low-dose dexamethasone test is generally used to rule out pseudo-Cushing's disease.

If the patient's cortisol concentration is higher than 50 µg/dL and the corticotropin concentration is lower than 5 pg/mL, the cortisol secretion is considered corticotropin independent; thus the patient has a primary adrenal problem. Conversely, if the patient's cortisol concentration is elevated and the plasma corticotropin concentration is higher than 50 pg/mL, the cortisol secretion is considered corticotropin dependent; thus the patient has Cushing's disease (a pituitary cause) or an ectopic secretion of corticotropin or CRH syndrome.

Transphenoidal pituitary tumor removal cures Cushing's disease in 67% to 91% of patients. Patients not cured by surgery may require irradiation or bilateral adrenalectomy [27]. Corticotropin levels higher than twice the upper limit of normal suggests either ectopic production of corticotropin or corticotropin-releasing factor (CRF). These patients should be evaluated for carcinoid, thymoma, oat cell carcinoma of the lung, medullary carcinoma of the thyroid, pheochromocytoma, islet cell tumor, and carcinoma of the prostate. Surgical treatment should be directed at the primary tumor if possible. Bilateral adrenalectomy should be considered in patients whose primary tumor cannot be located or in whom tumor cannot be cured but who require relief of hyperadrenocorticotropism [28].

Usually, computed tomography (CT) scanning of adrenal adenomas will demonstrate lesions that are larger than 2 cm, solitary, and associated with atrophy of the opposite gland. Adrenal carcinomas are often indistinguishable from adenomas except for their larger size (usually > 6 cm) [29]. MRI—magnetic resonance imaging.

FIGURE 7-7. Management of Cushing's syndrome. The characteristics of Cushing's syndrome include 1) pituitary hypersecretion of corticotropin (Cushing's disease), which accounts for 75% to 80% of such patients; 2) adrenal adenomas or carcinomas; and 3) ectopic secretion of corticotropin or corticotropin-releasing hormone (CRH) [24]. The evaluation of patients with possible Cushing's syndrome involves thorough questioning about the use of steroid-containing preparations.

The clinical manifestations of Cushing's syndrome include hypertension, diabetes, truncal obesity, moon face, red cheeks, proximal muscle weakness, thin skin, early bruising, increased supraclavicular and infrascapular fat pads, pendulous abdomen with striae, poor wound healing, hirsutism, menstrual abnormalities, sexual dysfunction, osteoporosis, and psychiatric illnesses [25]. Generally, the clinical findings do not distinguish patients with Cushing's disease from those with adrenal adenoma.

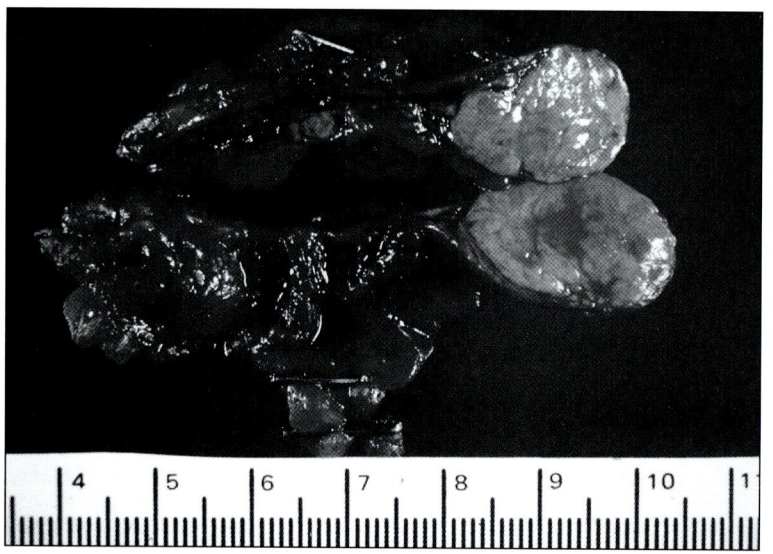

▶ FIGURE 7-8. (*See* Color Plate) Hyperaldosteronism. Hyperaldosteronism accounts for 1% to 2% of all hypertension [30]. The most common cause of aldosterone overproduction is idiopathic adrenal hyperplasia, followed by adrenal adenoma and, rarely, adrenal carcinoma. In 1955, Conn [31] described this syndrome in patients with elevated plasma aldosterone levels, hypertension, hypokalemia, and decreased plasma renin levels. Symptoms include headaches, proximal muscle cramps, polyuria, and nocturia, all of which are secondary to the hypokalemia. This metabolic syndrome can be caused by either a solitary adrenal adenoma or by bilateral adrenal zona glomerulosa hyperplasia.

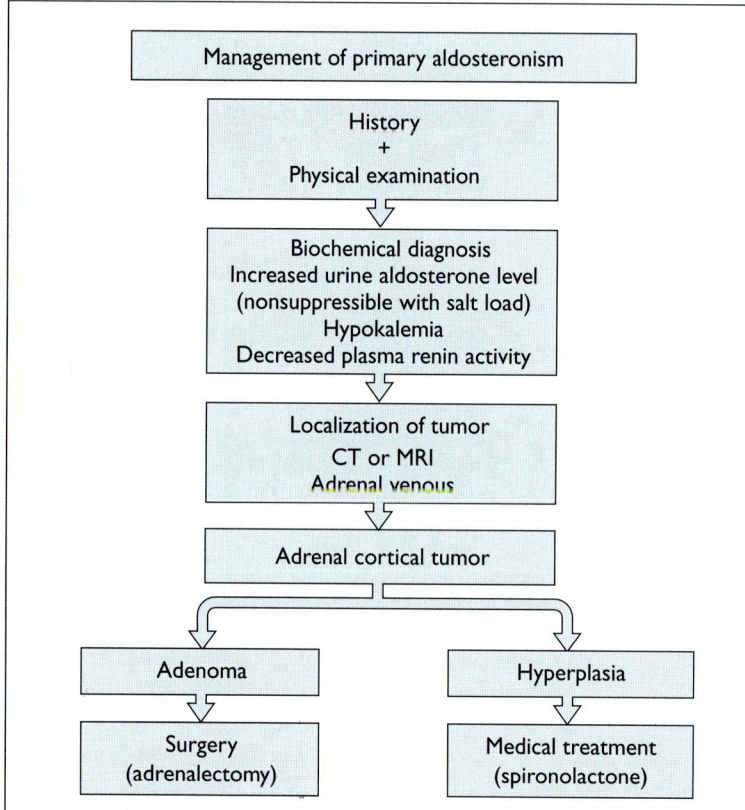

▶ FIGURE 7-9. Management of primary aldosteronism. The diagnosis of primary aldosteronism is based on the presence of hypokalemia (<3.5 mEq/L) and elevated urinary potassium in patients who are not taking antihypertensive medications (diuretics). Hypokalemia, however, may be absent in up to 38% of patients. Elevated aldosterone and decreased plasma renin levels indicate primary aldosteronism [32]. Currently, primary hyperaldosteronism is identified by the combined findings of hypokalemia, suppressed plasma renin activity (despite sodium restriction), and a high urinary and plasma aldosterone level after sodium repletion in hypertensive patients [33].

The control mechanisms of aldosterone secretion include corticotropin and potassium, but the primary physiologic control mechanism is angiotensin II. A clear detailed knowledge of the physiology of the renin-angiotensin-aldosterone system (RAAS) is mandatory to understand the pathophysiology and evaluate patients with primary hyperaldosteronism. The pivotal sensor in the RAAS resides in the juxtaglomerular apparatus within the kidney. Thus, in response to a variety of stimuli, but primarily decreased renal perfusion or a decreased intake of sodium, there is an increased renin release, formation of angiotensin II, and subsequent aldosterone secretion [34].

In contrast, an adrenal adenoma or adrenal hyperplasia is indicated by primary secretion of aldosterone and sodium retention, which leads to a suppression of plasma renin activity [35].

Therefore, the hallmark of primary hyperaldosteronism is hypokalemia, which is determined on sodium loading with 10 g of sodium a day for several weeks. MRI—magnetic resonance imaging.

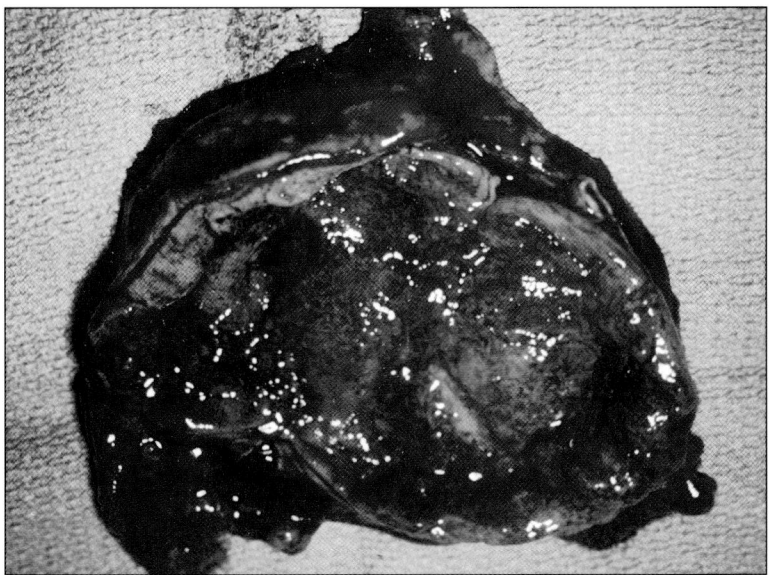

▶ **FIGURE 7-10.** (*See* color Plate) Pheochromocytoma. Pheochromocytomas usually are rounded and encapsulated by a compressed rim of adrenocortical tissue and a thin layer of vascularized fibrous tissue. On the cut surface, these lesions are gray to dusky red, and after formalin fixation are yellowish to brown. Some show cystic changes and hemorrhage and necrosis that may almost replace the neoplasm. The size can vary (1 to 16 cm in diameter). The larger tumors tend to be associated with cystic necrosis and hemorrhage into the central part of the lesion.

The exact incidence of pheochromocytoma is unknown but is estimated to occur in approximately 0.1% to 0.2% of all hypertensive patients in the United States. Approximately 20% of the adult population in the United States is hypertensive. Thus, there are approximately 35,000 to 70,000 persons in the United States who have pheochromocytomas [36].

Hypertension can be sustained (*eg,* in children with multiple endocrine adenomatosis II syndrome), paroxysmal (50% of cases, more common in women), or sustained with paroxysms [37]. Screening for pheochromocytoma is especially critical in patients with hypertension that is resistant to the usual treatment or who have other symptoms characteristic of pheochromocytoma.

Most pheochromocytomas occur in adults, but the ages of reported patients with this tumor have ranged from 5 months to 82 years (the peak incidence is in the fifth decade of life, and about 10% of cases may occur in children). Pheochromocytomas occur with nearly equal frequency in men and women (male-to-female ratio, 45:55), but the incidence of malignant tumors tends to be higher in women (male-to-female ratio, 25:75). In earlier reports from the Mayo Clinic, pheochromocytomas were present in the adrenal gland in 90%, extra-adrenal in 10%, bilateral within the adrenal gland in 4.4%, multiple in 7%, and malignant (as proven by metastases) in 13.4% of cases [36]. These figures suggested the "rule of 10s" (suggesting that roughly 10% of pheochromocytomas were extra-adrenal, malignant, or bilateral). More recently, Van Heerden *et al.* [38] at the Mayo Clinic noted that 13% of the tumors were bilateral within the adrenal gland, 68% were unilateral within the adrenal gland, and 19% had extra-adrenal tumors.

The clinical manifestations of pheochromocytoma are caused by the release of catecholamines from the tumor. Symptoms include headache, excessive sweating, heat intolerance, flushing, palpitations, chest pain, pallor, and anxiety. Headache caused by pheochromocytoma usually manifests as occipital pain, often waking patients from sleep. The headache can often be ameliorated by standing up.

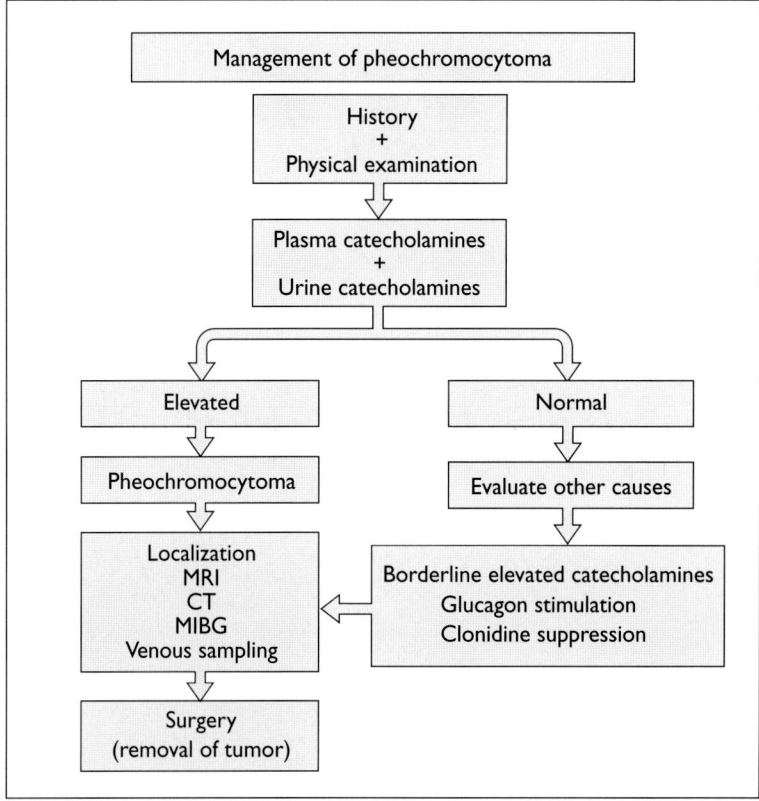

▶ **FIGURE 7-11.** Management of pheochromocytoma. The laboratory diagnosis of pheochromocytoma is now quite accurate with the availability of plasma and urinary measurements of catecholamines and their byproducts. Serum catecholamines are elevated in 95% to 99% of cases. Urinary catecholamines (total urinary catecholamines and metanephrines) may also be measured [39,40]. During the collection of the 24-hour urine sample, it is essential that the patient avoid stress, physical exertion, and all medications that might interfere with the results (*eg,* drugs containing catecholamines [nasal drops, L-dopa, and amphetamines]). Approximately 95% of patients will have elevated urinary levels of catecholamines and their byproducts. In the patient with severe paroxysmal hypertension who presents in the middle of hypertensive crisis, the plasma catecholamines are almost always elevated. In 10% of patients with pheochromocytoma, no hypertension is documented. Chromogranin A measurement has also been used to diagnose pheochromocytoma, with approximately 90% of patients demonstrating increased serum levels [41]. The test result may be falsely elevated in patients with decreased renal function (creatinine clearance <80 mL/min). Stimulation or suppression tests are generally not used. The one situation in which they may be useful is in the patient who appears to have essential hypertension but borderline elevated catecholamines. In this setting a clonidine suppression test may be useful [42,43]. Following a single 0.3-mg oral dose of clonidine, patients with essential hypertension at rest show a decrease in norepinephrine whereas patients with pheochromocytomas do not. CT—computed tomography; MIBG—meta-iodobenzyl guanidine; MRI—magnetic resonance imaging.

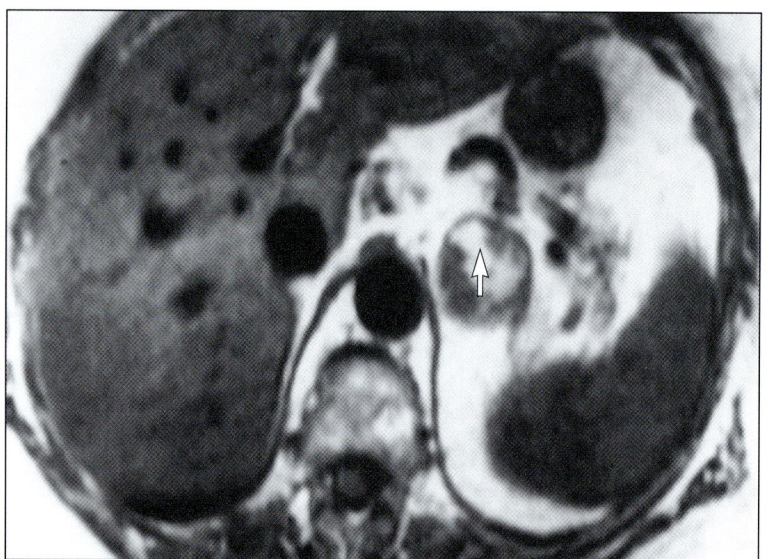

FIGURE 7-12. Magnetic resonance imaging (MRI) of pheochromocytoma (*arrow*). MRI is the most useful radiographic test in both identifying and characterizing pheochromocytoma and in identifying surrounding structures. This modality is as accurate as CT in identifying such lesions, which have a characteristic "bright light bulb" appearance on the T_2-weighted images. In addition, sagittal and coronal imaging can provide excellent anatomic information on the relationship between the tumor and the surrounding vasculature. Therefore, MRI should be the initial scanning procedure in patients with the biochemical findings of pheochromocytoma [19].

INCIDENTALLY DISCOVERED ADRENAL MASSES

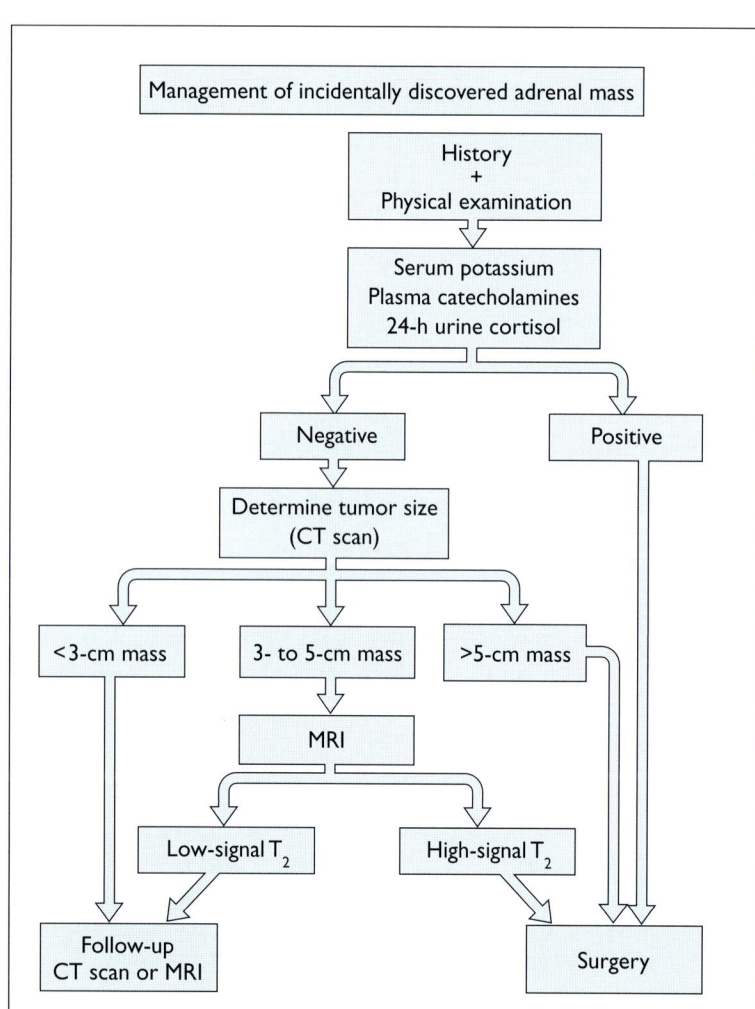

FIGURE 7-13. Management of the incidentally discovered adrenal mass. The increased use of abdominal ultrasound and CT has allowed the incidental discovery of unsuspected adrenal masses or "incidentalomas." These masses are detected in 0.6% to 1.3% of abdominal CT scans and in

3% (1.4% to 8.7%) of adults at autopsy [44]. Histologically, most of these tumors are benign, nonfunctional adrenocortical adenomas (86% of cases) without clinical significance [45]. Usually, the diagnosis of whether the adrenal mass requires therapy can be made by careful attention to the patient's history, physical examination, the radiographic appearance, and the biochemical profile. Hypertension is nonspecific and may be associated with Cushing's syndrome, aldosterone-secreting tumors, and pheochromocytoma. A detailed history of abdominal or flank trauma may suggest the presence of adrenal hemorrhage. Moreover, all patients with solid adrenal masses should undergo biochemical assessment [46]. If biochemical abnormalities are identified, the lesion should be surgically removed. A very limited biochemical evaluation is recommended, including only tests to rule out pheochromocytoma, a potassium level in hypertensive cases, and a glucocorticoid evaluation only in the presence of clinical signs of Cushing's syndrome or virilization. Moreover, because adrenal malignancies are almost always larger than 5 cm [47], any nonfunctioning solid lesions larger than 4 cm should be removed. If lesions are shown to be purely cystic by CT or magnetic resonance imaging (MRI), cyst puncture is often not necessary and these lesions can be followed up with radiologic imaging. Controversy still exists in the management strategy for the solid adrenal lesions that are smaller than 5 cm. MRI can distinguish between benign or malignant lesions. Most adenomas appear slightly hypo- or isointense relative to the liver or spleen on T_1-weighted images and slightly hyper- or isointense relative to the hepatic or splenic parenchyma on T_2-weighted images. Conversely, adrenal cortical carcinoma is hypointense relative to liver or spleen on T_1-weighted images and are hyperintense to the liver or spleen on T_2-weighted images. Thus, the lesion is more likely to be malignant if the mean signal intensity ratio between the lesion and the spleen is over 0.8 [17,18].

Although not commonly performed, fine-needle adrenal biopsy guided by ultrasound or CT scan may provide significant material for cytology. According to Tikkakoski *et al.* [48], the accuracy to differentiate benign from malignant disease is 85.7%; however, aspiration cytology requires an extremely experienced cytologist, and in some cases it is difficult to distinguish an adrenal adenoma from a carcinoma even on pathologic review of the entire specimen.

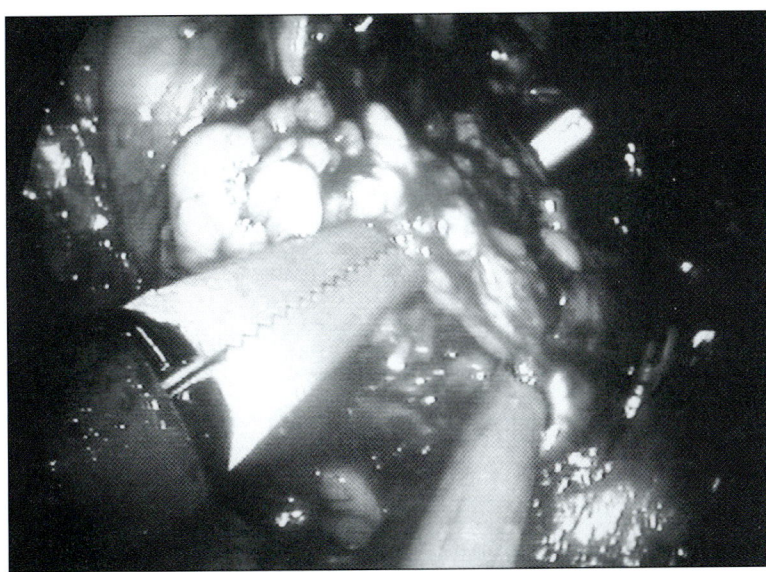

▶ **FIGURE 7-14.** (*See* Color Plate) Adrenalectomy using the laparoscopic approach. Adrenalectomy is indicated if there is any radiographic evidence that argues against a characteristic benign adenoma, if the mass is functional, or if there is any change in size of an adrenal lesion with repeated studies. This fairly aggressive approach is justified in view of the extremely poor prognosis of patients when adrenal carcinoma is diagnosed, even when the lesion is localized.

The adrenal gland can be approached surgically by several routes [49]. The proper approach depends on the underlying cause of adrenal pathology, the size of the adrenal gland, the side of the lesion, the body habitus of the patient, and the experience and preference of the surgeon.

In addition to open surgical options, the laparoscopic approach can be used, particularly for smaller adrenal tumors [50–55]. In most cases, several different options are available and a careful review of all the variables is required before a choice is made. Thus, each case should be considered individually, although some approaches are preferable for a given disease.

Two main anatomic points deserve emphasis. The right adrenal vein is very short and enters the posterolateral surface of the inferior vena cava [56]. The right adrenal gland, especially if neoplastic, may engulf the vein and obscure it from view. This short vein is easily torn, resulting in substantial hemorrhage; this problem is best avoided by dissecting the vena cava away from the adrenal, instead of pulling the adrenal inferolaterally to expose the vein. Another site that deserves particular care is the inferomedial junction of the left adrenal gland, where it may abut the vascular pedicle of the left kidney [57]. Finally, when dividing the arterial supply to the left adrenal (especially during a posterior left adrenalectomy), the renal vessels are more easily injured than would be expected.

Surgeons may choose their preferred approach but must follow a number of unifying concepts concerning surgical technique. First, adequate visualization is imperative. Second, proper hemostasis should be rigorously maintained. The adrenal glands lie high in the retroperitoneum and quite posterior. Therefore, the surgeon should bring the adrenal down by initially exposing the cranial attachments and dividing the rich blood supply between either right-angled clips or with a forceps cautery. It is often simplest to begin the dissection laterally, identifying the vascular supply and working around the cranial edge of the gland. The posterior surface is generally devoid of vasculature. After the gland is freed superiorly with gentle traction on the kidney, the gland can be brought inferiorly for control of the adrenal vein. The adrenal gland is extremely friable and fractures easily, causing troublesome bleeding. Therefore, tension or traction should be maintained on the kidney or surrounding structures and not on the adrenal itself. In patients with pheochromocytomas, the adrenal glands should not be manipulated and the adrenal vein should be controlled early to minimize the chance of a burst of catecholamine release during manipulation [58].

The anterior transperitoneal approach may be used in patients with pheochromocytoma because approximately 10% of these patients have either extra-adrenal tumors or malignancy not accessible through a retroperitoneal approach. Similarly, for large tumors (> 10 cm in diameter), an anterior abdominal incision is best used to obtain wide exposure and permit en-bloc excision when malignancy is encountered.

In capable hands, laparoscopic adrenalectomy has a success rate of approximately 90% [50–52,55]. Albala *et al.* [58] concluded that laparoscopy can be used successfully for adrenalectomy. The postoperative complications reported include anemia, colonic pseudoobstruction, and incisional hematoma. The median postoperative stay is shorter than open procedures (4 days) and the pain control requirements are less. This procedure also permits rapid return to normal activity.

REFERENCES

1. Vaughan ED, Jr., Carey RM: *Adrenal Disorders.* New York: Thieme Medical Publishers; 1989:241–252.

2. Howards SS, Carey RM: The adrenals. In *Adult and Pediatric Urology*, edn 2. Edited by Gillenwater JY, Grayhack JT, Howards SS, Duckett JW. Chicago: Year Book Medical Publishers; 1991:587–615.

3. Moore M, Amberson JB, Kazam E, Vaughan ED, Jr.: Anatomy, histology, embryology. In *Adrenal Disorders.* Edited by Vaughan ED, Jr., Carey RM. New York: Thieme Medical Publishers; 1989:187–201.

4. Bornstein SR, Ehrhart-Bornstein M, Usadel H, *et al.*: Morphological evidence for a close interaction of chromaffin cells with cortical cells within the adrenal gland. *Cell Tissue Res* 1991, 265:1–9.

5. Dolan LM, Carey RM: Adrenal cortical and medullary function: diagnostic tests. In *Adrenal Disorders.* Edited by Vaughan ED, Jr., Carey RM. New York: Thieme Medical Publishers; 1989:81–145.

6. Parker L, Odell W: Control of adrenal androgen secretion. *Endocr Rev* 1980, 1:392–410.

7. Orth DN, Kovacs WJ, DeBold CR: The adrenal cortex. In *Williams Textbook of Endocrinology*, edn 8. Edited by Wilson JD, Fister DW. Philadelphia: WB Saunders; 1992:489–619.

8. Lewis GP: Physiological mechanisms controlling secretary activity of adrenal medulla. In *Handbook of Physiology.* Edited by Blaschko H, Sayer G, Smith AD. Washington, DC: American Physiological Society; 1975:309–312.

9. Abrams HL, Siegelman S, Adams DF, *et al.*: Computed tomography versus ultrasound of the adrenal gland: a prospective study. *Radiology* 1982, 143:121–128.

10. Bilbey JH, McLoughlin RF, Kurkjian PS, *et al.*: MR imaging of adrenal masses: value of chemical-shift imaging for distinguishing adenomas from other tumors. *Am J Roentgenol* 1995, 164:637–642.

11. Huebener K-H, Treugut H: Adrenal cortex dysfunction: CT findings. *Radiology* 1994, 150:195–199.

12. White EA, Schambelan M, Rost LR, *et al.*: Use of computed tomography in diagnosing the cause of primary aldosteronism. *N Engl J Med* 1980, 303:1503–1507.

13. Geisinger MA, Zelch MG, Bravo EL, *et al.*: Primary hyperaldosteronism: comparison of CT, adrenal venography and venous sampling. *Am J Roentgenol* 1983, 141:299–309.

14. Lee MJ, Mayo-Smith WW, Hahn PF, *et al.*: State-of-the-art MR imaging of the adrenal gland. *Radiographics* 1994, 14:1015–1029.

15. Lubat E, Weinreb JC: Magnetic resonance imaging of the kidneys and adrenals. *Top Magn Reson Imaging* 1990, 2:17–36.

16. Newhouse JH: MRI of the adrenal gland. *Urol Radiol* 1990, 12:1–12.

17. Reinig JW, Doppelman JL, Dwyer AJ, *et al.*: Adrenal masses differentiated by MR. *Radiology* 1986, 158:81–87.

18. Campeau RJ, Garcia OM, Correa OA, Rege AB: Pheochromocytoma: diagnosis by scintigraphy using iodine 131-metaiodobenzyl-guanidine. *South Med J* 1991, 94:1221–1230.

19. Vaughan ED, Jr.: Imaging of the adrenal gland. *World J Urol* 1992, 10:190–194.

20. Liu L, Haskin ME, Rose LA, Beemus CE: Diagnosis of bilateral adrenalcortical hemorrhage by computerized tomography. *Ann Intern Med* 1982, 97:720–725.

21. Sroujieh AS, Farah GR, Haddad MJ, Abu-Khalaf MM: Adrenal cysts: diagnosis and management. *Br J Urol* 1990, 65:570–575.

22. Pasieka JL, McLeod MK, Tbompson NW, *et al.*: Adrenal scintigraphy of well-differentiated (functioning) adrenocortical carcinomas: potential surgical pitfalls. *Surgery* 1992, 12:884–890.

23. Kane NM, Korobkin M, Francis IR, *et al.*: Percutaneous biopsy of left adrenal masses: prevalence of pancreatitis after anterior approach. *Am J Roentgenol* 1991, 157:777–790.

24 Besser GM, Edwards CRW: Cushing's syndrome. *Clin Endocrinol* 1972, 1:451.

25. Howler TA, Rees LH, Besser GM: Cushing's syndrome. *J Clin Endocrinol Metab* 1985, 14:911–918.

26. Miller J, Crapo L: The biochemical analysis of hypercortisolism. *Endocrinologist* 1994, 4:7–16.

27. Jenkins PJ, Trainer PI, Plowman PN, *et al.*: The long-term outcome after adrenalectomy and prophylactic pituitary radiotherapy in adrenocorticotropin-dependent Cushing's syndrome. *J Clin Endocrinol Metab* 1995, 80:165–171.

28. Reyes L, Parvez Z, Nemoto P, *et al.*: Adrenalectomy for adrenal metastases from lung carcinoma. *J Surg Oncol* 1990, 44:32–37.

29. Sullivan M, Boileau M, Hodges CV: Adrenal cortical carcinoma. *J Urol* 1978, 120:600–665.

30. Vaughan ED Jr.: Diagnosis of adrenal disorders in hypertension. *World J Urol* 1989, 7:111–116.

31. Conn JW: Primary hyperaldosteronism: a new clinical syndrome. *J Lab Clin Med* 1955, 45.

32. Blumenfeld JD: Hypertension and adrenal disorders. *Curr Opin Nephrol Hypertens* 1993, 2:274–282.

33. Bravo EL, Tarazi RC, Dustan HP, *et al.*: The changing clinical spectrum of primary aldosteronism. *Am J Med* 1983, 74:641–649.

34. Weinberger MH, Grim CE, Hollifield JW, *et al.*: Primary aldosteronism: diagnosis, localization and treatment. *Ann Intern Med* 1979, 93:86–90.

35. Banks WA, Kastin HA, Biglieri EG, Ruiz EA: Primary adrenal hyperplasia: a new subset of primary hyperaldosteronism. *J Clin Endocrinol Metab* 1984, 58:783–789.

36. Bravo EL: Pheochromocytoma: new concepts and future trends. *Kidney Int* 1991, 40:544–556.

37. Larsson C, Nordenskjold M: Multiple endocrine neoplasia. *Cancer Surv* 1990, 9:703–723.

38. Van Heerden JA, Young WF, Jr., Grant CS, Carpenter PC: Adrenal surgery for hypercortisolism: surgical aspects. *Surgery* 1995, 117:466–472.

39. Kaplan NM, Kramer NJ, Holland OB, *et al.*: Single-voided urine metanephrine assays in screening for pheochromocytoma. *Arch Intern Med* 1977, 137:190–197.

40. Stridsberg M., Husebye ES: Chromogranin A and chromogranin B are sensitive circulating markers for pheochromocytoma. *Eur J Endocrinol* 1997, 136:28–29.

41. Kariberg BE, Hedman L: Value of clonidine suppression test in the diagnosis of pheochromocytoma. *Acta Med Scand* 1986, 714(suppl):15–18.

42. Rosen AE, Brown JJ, Lever AF: Treatment of pheochromocytoma and of clonidine withdrawal hypertension with labetalol. *Br J Clin Pharmacol* 1976, 3(suppl 3):809–812.

43. Vyberg M. Sestof TL: Combined adrenal myelolipoma and adenoma associated with Cushing's syndrome. *Am J Clin Pathol* 1986, 86:541–546.

44. Belldegrun A, Hussain S, Seltzer SE, *et al.*: The incidentally discovered adrenal mass: a therapeutic dilemma: BWH experience 1976–1983. *Surg Gynecol Obstet* 1986, 163:203–209.

45. Oselia G, Terzolo M, Borretta G, *et al.*: Endocrine evaluation of incidentally discovered adrenal masses (incidentalomas). *J Clin Endocrinol Metab* 1994, 79:1532–1539.

46. Ross NS, Aron DC: Hormonal evaluation of the patient with an incidentally discovered adrenal mass. *N Engl J Med* 1990, 323:1401–1409.

47. Angermeier KW, Montie JE: Perioperative complications of adrenal surgery. *Urol Clin North Am* 1989, 16:597–606.

48. Tikkakoski T, Taavitsainen M, Paivansato M, *et al.*: Accuracy of adrenal biopsy guided by ultrasound and CT. *Acta Radiol* 1991, 32:371–374.

49. Brunt LM, Doherty GM, Norton JA, *et al.*: Laparoscopic adrenalectomy compared to open adrenalectomy for benign adrenal neoplasms. *J Am Coll Surg* 1996, 183:1–10.

50. Gagner M, Lacroix A, Bolte E: Laparoscopic adrenalectomy in Cushing's syndrome and pheochromocytoma [letter]. *N Engl J Med* 1992, 327:1033.

51. Go H, Takeda M, Takahashi H, *et al.*: Laparoscopic adrenalectomy for primary aldosteronism: a new operative method. *J Laparoendosc Surg* 1993, 3:455–459.

52. Higashihara E, Tanaka Y, Horie S, *et al.*: Laparoscopic adrenalectomy: the initial 3 cases. *J Urol* 1993, 149:973–976.

53. Suzuki K, Ka-evama S, Ueda D, *et al.*: Laparoscopic adrenalectomy: clinical experience with 12 cases. *J Urol* 1993, 150:1099–1102.

54. Takeda M, Go H, Imai T, *et al.*: Laparoscopic adrenalectomy for primary aldosteronism: report of initial 10 cases. *Surgery* 1994, 115:621–625.

55. Anson BJ, Caldwell EW, Pick JW, Beaton LE: The blood supply of the kidney suprarenal gland and associated structures. *Surg Gynecol Obstet* 1947, 84:313–320.

56. Bianchi H, Ferrari A: The arterial circulation of the left suprarenal gland. *Surg Radiol Anat* 1991, 13:113–116.

57. Malhotra V (ed.): *Anesthesia for Renal and Genitourinary Surgery.* New York: McGraw-Hill; 1995.

58. Albala DM: Laparoscopic nephrectomy and adrenalectomy. *Sem Surg Oncol* 1994, 10:417–421.

Section II — Noncancerous Disease

Michael Marberger

Virtually no other field in surgery has seen such profound changes within such a short period of time as renal surgery for non-malignant disease. Dominated by incisional stone surgery just over a decade ago, which then accounted for about 25% of the surgical activity of most general urologists, the art of "cutting for the stone" has all but vanished. Upper tract urinary stones are today almost uniformly managed by extra corporeal shock-wave lithotripsy, endoscopic surgery or a combination thereof.

To offer the stone patient the full benefit of modern minimally invasive therapy the entire armamentarium of modern stone therapy is needed. The principles of shock-wave lithotripsy are well established, but technology is changing continuously. Modern shock-wave sources with improved focusing systems usually based on ultrasonography and fluoroscopy, and better delineated high-pressure focal zones today permit treating most patients on an outpatient basis without anesthesia. Nevertheless, the need to pass all stone debris after disintegration and the inverse relation in achieving this and stone mass and impaired urinary drainage render more invasive endoscopic approaches preferable in specific situations. Debate today mainly centers around the best choice of primary treatment in borderline cases. Percutaneous nephrolithotripsy has firmly established its position in the management of complex stones, in particular staghorn stones and calculi in obstructed urinary systems. Retrograde endoscopic techniques using semirigid, ultra-thin ureteroscopes and pneumatic or electrohydraulic lihtotripsy have severely narrowed the utilization of SWL in situ for distal and midureteric stones. Flexible ureteroscopy and laser lithotripsy are now challenging primary ESWL in situ in the upper ureter. Better flexible endoscopes and contact lithotripsy today even permit retrograde transureteric management of some difficult renal stones, such as in caliceal diverticula. The main difficulty in mastering these techniques today arises for many urologists from the relative paucity of cases, which concentrate at stone referral centers. A step-by-step guide with excellent illustrations helps overcome the dilemma.

The role of traditional incisional surgery is also increasingly being challenged by laparoscopic approaches. Laparoscopic removal of a kidney destroyed by benign pathology is standard today, but laparoscopic surgery is also becoming more attractive for reconstructive procedures. Although manipulations as simple as tying a surgical knot are extremely tedious though an endoscope, technical innovations are rapidly helping to overcome the problems. Pyeloplasty, the most common reconstructive procedure today, reflects the development. Laparoscopic pyeloplasty is becoming a valid option. Together with retrograde or antegrade endopyelotomy, it may replace another "classical" incisional procedure in the near future. The main limiting factor for this development appears to be the age of the patients. By far most pyeloplasties are today performed to correct severe ureteropelvic obstruction in babies, usually already detected by fetal ultrasonography.

The trend towards minimally invasive "key-hole" surgery for benign pathology of the kidney not only results in the need to master the new techniques, but also in a teaching deficit in traditional kidney surgery. Most urologists in training today have learned to master ablative renal surgery for malignant disease before they ever do an incisional procedure for a benign condition. There is no need to preserve and teach procedures of historical value only. This is not so, however, in this situation. Albeit the indications for "open" surgery for non-malignant disease of the kidney are rare today, they still exist, often even on an emergency basis. It therefore appears important to preserve some of the essential tricks-of-the-trade developed by generations of kidney surgeons, such as the posterior lumbotomy approach.

Extracorporeal Shock Wave Lithotripsy of Renal Calculi

Francis X. Keeley, Jr.
David A. Tolley

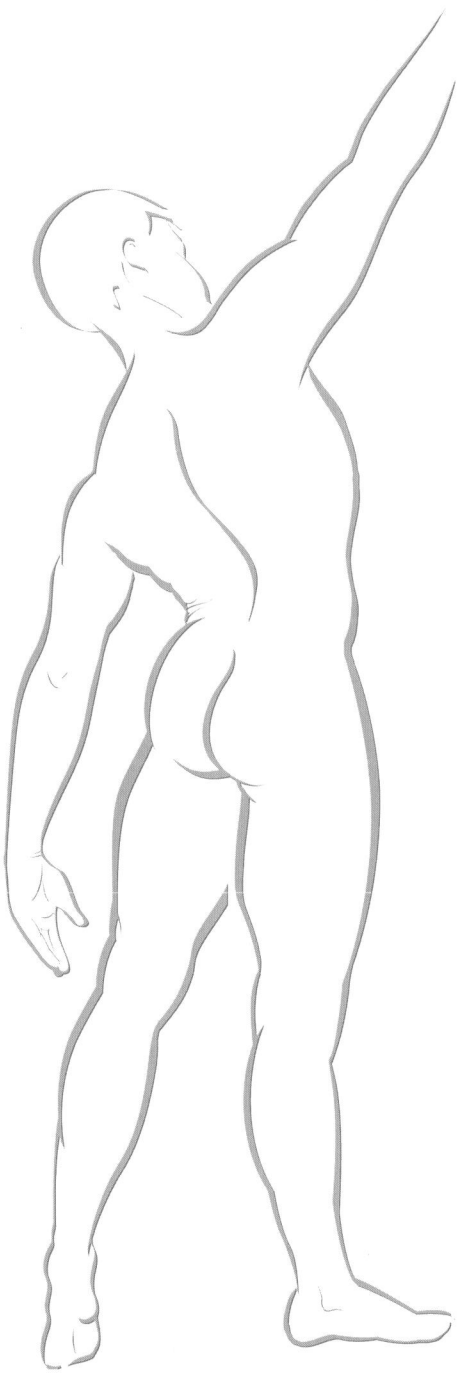

Extracorporeal shock wave lithotripsy (ESWL) has revolutionized the treatment of renal calculi since the first patient was treated in 1980 [1]. ESWL has set the standard for effective noninvasive treatment. In doing so, it has become an indispensable part of modern urologic practice.

Athough the clinical use of ESWL is familiar to most clinicians, the mechanism by which it achieves its effects is well worth reviewing. A lithotriptor consists of three essential components: an *energy source* produces shock waves, which are transmitted through a *coupling medium* and focused on a target by means of a *localization apparatus.* The energy source for a particular lithotriptor may be electrohydraulic (spark-gap), piezoelectric, or electromagnetic. The coupling medium may be a water bath or an enclosed water cushion. Finally, localization may be accomplished with fluoroscopy or ultrasonography. The basic principle remains the same: shock waves are applied repeatedly to a stone to reduce it to fragments small enough to pass spontaneously.

Modifications in lithotriptor design have reduced or, in some cases, eliminated the need for anesthesia; however, the number of shocks and the need for retreatment sessions have increased. The water bath of the Dornier HM-3 (Dornier Med Tech, Kennesaw, GA), the original lithotriptor, has been largely replaced by therapy heads. Finally, fluoroscopic localization is now complemented by ultrasonography, which can provide continuous localization without the hazards of radiation exposure. The choice of a lithotriptor must take into account the strengths and weaknesses of each machine. For example, lack of the need for anesthesia is often associated with decreased efficiency in fragmentation, especially for large stones.

The role of ESWL in the treatment of renal and ureteral calculi has been well established for over a decade. Effective fragmentation and clearance of most small renal calculi with ESWL have been reported using a variety of lithotriptors [2–4]. Although the results of treatment for ureteral stones were initially thought to be poor [1], multiple reports have established ESWL as a safe first-line treatment [5–7]. Initial enthusiasm for ESWL monotherapy for staghorn calculi has been tempered by generally disappointing results [8]; nevertheless, ESWL combined with percutaneous nephrolithotomy, the so-called "sandwich" treatment, has become the recommended treatment for staghorn calculi [9,10].

The early history of ESWL saw a gradual broadening of clinical indications as its capabilities became more apparent. Its clinical use expanded rapidly as many urologists began to rely on it as monotherapy for even complex stones. The recent literature on ESWL, however, has stressed its limitations [8,11,12].

For example, the term "clinically insignificant residual fragments," which has been used to describe small fragments remaining following ESWL, has been largely discredited by recent reports demonstrating that they are, in fact, clinically significant [13,14]. To ensure that ESWL is used properly along with other endourologic procedures, guidelines have been drawn up by the American Urological Association (AUA) Guidelines Panel for the treatment of ureteral stones and staghorn calculi [10,15]. The rapid evolution of ESWL during the 1980s slowed perceptibly by the late 1990s, demonstrating that the field has reached a fairly mature stage.

PRINCIPLES OF SHOCK WAVE LITHOTRIPSY

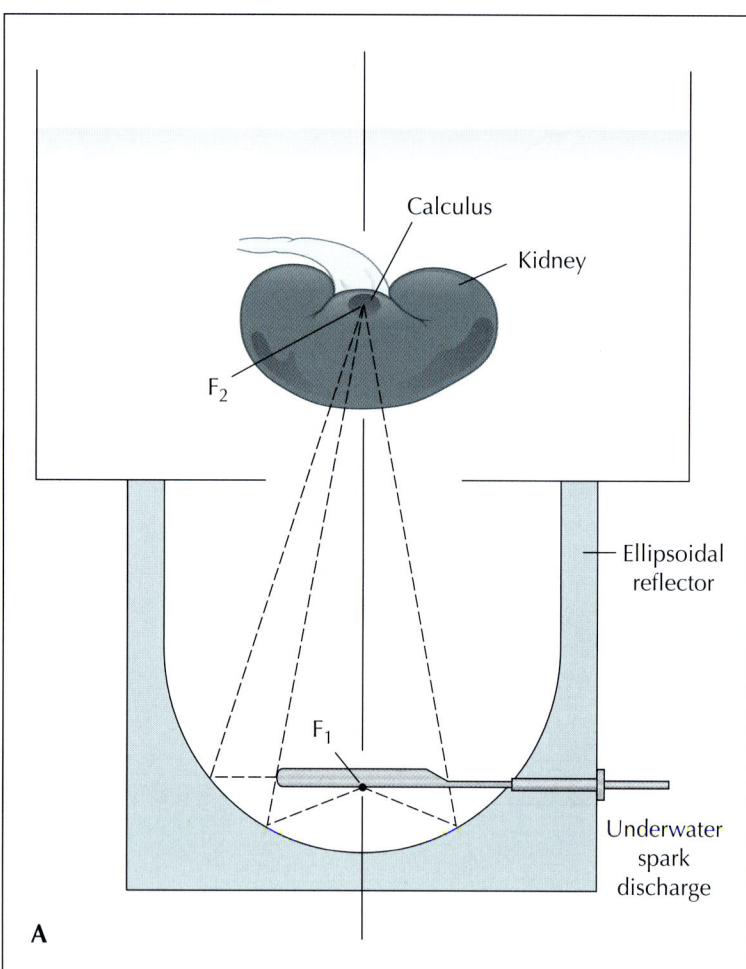

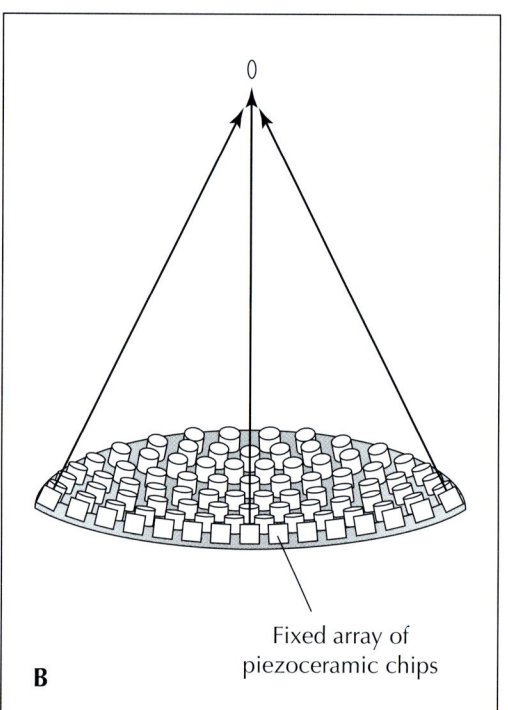

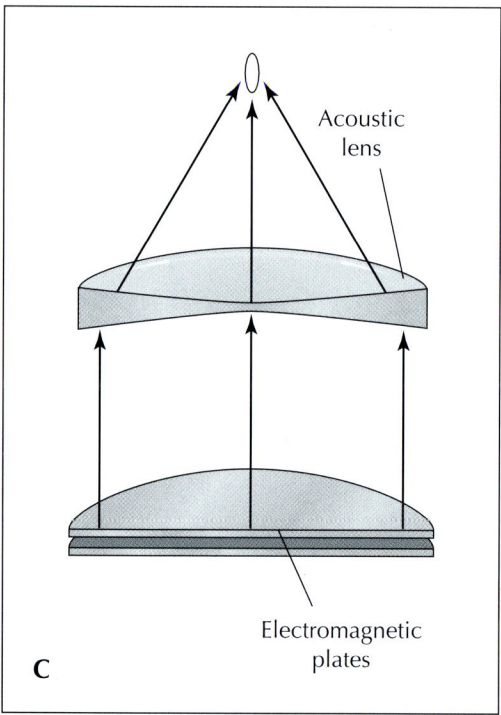

▶ **FIGURE 8-1.** Focusing of the shock wave. Regardless of their source, extracorporeal shock waves must be focused inside a patient's body to produce the intended clinical effect. Focusing produces the high pressures required to fragment a stone while allowing the shock wave to pass through the patient's skin over a large area (*ie*, at a relatively low energy density). **A,** Electrohydraulic lithotriptors use a spark-gap energy source and an ellipsoidal reflector. **B** and **C,** In an effort to reduce the need for anesthesia, subsequent lithotriptors have used lower-energy sources combined with a piezoelectric spherical dish or an acoustic lens combined with an electromagnetic energy source. This lower-energy source enables them to generate high focal pressures with smaller pulse energies; however, more shock waves are required. In addition, patients require more sessions of treatment, and lower stone-free rates are achieved [4,16]. F1—focal point shock 1, shock wave source; F2—focal point shock 2, kidney stone. (Panel A *adapted from* Chaussy and Fuchs [17]; panel B *adapted from* Harrison *et al.* [18].)

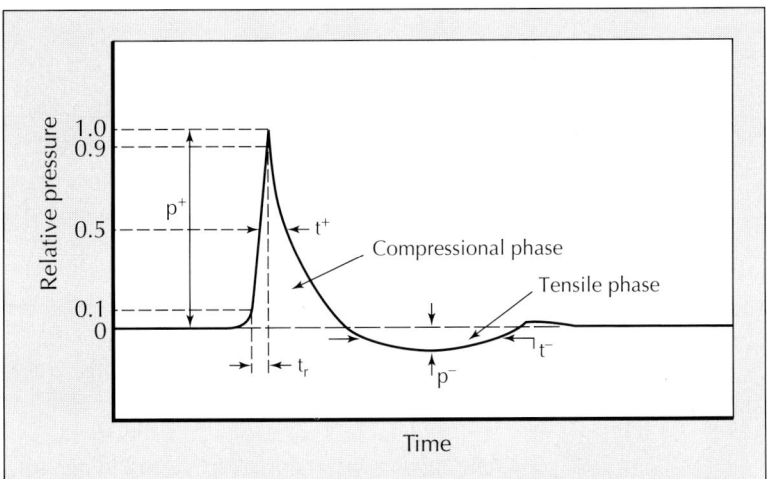

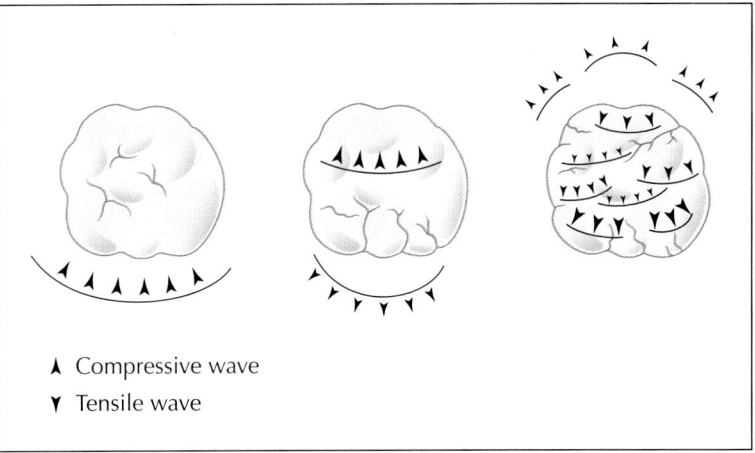

▶ **FIGURE 8-2.** Pressure course at the focal zone. The shock wave as it reaches the focal zone consists of a compressive (positive) phase with a rapid rise followed by a tensile (negative) phase. The acoustic energy of the shock wave can be estimated from the pressure waveforms, which vary from lithotriptor to lithotriptor. Originally, the peak pressure, which is highest in piezoelectric lithotriptors, was thought to be the most important parameter, but recent work suggests that the total acoustic energy delivered is more significant [19,20]. (*Adapted from* Zhong and Preminger [21].)

▶ **FIGURE 8-3.** Shock-wave–induced spallating of a stone. As the shock wave reaches the surface of a stone, the leading edge of the pressure wave is partially reflected, leading to the formation of a tensile shock wave. The large compressive and tensile forces can overcome the tensile strength of the stone to tear a layer of stone free from its surface. The shock wave then passes through the stone, and an identical process occurs at the back surface of the stone, leading to fragmentation of both surfaces. This phenomenon is called spallating. Although this mechanism occurs in a predictable fashion in vitro, the exact effect of shock waves on a stone in vivo is more complex, depending in part on the internal architecture of the stone, which may have a number of interfaces within it [22]. (*Adapted from* Chaussy and Fuchs [17].)

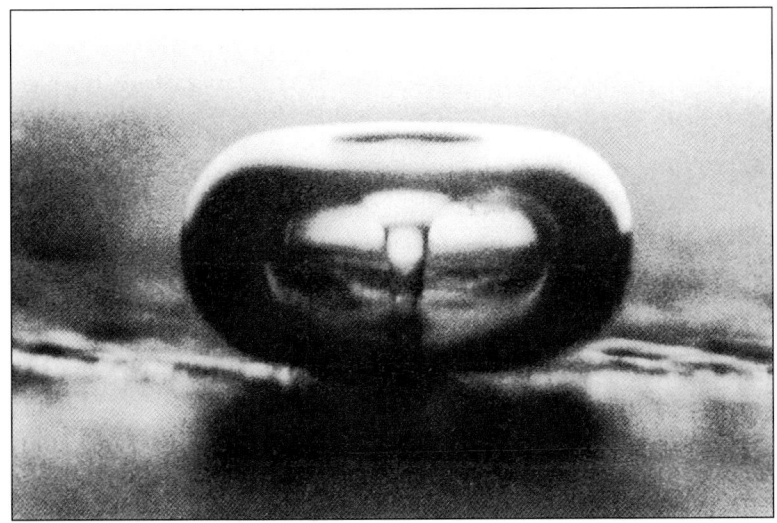

▶ **FIGURE 8-4.** Cavitation. Another mechanism of stone fragmentation is the formation and collapse of cavitation bubbles [23,24]. The large (negative) tensile force generated by the shock wave can create cavitation bubbles. When a bubble is formed close to a surface, it tends to collapse with a microjet passing through its center, directed at that surface. The forces created have been shown to damage hard materials [23]. Cavitation may also be responsible for tissue damage associated with extracorporeal shock wave lithotripsy. (*From* Crum [23]; with permission.)

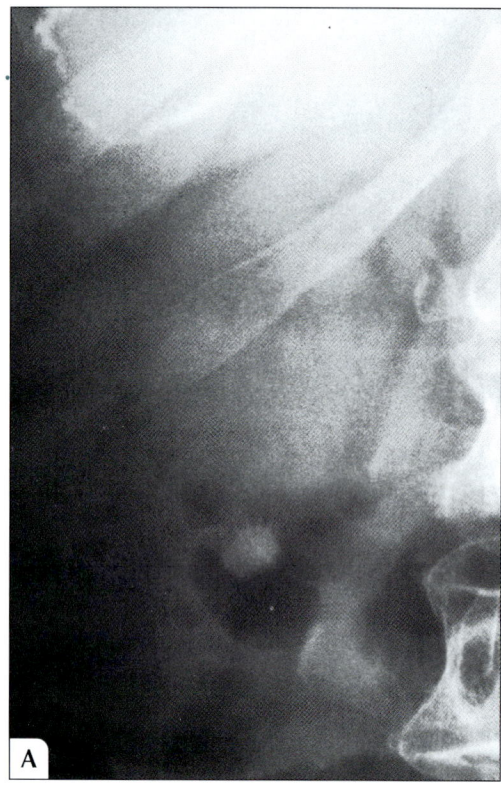

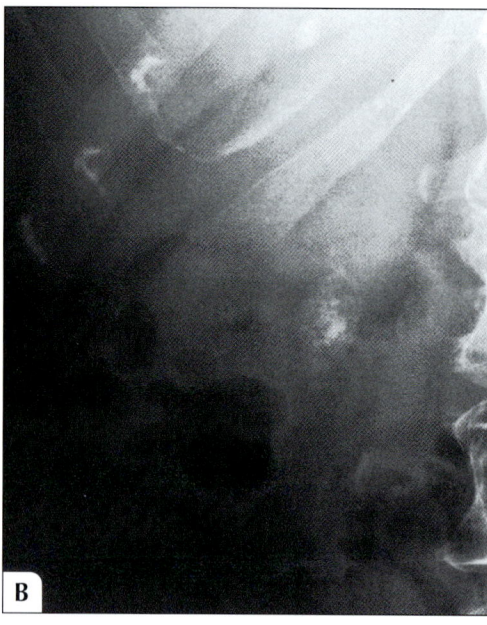

▶ **FIGURE 8-5. A** and **B**, Treatment of small renal calculi. Patients with stones less than 1.5 cm in diameter are ideal candidates for lithotripsy (**A**). Stones that are situated in the upper or middle calyces or the renal pelvis clear more rapidly than stones in the lower calyces, and these patients are much more likely to become stone free. Fragmentation will occur in more than 98% of patients irrespective of the lithotriptor used [16], and the treatment should be continued until fine fragmentation of the stone is achieved (**B**). Stone-free rates of 78% to 91% can be achieved with a retreatment rate of 9% to 16% [2,25,26]. Factors that reduce the stone-free rate following extracorporeal shock wave lithotripsy are the presence of multiple stones, stone composition of cystine or brushite, and location in the lower-pole calyces [25,26].

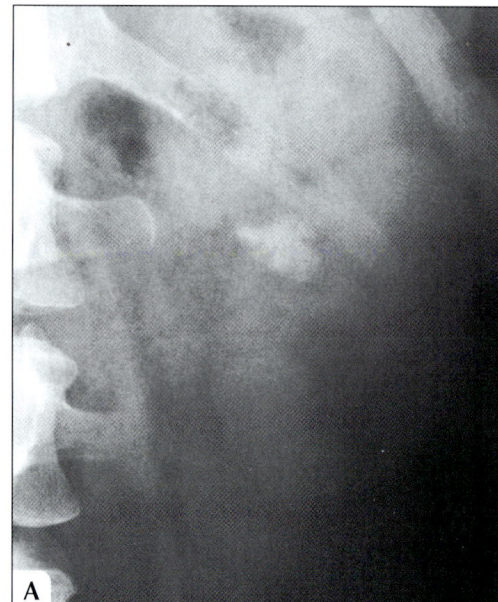

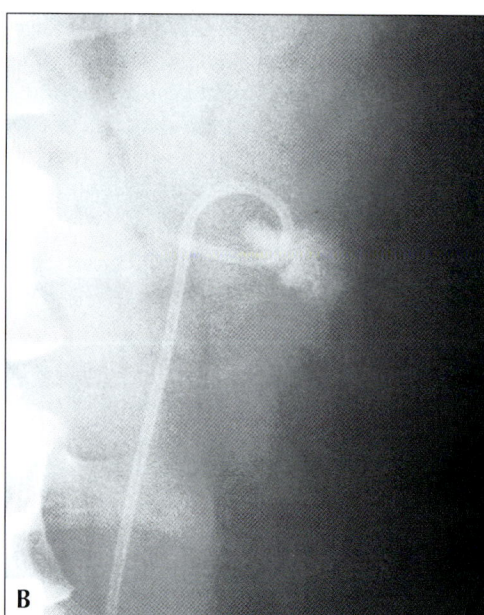

▶ **FIGURE 8-6.** Treatment for larger renal calculi. Stones greater than 2 cm in diameter can also be treated with lithotripsy (**A**), but because of the increased risk of steinstrasse, such patients are better treated following the insertion of a ureteral stent (**B**). This stent allows dilation of the ureter to occur, thus increasing the capacity of the ureter, which allows the fragments to pass. Stones greater than 3 cm in diameter or complex stones occupying multiple calyces are best treated with percutaneous surgery because of the unacceptably high risk of steinstrasse, obstruction, and failure to clear stone fragments.

The best stone-free results for the treatment of large stones are achieved with the Dornier HM-3 (Dornier Med Tech, Kennesaw, GA). The results using piezoelectric lithotriptors are significantly worse for these large stones [16]. Stone-free rates with electromagnetic lithotriptors are generally 10% less than for the HM-3 for any given stone size, and the difference increases with the size of the stone [27].

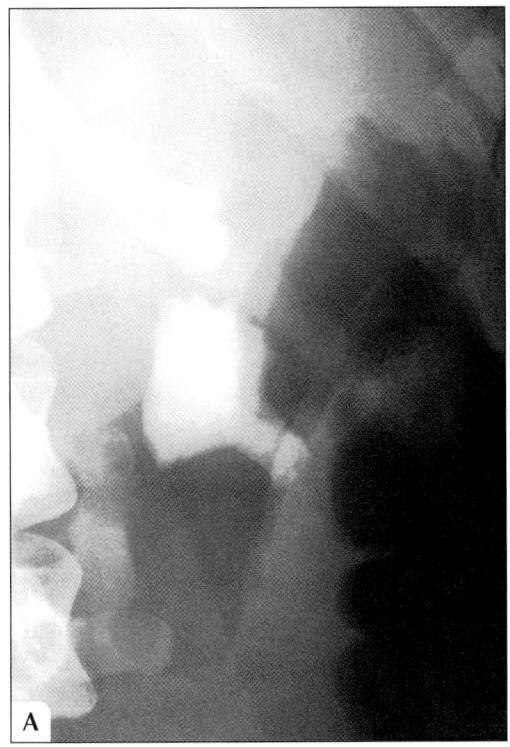
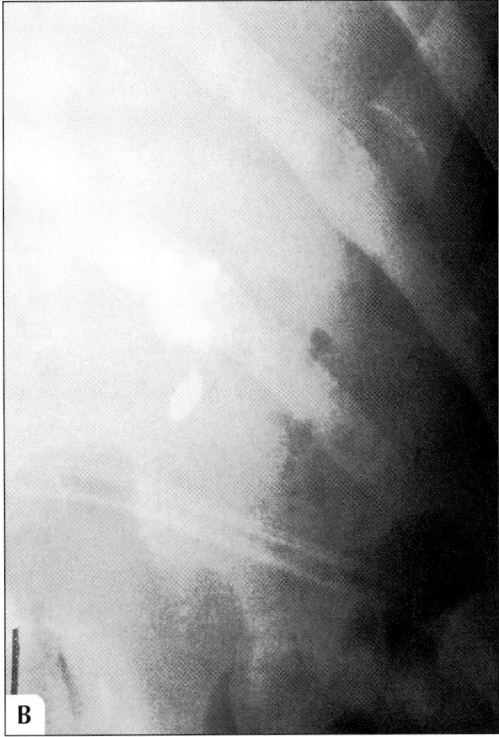
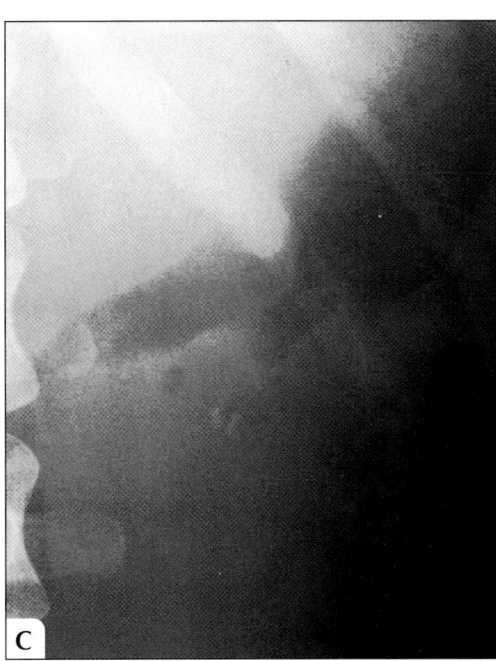

▶ **FIGURE 8-7.** Treatment of staghorn calculi (**A–C**). Lithotripsy may be used in combination with other techniques such as percutaneous stone extraction to treat patients with complex stone disease more efficiently. The stone is debulked by preliminary percutaneous surgery, and any residual fragments are then treated with extracorporeal shock wave lithotripsy (ESWL) [28]. A "second-look" procedure may be needed following ESWL as part of a "sandwich" technique [9], which is considered the recommended treatment for staghorn calculi by the American Urological Association Guidelines Panel [10].

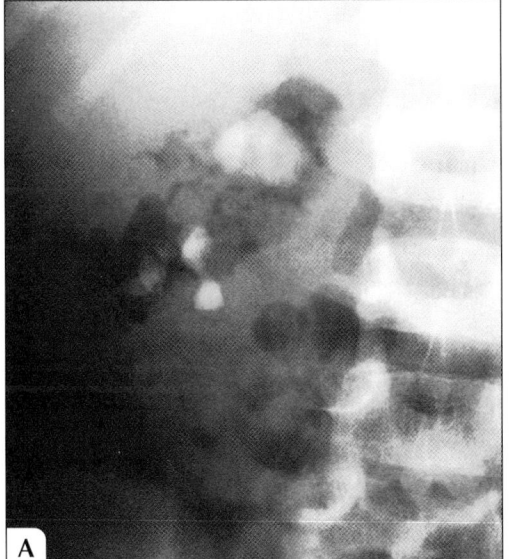
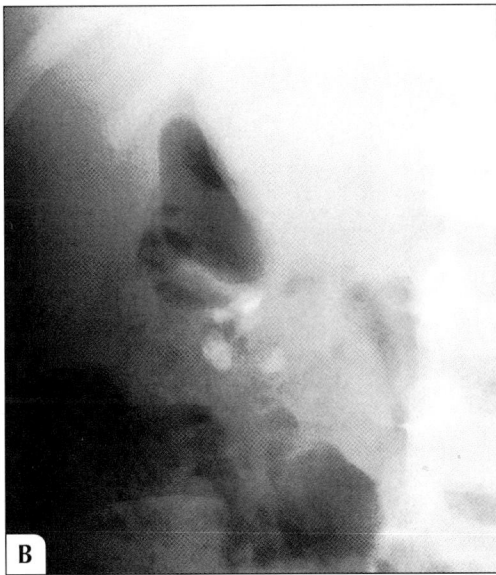
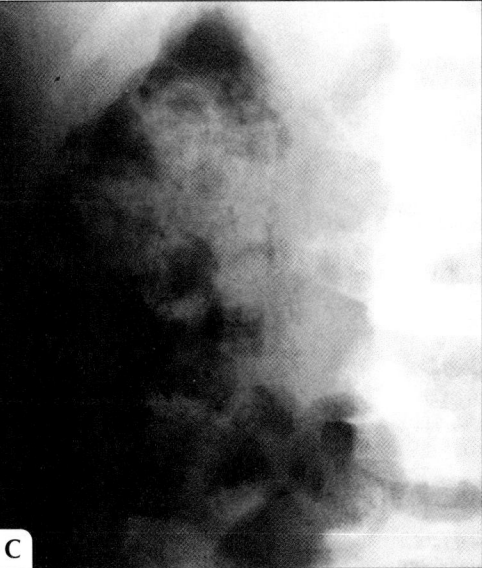

▶ **FIGURE 8-8.** Extracorporeal shock wave lithotripsy (ESWL) in children. Successful treatment of stones with lithotripsy in children has also been reported with stone-free rates reported as high as 96% (**A**) [29]. It is possible to treat larger stones in children than in adults because of the relative softness of the stone and the greater capacity of the child's ureter. Thus, quite complex stones can be successfully treated with one or two sessions of lithotripsy without the need for stenting or postoperative intervention (**B**). Piezoelectric lithotriptors are particularly well suited for children because the smaller focal area minimizes the risk of damage to surrounding tissue (**C**). Approximately 50% of children can be treated without general anesthesia [29]. Concerns regarding the potential risks of ESWL in children have been allayed by prospective studies showing no change in growth parameters as well as improvement in renal function following ESWL [30].

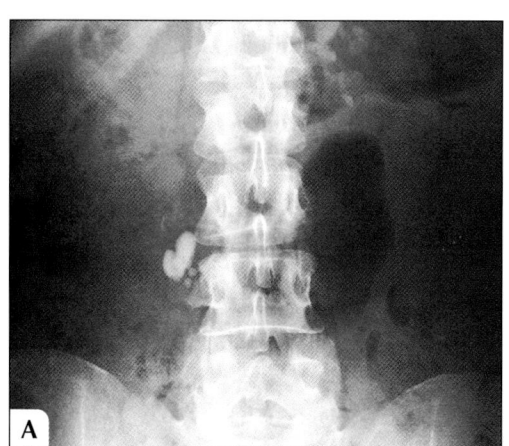

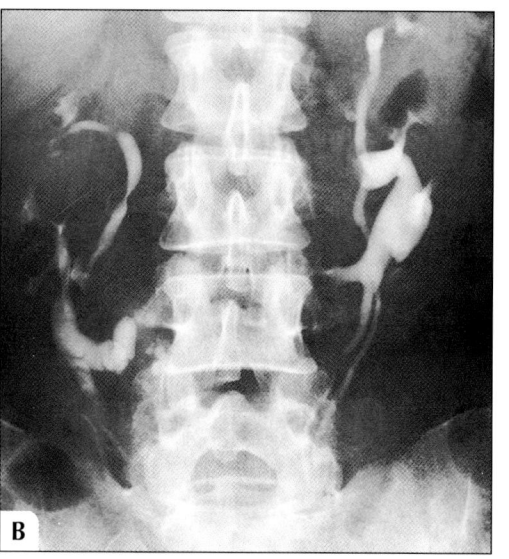

FIGURE 8-9. Extracorporeal shock wave lithotripsy (ESWL) in the presence of anatomic abnormalities (A–C). Lithotripsy is less efficient when used to treat patients with anatomic abnormalities or drainage problems. In cases of horseshoe kidney, there may be problems with localization as well as subsequent drainage of the fragmented stone [31]. Outflow obstruction (whether from the calyx or the ureteropelvic junction) is also a contraindication to lithotripsy.

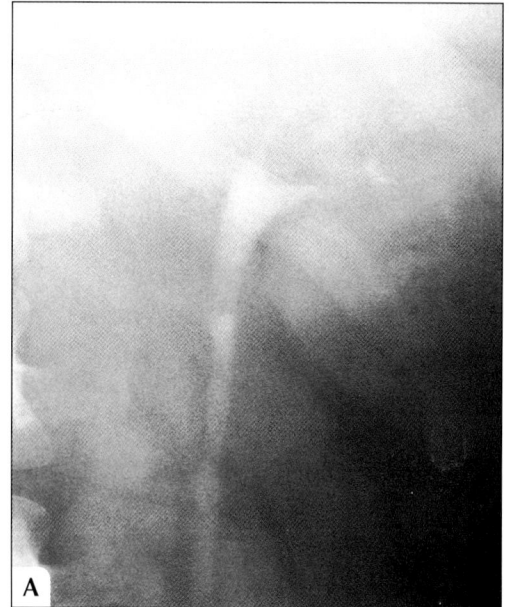

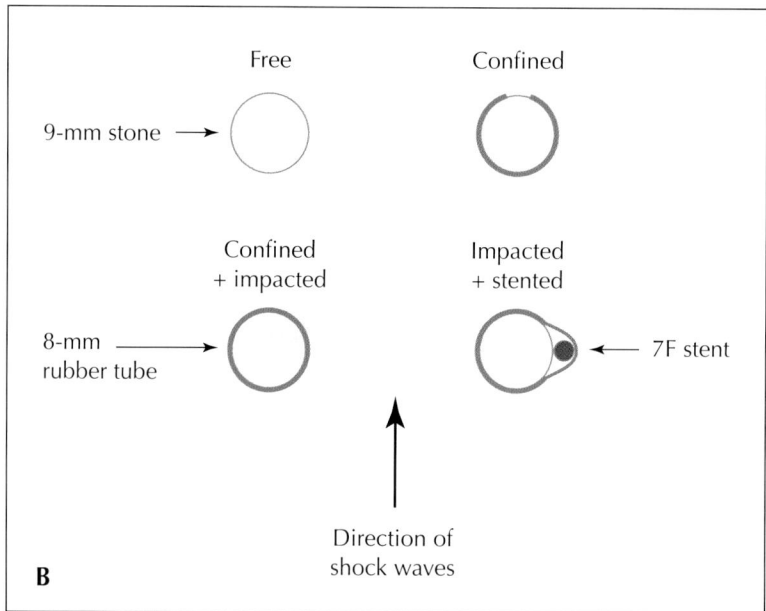

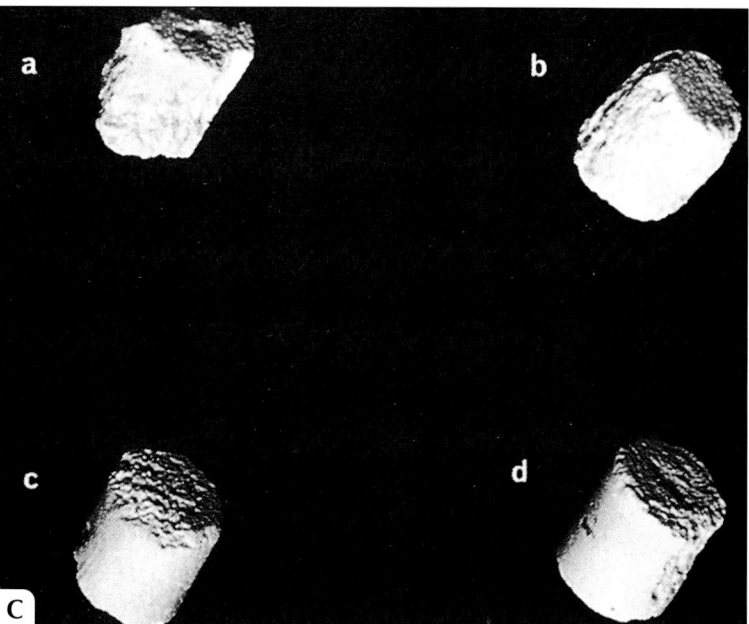

FIGURE 8-10. Treatment of ureteral stones. **A**, Early reports on the treatment of patients with ureteral stones suggested that lithotripsy was relatively inefficient [1]. This was thought to be due to the lack of an expansion chamber and possibly to the presence of obstruction. Work by Parr *et al.* [32] suggested that complete impaction of the stone rendered lithotripsy ineffective. **B** and **C**, Their work also showed that the presence of an expansion chamber produced by a stent caused fragmentation of the stone in close proximity to the stent, but the remainder of the stone remained intact. Another factor thought to reduce fragmentation is the development of multiple interfaces caused by fragmentation of the outer layers of the stone, which may cushion the impact of subsequent shock waves on the inner aspect of the stone.

The ability to localize the stone with either fluoroscopy or ultrasonography is one of the determining factors in the choice of treatment. Thus, for stones in the upper third of the ureter, which can usually be visualized with either imaging modality, extracorporeal shock wave lithotripsy in situ remains the first choice [15]. It is also suitable for treatment of many stones in the lower third of the ureter [33]. For most stones overlying the bony pelvis, however, which are particularly difficult to localize with either imaging modality, ureteroscopy and endoscopic lithotripsy are the first-line treatment. (Panels B and C *from* Parr *et al.* [32]; with permission.)

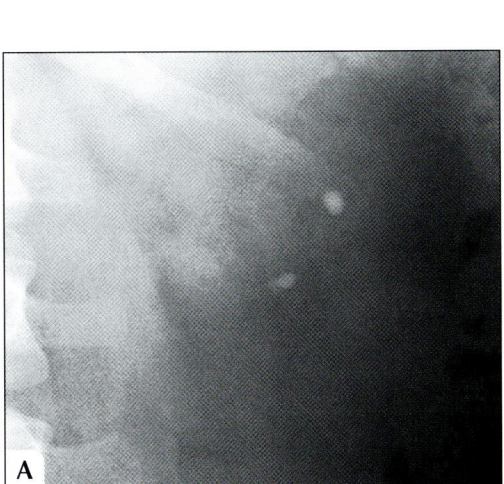

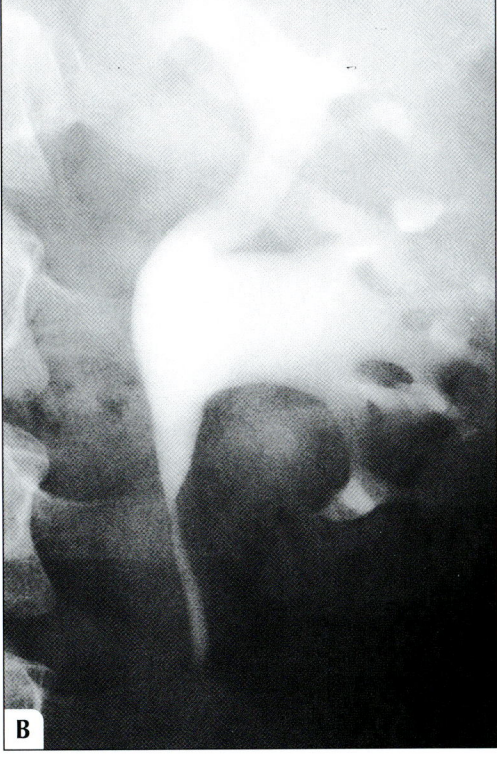

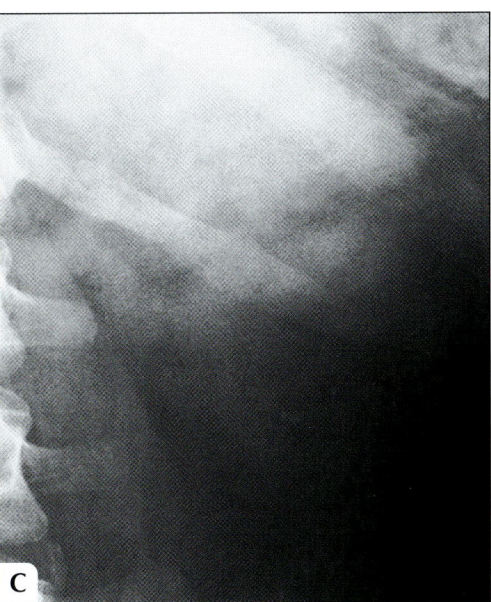

FIGURE 8-11. A–C, The effect of calyceal anatomy on stone clearance after extracorporeal shock wave lithotripsy (ESWL). Factors influencing stone clearance include outflow obstruction (see Fig. 8-9), scarring, and poor renal function. Recent work has attempted to identify the relationship between stone clearance and the anatomy of the lower-pole calyces [12,34–36]. The goal is to define the relative risk of ESWL failure associated with acute angles so as to choose appropriate patients for primary percutaneous nephrolithotomy (PCNL). These studies tie in well with an ongoing debate about the optimal treatment for lower calyceal stones greater than 1 cm in diameter. The Lower Pole Study Group in the United States is conducting a randomized study that compares the outcomes of patients with lower-pole stones treated with ESWL or with PCNL.

COMPLICATIONS

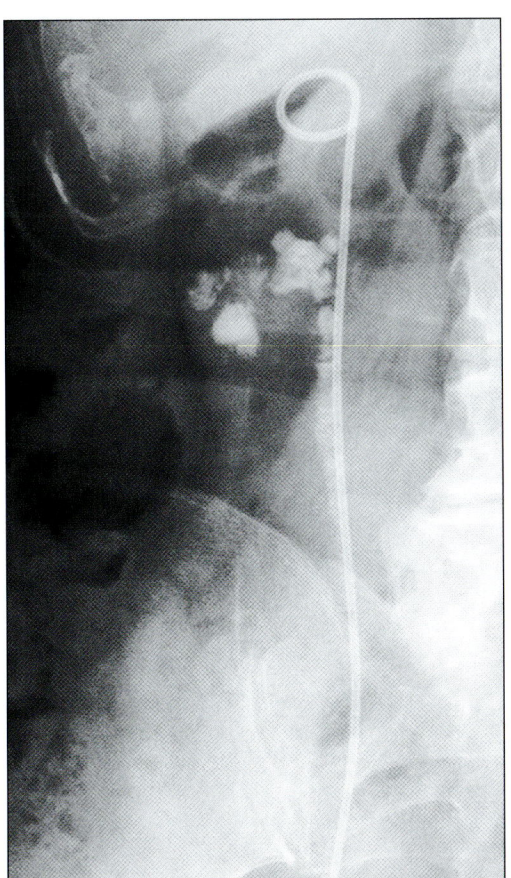

FIGURE 8-12. Steinstrasse. The principal adverse event following lithotripsy is the development of steinstrasse. This occurs if the stone is incompletely fragmented, resulting in a lead fragment obstructing the ureter. Many cases of steinstrasse will resolve spontaneously, but in the presence of obstruction or failure of the fragments to progress, the lead fragment may require further lithotripsy or ureteroscopic extraction. Acute obstruction can be relieved by the insertion of a stent or nephrostomy tube. Some centers prefer the use of a nephrostomy tube, because this allows peristalsis to return to normal, thus increasing the likelihood of spontaneous resolution of the steinstrasse.

Other complications of extracorporeal shock wave lithotripsy (ESWL) include ureteral obstruction, pyelonephritis, and perinephric hematoma, which is more common in patients with uncontrolled hypertension [37]. The vast majority of perirenal hematomas eventually settle with no long-term sequelae [38]. The relationship of ESWL to the onset of hypertension continues to be the subject of research. Although large studies have shown no association between ESWL and hypertension [39], recent reports suggest that elderly patients may be at risk [40].

ACKNOWLEDGEMENT

The authors would like to acknowledge the assistance of Steven D. Pye, PhD, Physicist in the Department of Medical Physics and Medical Engineering, Western General Hospital, Edinburgh, Scotland, UK.

REFERENCES

1. Chaussy C, Schmeidt E, Jocham D, *et al.*: First clinical experience with extracorporeally induced destruction of kidney stones by shock waves. *J Urol* 1982, 127:417–420.

2. Drach GW, Dretler S, Fair W, *et al.*: Report of the United States cooperative study of extracorporeal shock wave lithotripsy. *J Urol* 1986, 135:1127–1133.

3. Marberger M, Turk C, Steinkogler I: Painless piezoelectric extracorporeal lithotripsy. *J Urol* 1988, 139:695–697.

4. Bierkins AF, Hendrkx AJM, DeKort WJW, *et al.*: Efficacy of second generation lithotriptors: a multicenter comparative study of 2206 extracorporeal shock wave lithotripsy treatments with the Siemens Lithostar, Dornier HM4, Wolf Piezolith 2300, Direx Tripter XI, and Breakstone lithotriptors. *J Urol* 1992, 148:1052–1058.

5. Tiselius H-G: Anesthesia-free in situ extracorporeal shock wave lithotripsy of ureteral stones. *J Urol* 1991:146:8–11.

6. Albala DM, Clayman RV, Meretyk S: Extracorporeal shock wave lithotripsy for proximal ureteral calculi: to stent or not to stent? *J Endourol* 1991, 5:277–282.

7. Mobley TB, Myers DA, Jendins JM, *et al.*: Effects of stents on lithotripsy of ureteral calculi: treatment results with 18,825 calculi using the Lithostar lithotriptor. *J Urol* 1994, 152:53–56.

8. Beck EM, Riehle RA, Jr.: The fate of residual fragments after extracorporeal shock wave lithotripsy monotherapy of infection stones. *J Urol* 1991, 145:6–11.

9. Streem SB, Yost A, Dolmatch B: Combination "sandwich" therapy for extensive renal calculi in 100 consecutive patients: immediate, long-term and stratified results from a 10-year experience. *J Urol* 1997, 158:342–345.

10. Segura JW, Preminger GM, Assimos DG, *et al.*: Nephrolithiasis Clinical Guidelines Panel summary report on the management of staghorn calculi. *J Urol* 1994, 151:1648–1653.

11. Lingeman JE, Siegel YI, Steele B, *et al.*: Management of lower pole nephrolithiasis: a critical analysis. *J Urol* 1994, 151:663–667.

12. Sampaio FJB, Aragao AHM: Limitations of extracorporeal shock wave lithotripsy for lower caliceal stones: anatomic insight. *J Endourol* 1994, 8:241–247.

13. Streem SB, Yost A, Mascha E: Clinical implications of clinically insignificant stone fragments after extracorporeal shock wave lithotripsy. *J Urol* 1996, 155:1186–1190.

14. Zanetti G, Seveso M, Montanari E, *et al.*: Renal stone fragments following shock wave lithotripsy. *J Urol* 1997, 158:352–355.

15. Segura JW, Preminger GM, Assimos DG, *et al.*: Ureteral Stones Clinical Guidelines Panel summary report on the management of ureteral calculi. *J Urol* 1997,158: 1915–1921.

16. Sofras F, Karayannis A, Kastriotis J, *et al.*: Extracorporeal shockwave lithotripsy or extracorporeal piezoelectric lithotripsy? Comparison of costs and results. *Br J Urol* 1991, 68:15–17.

17. Chaussy C, Fuchs G: Extracorporeal shock wave lithotripsy (ESWL) for the treatment of upper urinary stones. In *Adult and Pediatric Urology*. Edited by Gillenwater J, Grayhack J, Howards S, *et al.* Chicago: Year Book Medical Publishers; 1987: 605–619.

18. Harrison (ed.): *Campbell's Urology*, edn 5. Philadelphia: WB Saunders; 1992.

19. Granz B, Kohler G: What makes a shock wave efficient in lithotripsy? *J Stone Dis* 1992, 4:123–129.

20. Chuong CJ, Zhong P, Preminger GM: A comparison of stone damage caused by different modes of shock wave generation. *J Urol* 1992, 148:200–204.

21. Zhong P, Preminger GM: Physical principles of extracorporeal shock wave lithotripsy. In *Textbook of Endourology*. Edited by Sosa RE, Albala DM, Jenkins AD, *et al.* Philadelphia: WB Saunders; 1997: 569–585.

22. Zhong P, Preminger GM: Mechanisms of differing stone fragility in extracorporeal shock wave lithotripsy. *J Endourol* 1994, 8:263–270.

23. Crum LA: Cavitation microjets as a contributory mechanism for renal calculi disintegration in ESWL. *J Urol* 1988, 140:1587–1590.

24. Zhong P, Cocks FH, Cioanta I, *et al.*: Controlled, forced collapse of cavitation bubbles for improved stone fragmentation during shock wave lithotripsy. *J Urol* 1997, 158:2323–2328.

25. Graff J, Diedrichs W, Schulze H: Long-term follow up in 1003 extracorporeal shock wave lithotripsy patients. *J Urol* 1988, 140:479–483.

26. Lingeman JE, Newman DM, Mertz JHO, *et al.*: Extracorporeal shock wave lithotripsy: the Methodist Hospital of Indiana experience. *J Urol* 1986, 135:1134–1137.

27. Lingeman JE: Extracorporeal shock wave lithotripsy. *Urol Clin North Am* 1997, 24:192–211.

28. Lam HS, Lingeman JE, Mosbaugh PG, *et al.*: Evolution of the technique of combination therapy for staghorn calculi: a decreasing role for extracorporeal shock wave lithotripsy. *J Urol* 1992, 148:1058–1062.

29. Marberger M, Turk C, Steinkogler I: Piezoelectric extracorporeal lithotripsy in children. *J Urol* 1989, 142:349–350.

30. Thomas R, Frentz JM, Harmon E, *et al.*: Effect of extracorporeal shockwave lithotripsy on renal function and body height in pediatric patients. *J Urol* 1992, 148: 1064–1067.

31. Lampel A, Hohenfellner M, Schultz-Lampel D, *et al.*: Urolithiasis in horseshoe kidneys: therapeutic management. *Urology* 1996, 47:182–186.

32. Parr NJ, Pye SD, Ritchie WS, Tolley DA: Mechanisms responsible for diminished fragmentation of ureteral calculi: an experimental and clinical study. *J Urol* 1992, 148:1079–1083.

33. Keeler LL, McNamara TC, Dorey FO, Milstein RE: De novo extracorporeal shock wave lithotripsy for lower ureteral calculi: treatment of choice. *J Endourol* 1990, 4:71–74.

34. Sabnis RB, Naik K, Patel SH, *et al.*: Extracorporeal shock wave lithotripsy for lower calyceal stones: can clearance be predicted? *Br J Urol* 1997, 80:853–857.

35. Elbahnasy AM, Shalhav AL, Hoenig DM, *et al.*: Lower caliceal stone clearance after shock wave lithotripsy or ureteroscopy: the impact of lower pole radiographic anatomy. *J Urol* 1998, 159:676–682.

36. Keeley FX, Jr., Moussa SA, Smith G, *et al.*: Clearance of lower pole stones following SWL: the effect of infundibulopelvic angle. *Eur Urol* 1999, 33:371–375.

37. Knapp PM, Kulb TB, Lingeman JE, *et al.*: Extracorporeal shock wave lithotripsy induced perirenal hematomas. *J Urol* 1988, 139:700–705.

38. Krishnamurthi V, Streem SM: Long term anatomic and functional sequelae of post-ESWL hematomas [abstract]. *J Urol* 1997, 153:510A.

39. Lingeman JE, Woods JR, Toth PD: Blood pressure changes following shock wave lithotripsy and other forms of treatment for nephrolithiasis. *JAMA* 1990, 263:1789–1793.

40. Knapp R, Frauscher F, Helweg G, *et al.*: Age-related changes in resistive index following extracorporeal shock wave lithotripsy. *J Urol* 1995, 154:955–958.

Percutaneous Nephrolithotomy

John W. Dushinski
James E. Lingeman

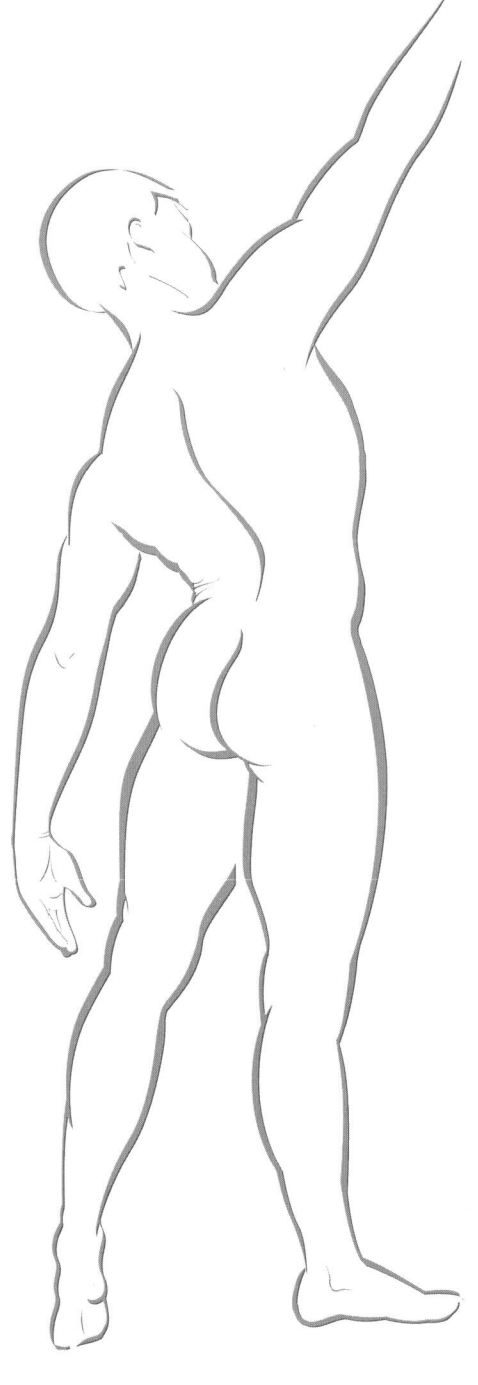

Percutaneous nephrolithotomy (PNL) was first described by Fernstrom and Johansson in 1976 [1]. Improved surgical instruments and endourologic techniques developed in the ensuing decade allowed the procedure to gain widespread acceptance [2,3]. Today, PNL in conjunction with shock wave lithotripsy (SWL) has replaced open-stone surgery at most institutions. Patient comfort has been improved by combining previously separate steps in the PNL procedure into a single setting. Retrograde placement of a ureteral catheter, percutaneous access, and stone removal are all performed in the operating room under a single anesthetic by the urologist. This also avoids becoming dependent on another person's skill and schedule and allows the flexibility to perform additional renal access procedures when required. Although other specialists may be capable of performing renal access, it is the urologist who should decide which site provides the best access to the stone.

The indications for removal of renal stones have not changed since the introduction of PNL and SWL. The stone should be symptomatic, obstructing (or in danger of becoming so), or a source of infection. Once it has been decided that a stone should be treated, a technique must be chosen.

There is no single technique suitable for the removal of all renal stones. Urologists must be able to use a variety of techniques if they are going to treat all patients with stone disease. Although renal stones can be treated with either PNL or SWL, urologists must decide which stones can be treated safely, expeditiously, and economically with SWL, and which stones are more appropriately treated with PNL. PNL is also the main treatment option for renal stones for which SWL has failed.

Percutaneous nephrolithotomy and SWL have also been used in combination as part of a "sandwich therapy" to remove complex stone burdens. This technique involves a primary procedure followed by SWL for residual fragments, followed by a second PNL procedure to clear the system of all fragments. Recent advances in flexible instrumentation and intracorporeal lithotripsy devices have greatly improved our ability to remove complex staghorn stones completely in one or two percutaneous procedures without resorting to SWL [4].

INDICATIONS AND PREOPERATIVE PREPARATION

Indications for Percutaneous Nephrolithotomy

Large stone burden (>2 cm)
Cystine stone (>1 cm or multiple stones)
Urinary obstruction distal to the stone
  Stone in calyceal diverticulum
  UPJ obstruction
  Horseshoe kidney (fragments unlikely to pass because of high insertion)

▶ **FIGURE 9-1.** Indications for percutaneous nephrolithotomy (PNL). The indications are similar to the contraindications for shock wave lithotripsy (SWL). Patients with a large stone burden are more suitably treated with PNL because SWL may cause incomplete fragmentation, multiple planned and unplanned procedures, and considerable illness due to obstructing fragments. Cystine calculi fragment poorly with SWL; however, fragmentation of solitary cystine stones smaller than 1 cm in diameter may be attempted. Obstruction distal to the stone is also a contraindication to SWL because fragments may not pass and may cause acute obstruction. Stones in calyceal diverticuli and found in association with ureteropelvic junction (UPJ) obstruction are more appropriately treated with PNL, because fulguration of the diverticulum and endopyelotomy may be performed in conjunction with PNL.

Contraindications to Percutaneous Nephrolithotomy

Uncorrected bleeding disorder
Acute urinary tract infection

Preoperative Preparation

Urine culture and sensitivity testing
Antibiotic coverage
Coagulation profile, CBC, type and screen

▶ **FIGURE 9-2.** Preoperative preparation. The goal of the preoperative evaluation is to minimize complications. Urine culture and sensitivity testing are performed to tailor perioperative antibiotic therapy. Negative culture results do not preclude perioperative parenteral antibiotic therapy because stone material may still harbor bacteria. Patients with staghorn calculi are treated preoperatively with 2 weeks of oral ciprofloxacin unless culture and sensitivity test results suggest an alternative antibiotic choice. A coagulation profile is performed to rule out bleeding diathesis. The complete blood count (CBC) and blood typing and screening are performed to assess and prepare for transfusion; however, routine cross-matching is not necessary because transfusion is rarely required for a routine case.

▶ **FIGURE 9-3** Absolute contraindications to percutaneous nephrolithotomy (PNL) are relatively few. All bleeding disorders must be corrected before PNL to prevent massive hemorrhage. Acute urinary tract infections must be treated with antibiotics, although insertion of a percutaneous nephrostomy tube may on occasion be required in an obstructed urinary system.

PATIENT POSITIONING AND NEEDLE PLACEMENT

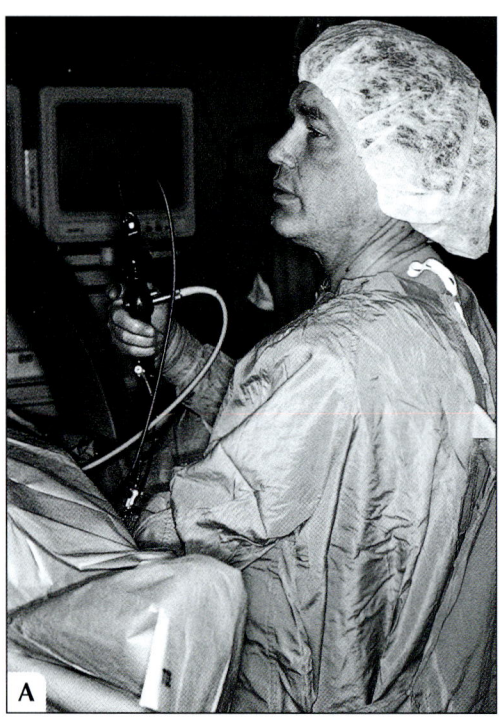
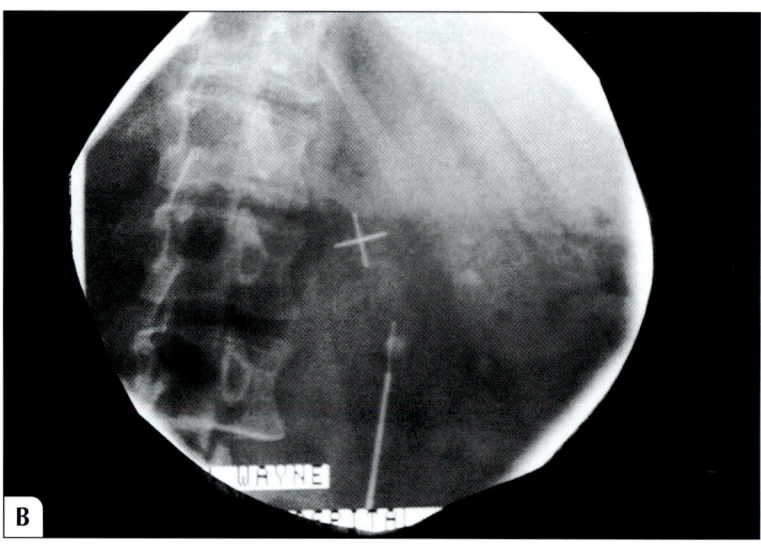

▶ **FIGURE 9-4.** Patient positioning for percutaneous nephrolithotomy (PNL). **A,** The patient is initially placed in the lithotomy position and a guidewire is passed up the ureter to the affected kidney under fluoroscopic guidance. **B,** A 5-F open-ended ureteral catheter is then advanced over the wire to the renal pelvis, and the wire is removed.

(Continued on next page)

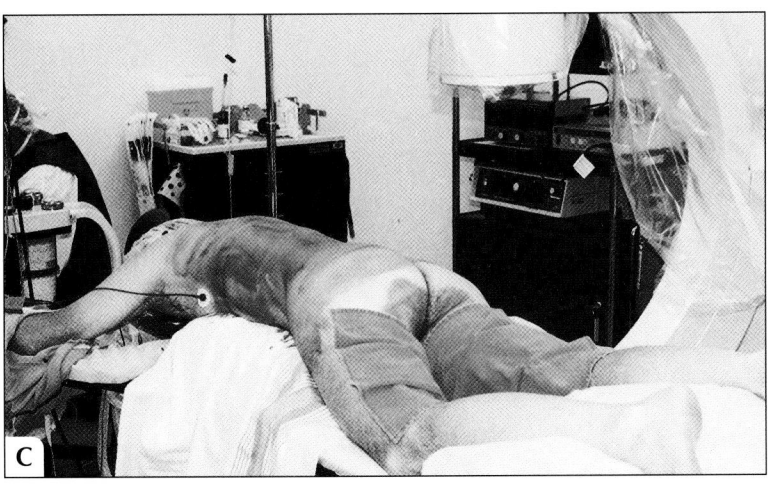

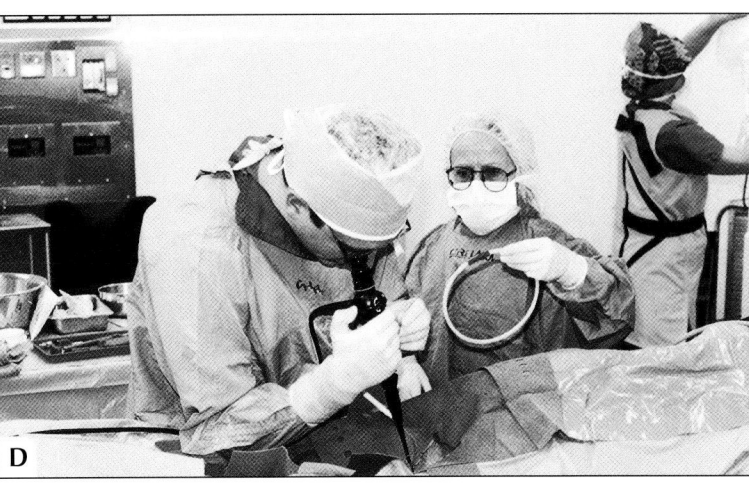

▶ **FIGURE 9-4.** (*Continued*) **C,** A Foley catheter is inserted before turning the patient over into the modified prone position (affected side elevated approximately 30°). **D,** As an alternative, the wire and ureteral catheter may be inserted with a flexible cystoscope with the patient in the modified prone position, thereby avoiding the need to reposition the patient.

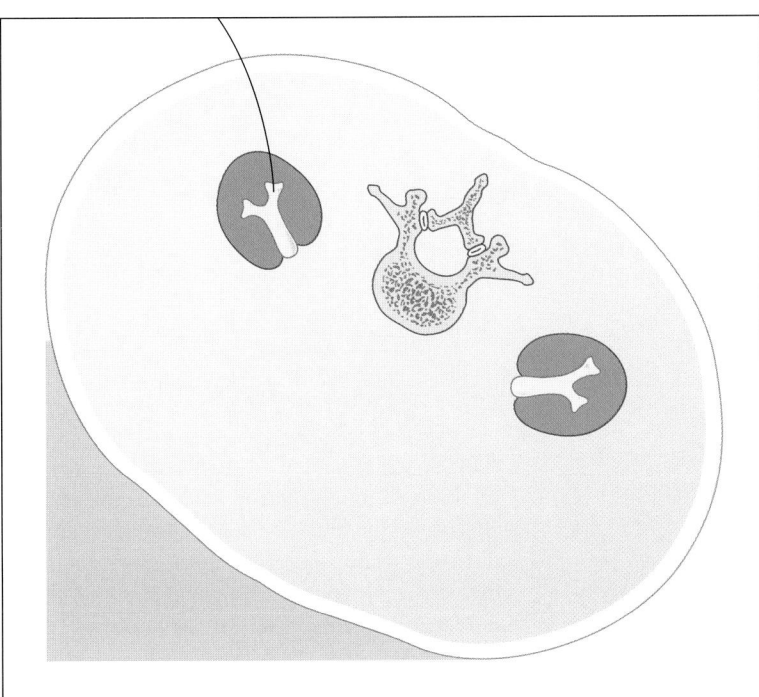

▶ **FIGURE 9-5.** Placement of the access needle for percutaneous renal access. The affected side is elevated approximately 30° by use of a foam wedge. Access is then gained into the posterior calyx of choice along the line of the infundibulum using biplanar C-arm fluoroscopy. Injury to intra-abdominal structures is unusual so long as the puncture is kept medial to the posterior axillary line because peritoneum rarely extends around to the posterior kidney.

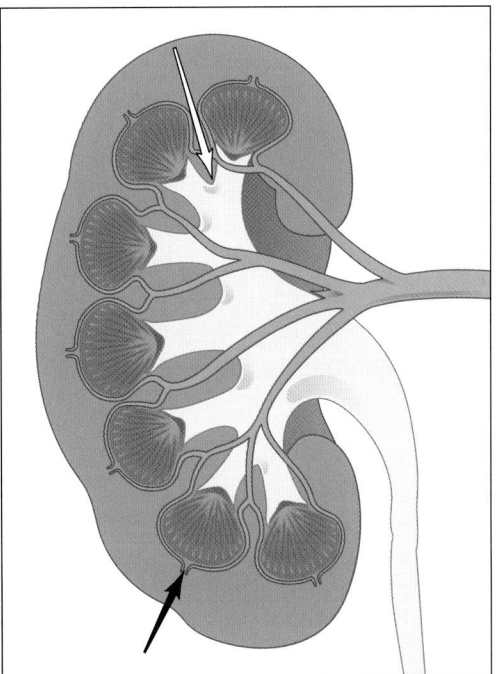

▶ **FIGURE 9-6.** Percutaneous needle placement. This anterior view of the right kidney shows the collecting system and major arterial branches. Major intrarenal veins have a distribution similar to the arteries. Percutaneous renal access is best performed directly through a papilla along the line of the infundibulum (*solid arrow*) to minimize hemorrhage. Access directly into an infundibulum (*open arrow*) or the renal pelvis risks damage to major vessels and subsequent hemorrhage.

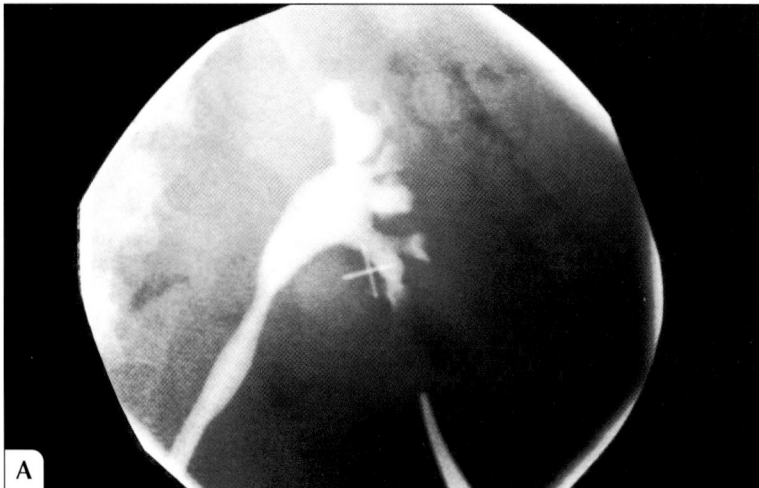

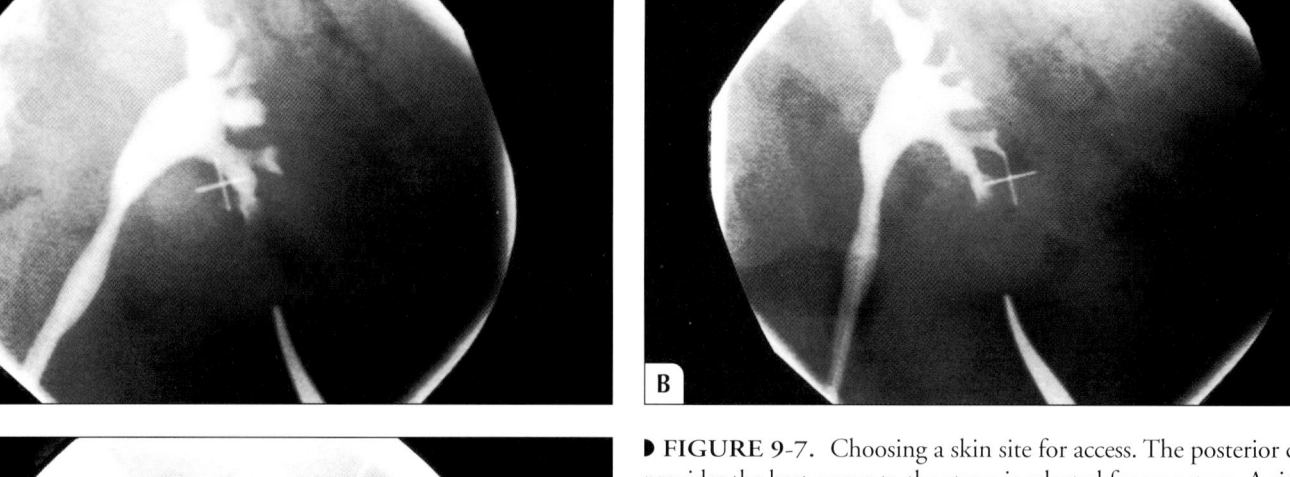

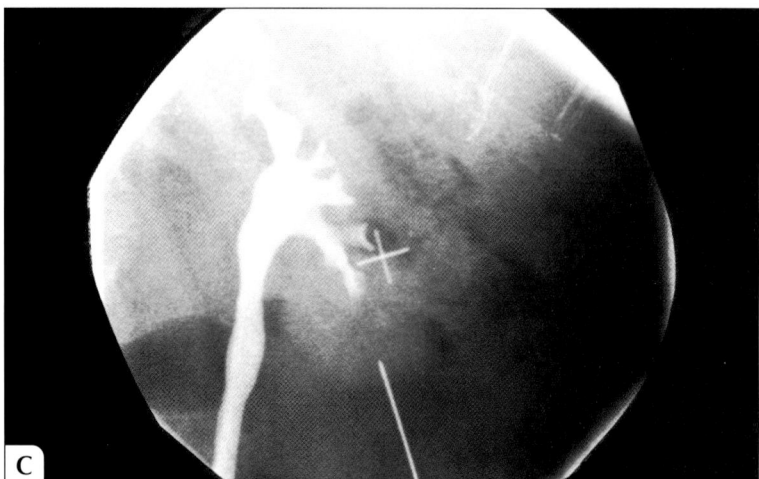

▶ **FIGURE 9-7.** Choosing a skin site for access. The posterior calyx that provides the best access to the stone is selected for puncture. A site on the skin is then selected that appears in line with the infundibulum on two different projections on C-arm fluoroscopy (**A** and **B**). A hemostat is placed on the skin and moved into position with fluoroscopic guidance. Biplanar C-arm fluoroscopy is then used to perform precise calyceal puncture along the line of the infundibulum with an 18-gauge needle (**C**).

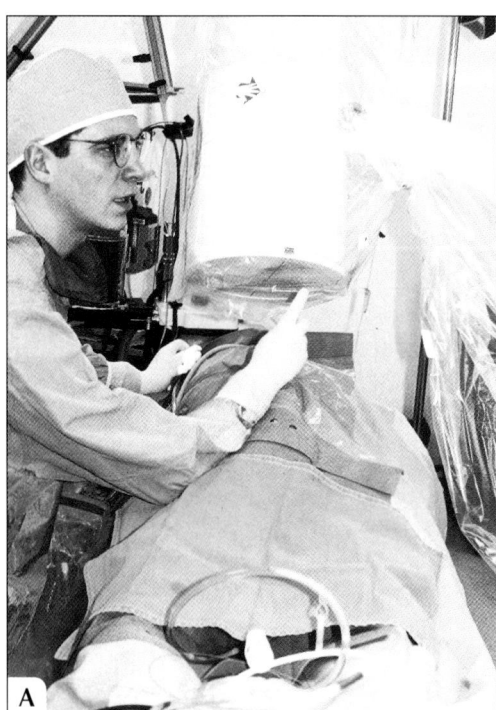

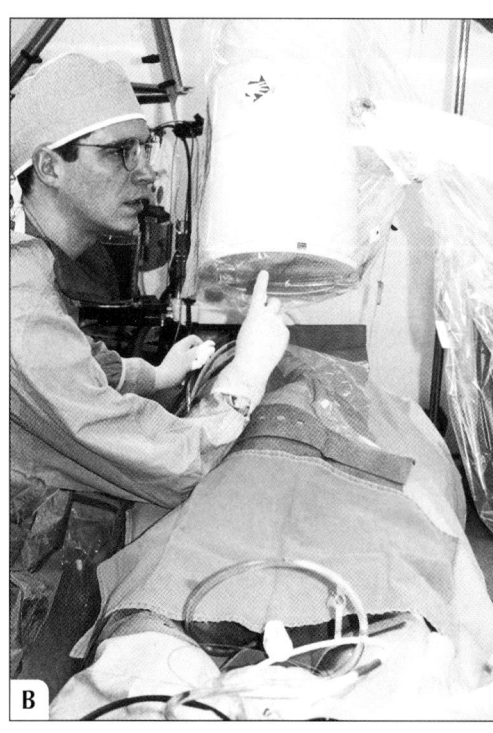

▶ **FIGURE 9-8.** Use of the C-arm during puncture. **A** and **B**, Medial-lateral (right-left) adjustments to the needle angle are made with the x-ray beam parallel to the sagittal plane of the needle. Note change in angle of the hand holding the needle.

(*Continued on next page*)

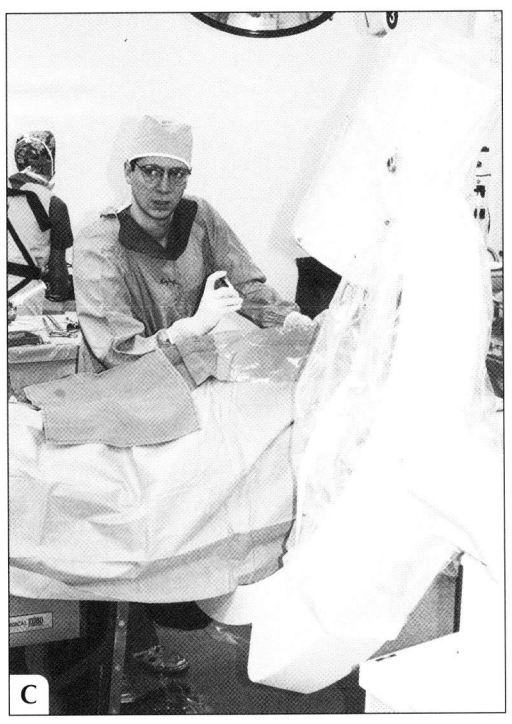

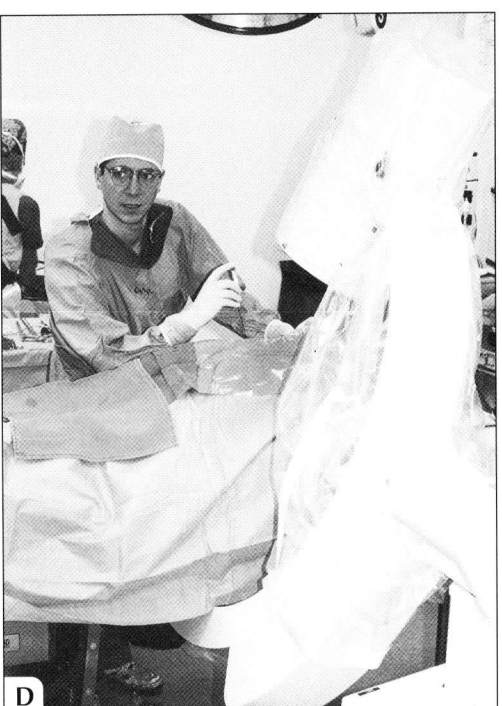

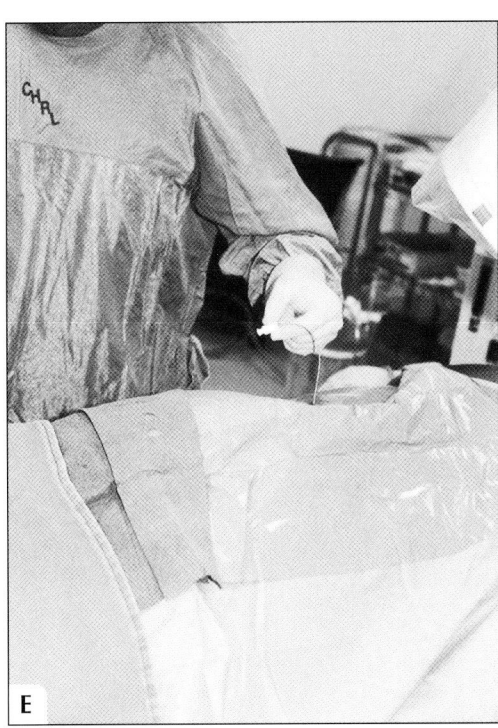

▶ **FIGURE 9-8.** (*Continued*) **C** and **D**, Cephalad-caudad (up-down) adjustments to the needle angle are made with the C-arm rotated as far laterally as possible. Again note change in needle angle. The orientation in one plane must not be changed when making adjustments in the opposite plane. Needle advancement into the collecting system can be performed only when the needle angle is correct in both planes. Accurate puncture is facilitated by temporary suspension of respirations. Advancement is monitored with the C-arm in the lateral position because this provides a better view of needle depth. **E**, Access is confirmed by aspirating urine through the needle.

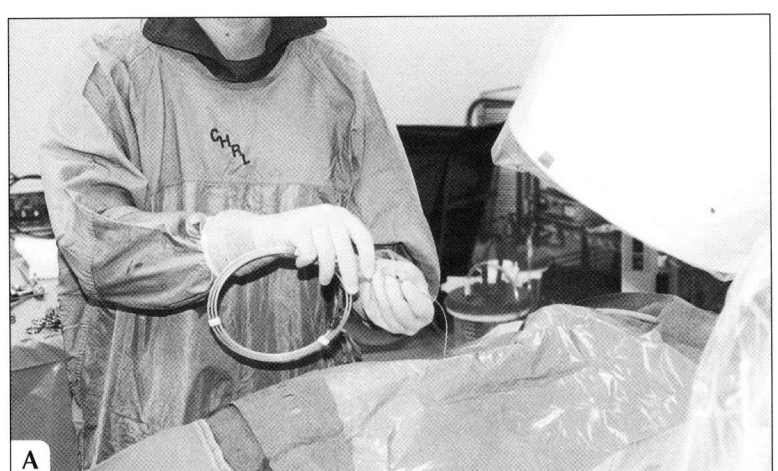

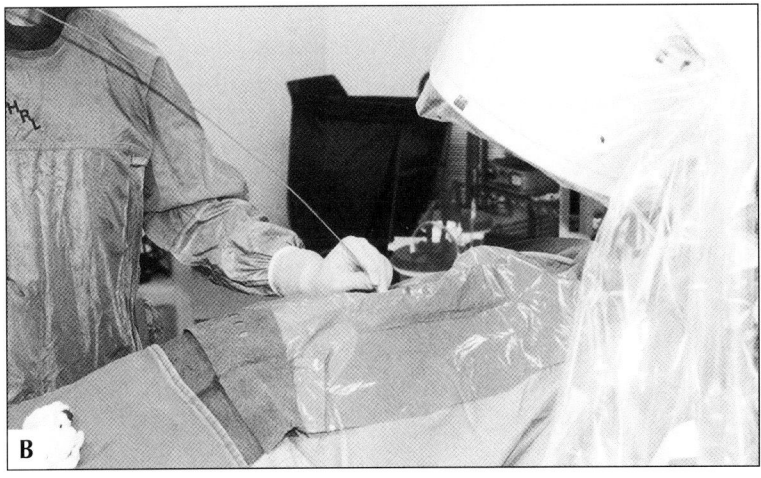

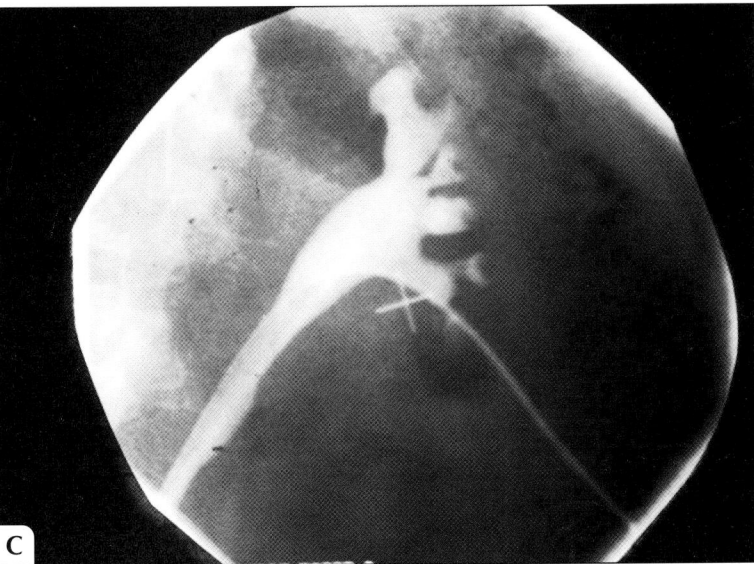

▶ **FIGURE 9-9.** Guidewire placement. **A**, Once access is confirmed, a hydrophilic guidewire is passed into the collecting system and down the ureter. **B** and **C**, A cobra-head angiographic catheter is useful in manipulating the wire down the ureter, particularly with lower pole punctures. The hydrophilic guidewire is then exchanged for a stiff wire (Amplatz superstiff).

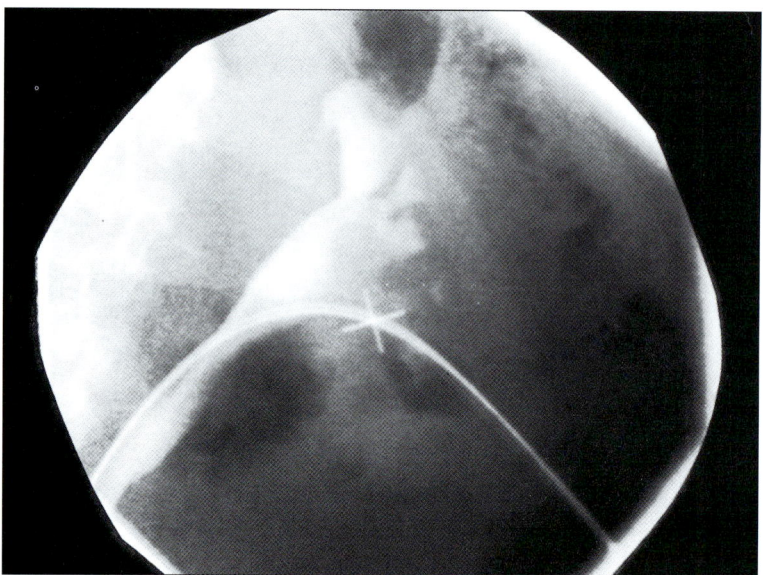

▶ FIGURE 9-10. Safety wire. An ordinary Bentson-type wire is also passed down the ureter using the 10-F coaxial Amplatz dilators. The Bentson wire is snapped to the drapes as a safety wire, and a stiff wire is used to dilate the access tract.

DILATION AND STONE REMOVAL

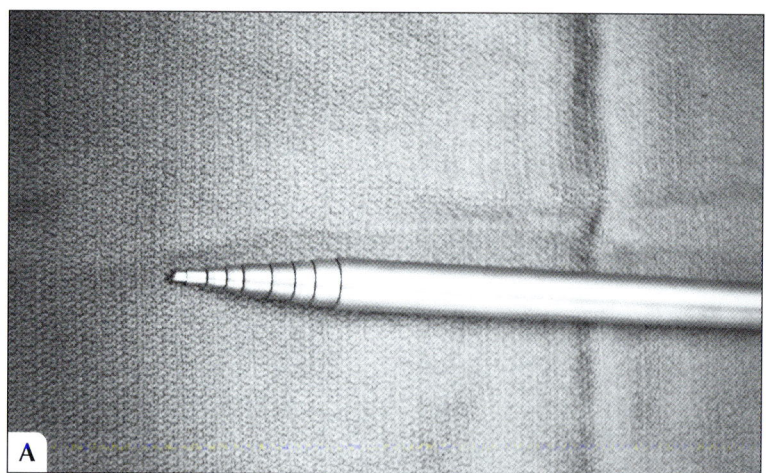

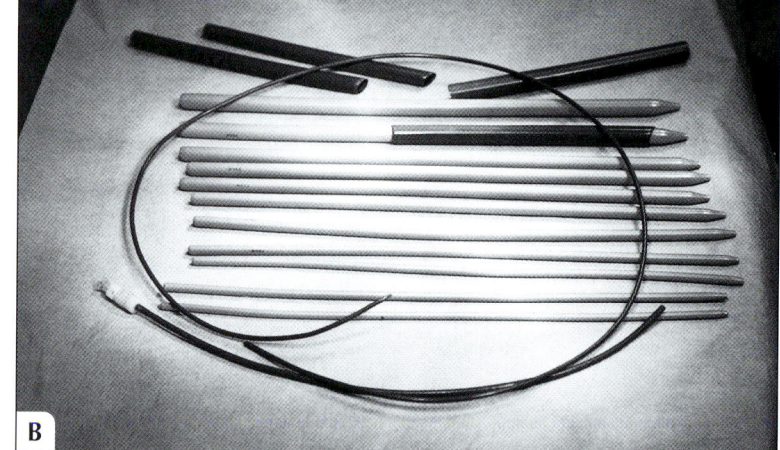

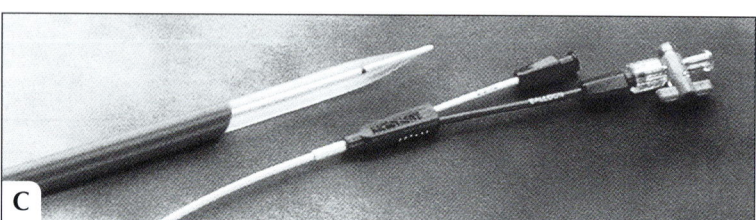

▶ FIGURE 9-11. Tract dilation. Telescoping metal dilators (**A**), sequential Amplatz dilators (**B**), and high-pressure balloons (**C**) are the three types of instruments available for tract dilation. The high-pressure balloons are fastest and simplest to use because the radial spreading action results in less bleeding than the shearing effect of the other techniques [5]. The surgeon must avoid over-advancement of the dilators because this may rupture the infundibulum, causing hemorrhage and limiting visualization.

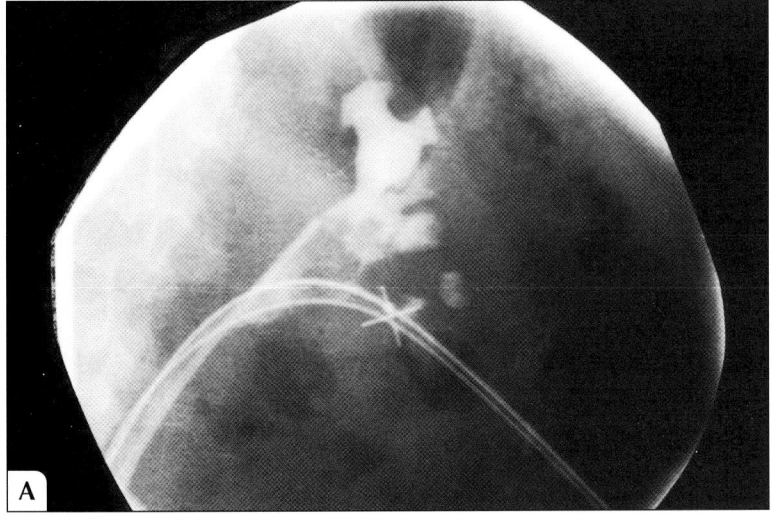

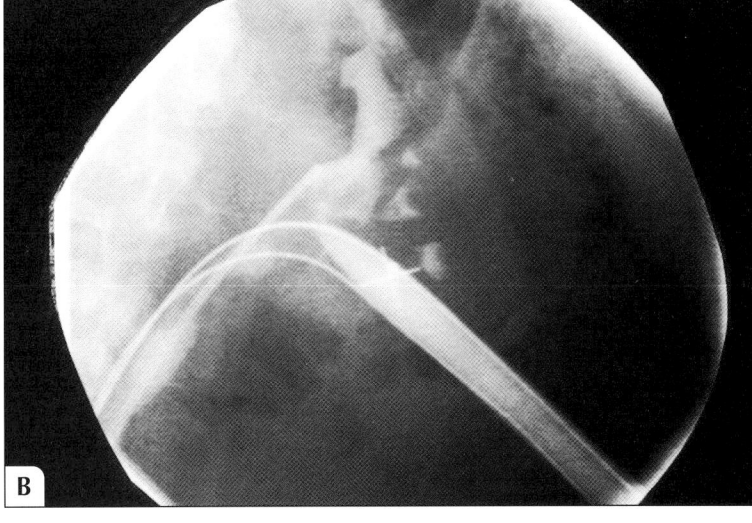

▶ **FIGURE 9-12.** Balloon dilation. The empty balloon is advanced over the stiff wire until the radiopaque tip is located in the punctured calyx (**A**). The balloon is then inflated with a high-pressure syringe (**B**), and a working sheath is advanced over the balloon (**C**). The balloon is deflated and removed once the working sheath has been advanced into the calyx.

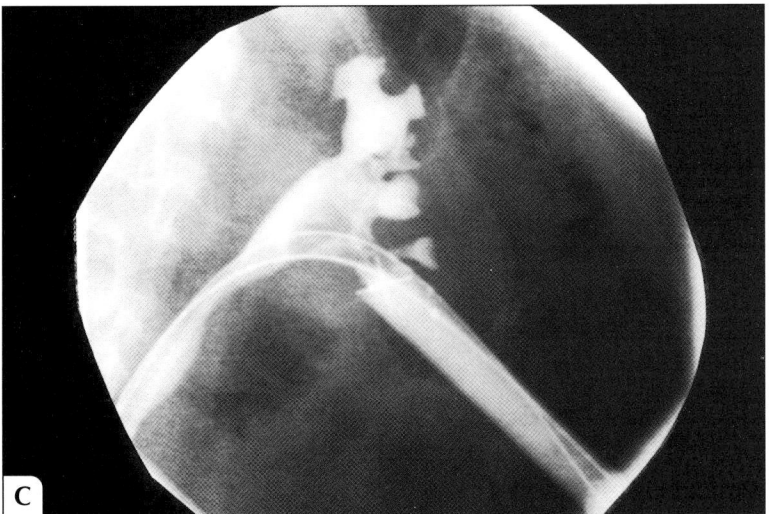

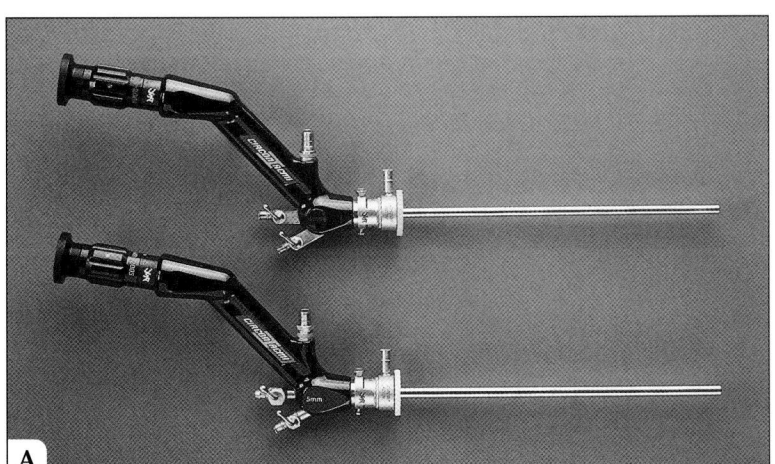

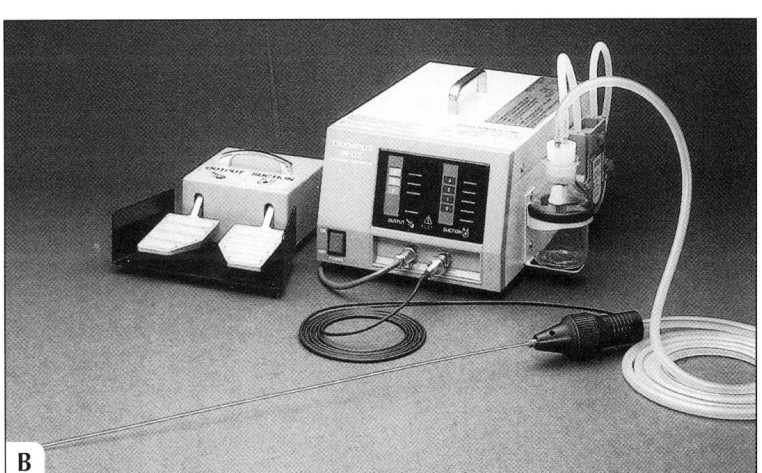

▶ **FIGURE 9-13.** Rigid nephroscopy. **A,** The bulk of the stone is removed initially with the rigid nephroscope. **B,** The ultrasonic lithotripsy device is useful because it rapidly fragments and evacuates stone material and blood clots via suction. **C,** A pneumatic device is also useful, particularly for very hard stones. Larger fragments are grasped and sent for stone analysis.

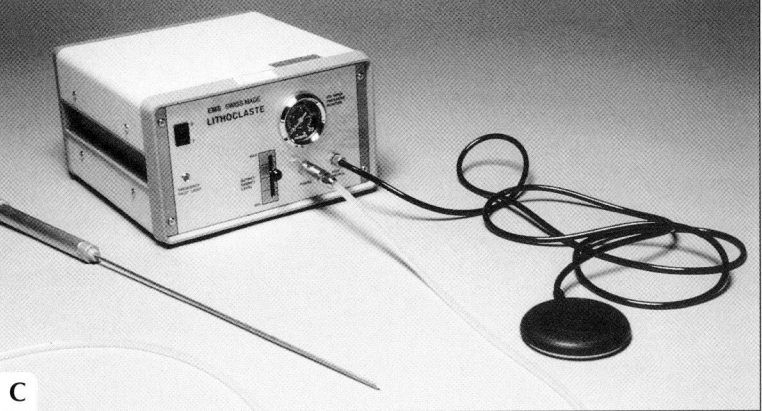

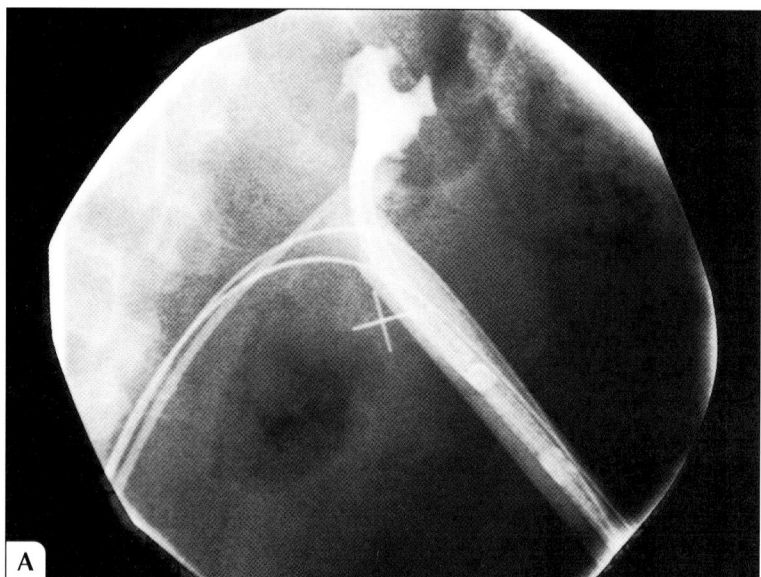

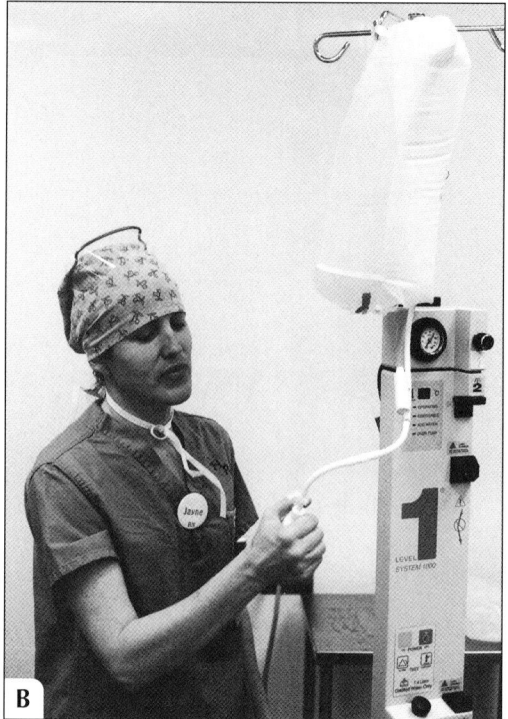

▶ **FIGURE 9-14.** Flexible nephroscopy. The flexible nephroscope is used to examine each calyx and ensure that the collecting system is stone-free. **A,** Radiographic contrast is injected through the irrigation port to guide the scope and ensure that each calyx is examined. **B,** Visualization is enhanced by pressurizing the irrigant fluid to 200 to 300 mm of water. When a calyceal stone is encountered, it can be removed with a basket or grasping forceps or simply manipulated into the renal pelvis with irrigation or wire manipulation, to be evacuated later with the rigid scope and ultrasonic device. It is often necessary to switch from flexible to rigid nephroscopy several times before the kidney appears stone-free.

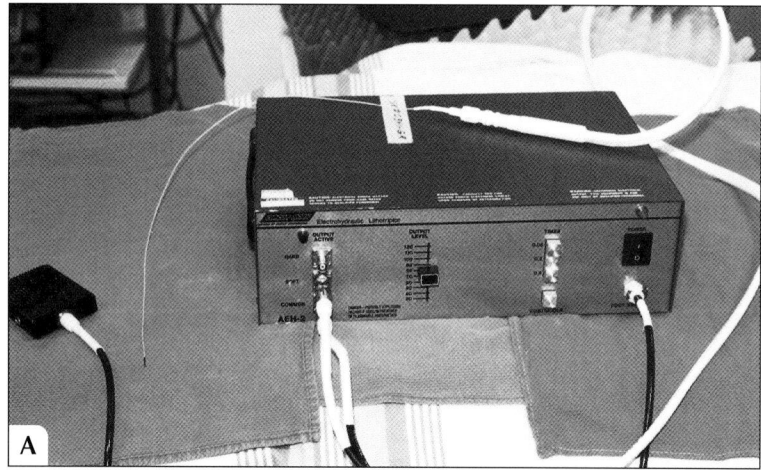

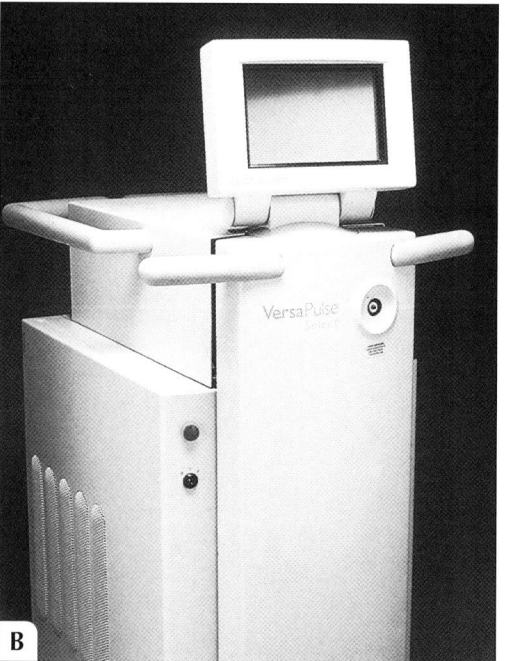

▶ **FIGURE 9-15.** Stone fragmentation with a flexible nephroscope. Larger calyceal stones encountered with a flexible scope may require fragmentation before retrieval. **A,** Traditionally, this was performed with the electrohydraulic lithotripsy device. **B,** The holmium laser more recently has been shown to fragment even the hardest calculi with probes as small as 200 μm in diameter, allowing maximal irrigant flow [6,7].

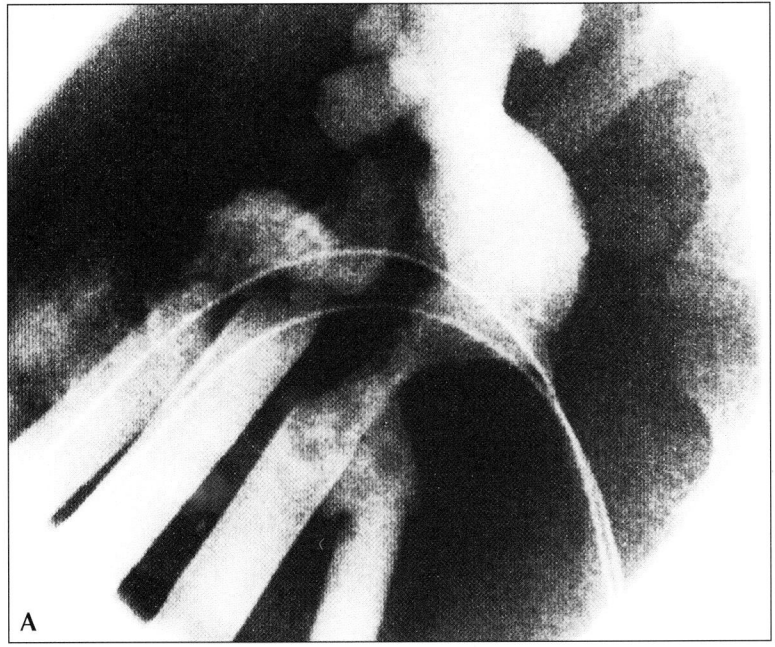

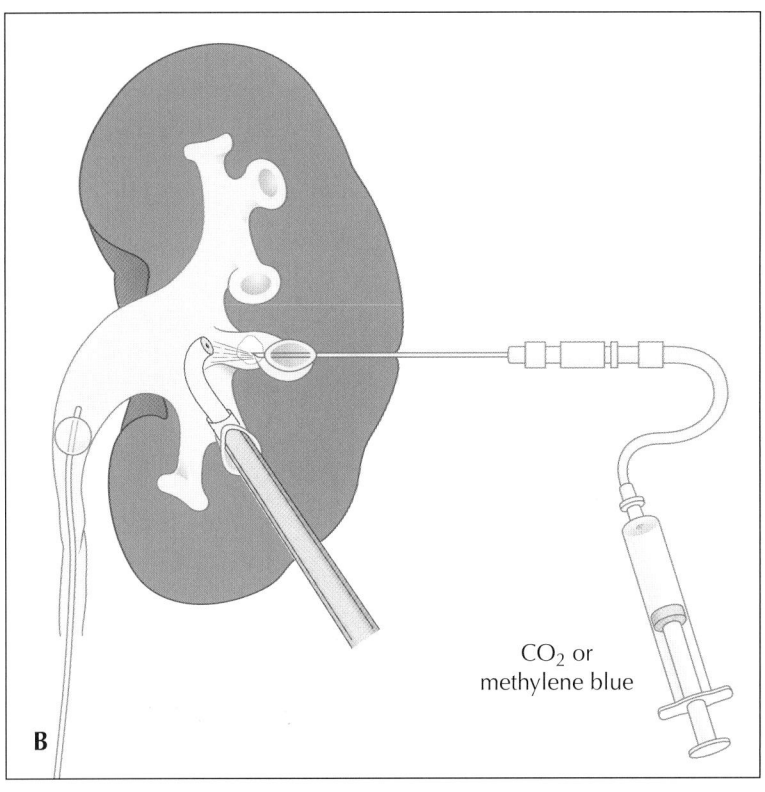

FIGURE 9-16. Additional access tracts. **A,** Additional access tracts may be required when there is a large staghorn stone or a complex collecting system. Multiple access sites can expedite the procedure without causing a significant increase in morbidity [8]. **B,** Nondilated punctures are occasionally used to aid in the localization of stones that cannot be located nephroscopically [4]. Both dilated and nondilated tracts are accessed using the same techniques discussed earlier in this chapter.

CO_2 or methylene blue

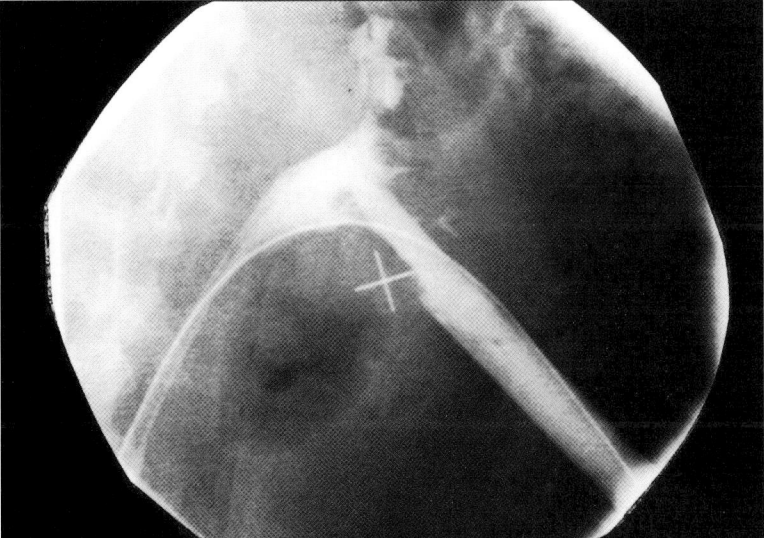

FIGURE 9-17. Nephrostomy tube placement. A nephrostomy tube is placed through the working sheath when the kidney appears stone-free, both fluoroscopically and nephroscopically, or when a secondary procedure is planned. Nephrostomy tube placement is confirmed with an intraoperative nephrostogram before suturing the tube to the skin. The safety wire is not removed until the tube is in good position and bleeding from the tract has subsided.

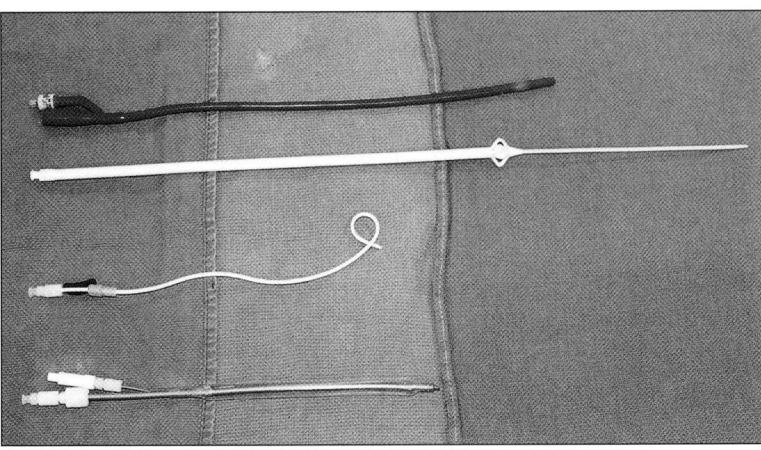

FIGURE 9-18. Nephrostomy tubes. Various nephrostomy tubes are available for use after percutaneous nephrolithotomy (PNL), and the specific type used varies with the clinical situation. For routine use, a regular 18-F Foley catheter (*top*) may be used, in which case the working sheath must be cut off from around the tube. The Malecot re-entry tube (*second from top*) is a good choice when a secondary procedure is planned (or likely) or if there is considerable edema at the ureteropelvic junction (UPJ). The ureteral tail at the distal end facilitates guidewire placement during secondary procedures, and it allows UPJ edema to subside before tube removal. For uncomplicated cases in which blood loss is minimal, a 10-F Cope tube (*third from top*) may be used. A Kaye nephrostomy tamponade balloon catheter (*bottom*) is placed over a guidewire and is inflated to tamponade bleeding from the nephrostomy tract if bleeding does not subside 5 minutes after removal of the working sheath.

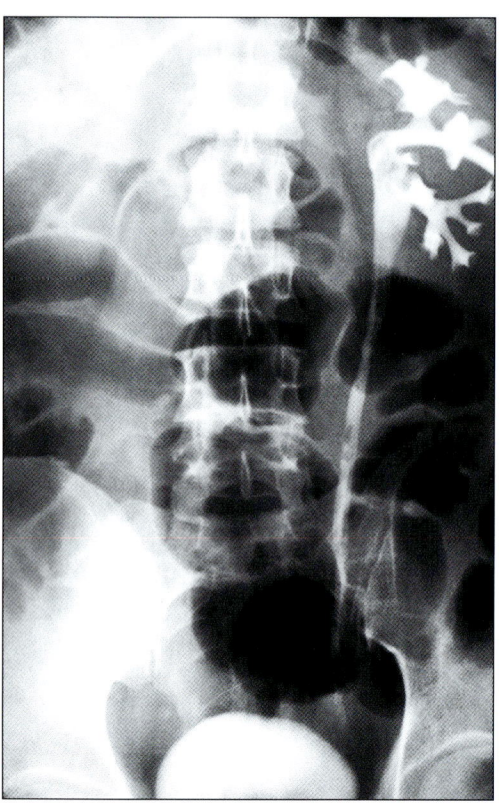

▶ **FIGURE 9-19.** Postoperative care. Nephrostograms and nephrotomograms are performed 24 to 48 hours after percutaneous nephrolithotomy (PNL). In patients with radiolucent stones or whose body habitus precludes adequate imaging, a noncontrast CT scan may be performed as an alternative. Nephrostomy tubes are removed after 48 hours if the imaging studies reveal no residual stones, an intact collecting system, and antegrade flow of contrast into the bladder. Patients with residual fragments are scheduled for secondary flexible nephroscopy.

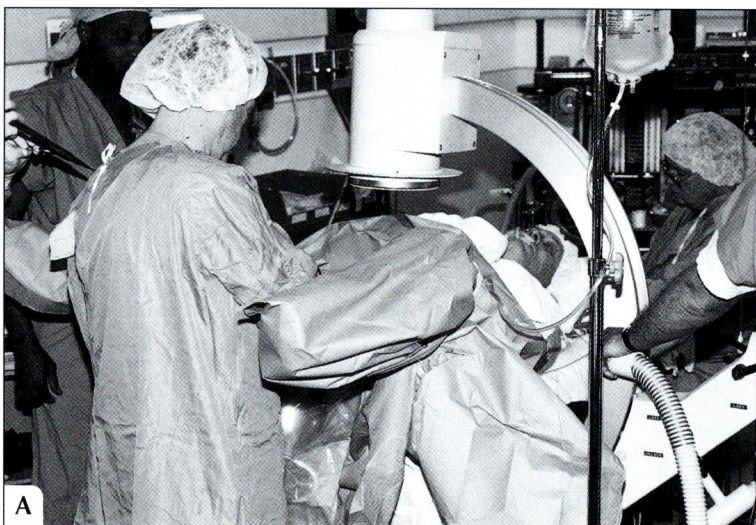
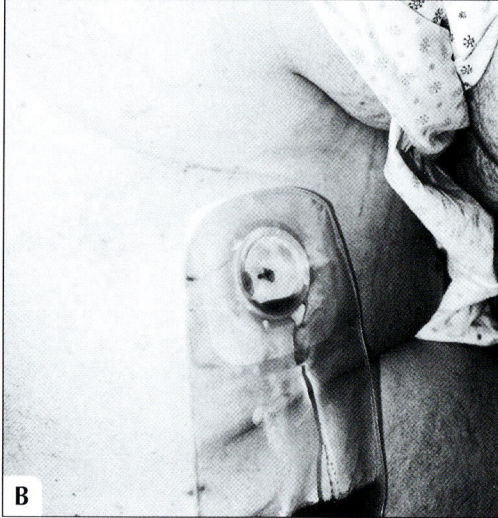

▶ **FIGURE 9-20.** Secondary flexible nephroscopy. **A,** The nephrostomy tract matures quickly so that after 48 hours, flexible nephroscopy can be performed without a working sheath in a nearly bloodless field. The secondary procedure is generally performed under intravenous sedation, unless additional access tracts are required. Stone fragmentation and extraction techniques are identical to those described previously for the primary procedure.

B, If the patient is stone-free, no additional access tracts are required during secondary nephroscopy, and bleeding is minimal, a collection bag is placed on the flank and the patient is discharged. Drainage from the tract typically stops within 24 hours, and patients are instructed to contact the urologist if drainage has not stopped in 1 week.

Complications of Percutaneous Nephrolithotomy

Bleeding: arteriovenous fistula, false aneurysm
Perforation or extravasation
Adjacent organ injury to colon, pleural cavity, liver, spleen, duodenum
Ureteral obstruction
Water intoxication
Infection: fever or urosepsis

▶ **FIGURE 9-21.** Complications of percutaneous nephrolithotomy (PNL). Some bleeding from the renal parenchyma occurs during every PNL procedure; however, transfusion is required in fewer than 2% of patients in the absence of pre-existing factors such as anemia. A Kaye nephrostomy tamponade balloon catheter is kept in the operating room to tamponade undue heavy bleeding that may occur following working sheath removal. Delayed bleeding should prompt concern about the presence of an arteriovenous fistula or a false aneurysm. Perforation and extravasation are managed by nephrostomy tube drainage alone. Virtually all perforations will heal with time, and closure is confirmed with a nephrostogram. The pleural cavity is commonly transversed during upper pole punctures; however, lung injury is extremely rare provided the puncture is performed in full expiration. Placing a working sheath into the upper pole during PNL minimizes the likelihood of hydrothorax. Fluoroscopic evaluation of the chest is performed in all patients with supracostal punctures to rule out pneumo- and hydrothoraces. Hydrothoraces are drained in the operating room with an 8-F ureteral catheter before waking the patient, and a chest tube is not left in place. Bowel injury during PNL occurs in fewer than one in 1000 cases and is usually heralded by high fever resistant to postoperative antibiotic therapy. Confirmation is via nephrostogram. In the absence of overwhelming sepsis or intraperitoneal extravasation, these injuries are managed simply by ureteral stent insertion, prolonged nephrostomy tube drainage, and antibiotic therapy. Open surgical repair is generally not recommended or necessary. Ureteral obstruction by fragment migration does occasionally occur and is managed ureteroscopically or with shock wave lithotripsy. Water intoxication should not occur so long as saline is used as the irrigant, but fluid overload may occur with large collecting system perforations. Management is diuretic correction in symptomatic patients. Fever commonly occurs postoperatively because many stones are infected. Urosepsis is uncommon provided patients are adequately treated with preoperative and perioperative antibiotics.

REFERENCES

1. Fernstrom I, Johansson B: Percutaneous pyelolithotomy: a new extraction technique. *Scand J Urol Nephrol* 1976, 10:257–259.

2. Segura JW, Patterson DE, LeRoy AJ, *et al.*: Percutaneous removal of kidney stones: preliminary report. *Mayo Clin Proc* 1982, 57:615–619.

3. Clayman RV, Surya V, Miller RP, *et al.*: Percutaneous nephrolithotomy: extraction of renal and ureteral calculi from 100 patients. *J Urol* 1984, 131:868–871.

4. Lam HS, Lingeman JE, Mosbaugh PM, *et al.*: Evolution of the technique of combination therapy for staghorn calculi: a decreasing role for extracorporeal shock wave lithotripsy. *J Urol* 1992, 148:1058–1062.

5. Davidoff R, Bellman GC: Influence of technique of percutaneous tract creation on incidence of renal hemorrhage. *J Urol* 1997, 157:1229–1231.

6. Denstedt JD, Razvi HA, Sales JL, *et al.*: Preliminary experience with holmium:YAG laser lithotripsy. *J Endourol* 1995, 9:255–258.

7. Grasso M: Experience with the holmium laser as an endoscopic lithotrite. *Urology* 1996, 48:199–206.

8. Lingeman JE, Newmark JR, Wong MR: Classification and management of staghorn calculi. In *Controversies in Endourology*. Edited by Smith AD. Philadelphia: WB Saunders; 1995:136–145.

Ureteroscopic Management of Renal Stones

Demetrius H. Bagley

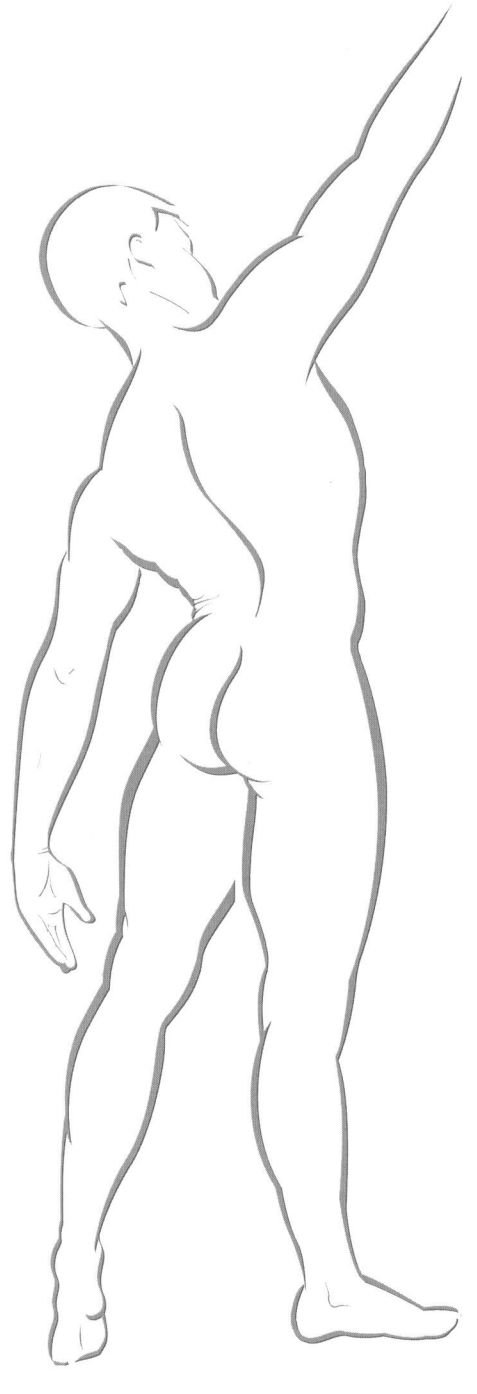

Ureteroscopy has been extremely successful in the treatment of ureteral calculi. Distal ureteral stones have been treated with a wide variety of ureteroscopes and endoscopic lithotriptors. Recent development of small-diameter rigid and flexible endoscopes and more effective lithotriptors has allowed extension of these same techniques into the mid- and proximal ureter with excellent results. Application of the techniques to the renal pelvis and intrarenal collecting system is a reasonable next step.

The primary methods of treating renal calculi have been shock-wave lithotripsy (SWL) and percutaneous nephrostolithotomy [1–3]. SWL has been widely applied for renal calculi but now is more selectively used for smaller or more fragile stones. Large stones (> 2.5 cm) and branched stones are more effectively treated with percutaneous nephrostolithotomy [4]. Initially, ureteroscopy was used for renal stones in patients who had a ureteral stone treated with ureteroscopy or proximal ureteral calculi that had moved retrograde into the intrarenal collecting system. Successful treatment of those patients prompted the application of the ureteroscopic techniques to patients in whom shock-wave lithotripsy has failed or those who have a contraindication to SWL or percutaneous nephrostomy, such as massive obesity or an uncorrectable bleeding disorder [5,6].

Several advances have rendered ureteroscopic stone management both technically easier and more effective. Small-diameter ureteroscopes, which are approximately 7 to 8 F in diameter, are available in both rigid and flexible designs [7,8]. These endoscopes can usually enter the ureteral orifice without dilation, and there is room between the instrument itself and the ureteral wall for drainage of irrigant, stone, or tissue fragments into the bladder. These instruments are easier to insert into the ureter and easier to manipulate within the collecting system. More effective small-diameter grasping devices have also become available. There are numerous styles of baskets, each of which has a particular purpose and advantage related to its design. One of the major advances that has allowed effective fragmentation of large calculi is the holmium yttrium-aluminum-garnet (YAG) laser [9–11]. This instrument has been effective in fragmenting all types of calculi and has an ablative effect. Using the holmium laser, the largest volume of stone is removed as tiny fragments in the irrigant. Although other larger fragments remain, much of the stone volume is removed during the laser lithotripsy.

The very high success rate for ureteroscopy in treating ureteral stones has been achieved in the kidney as well [5,12]. The same endoscopes, lithotriptors, and grasping devices are just as successful a few centimeters more proximally within the intrarenal collecting system as they are within the ureter. Numerous advantages can be seen with this approach. As noted, higher-risk patients can be treated in this way. The volume and size of fragments remaining can be estimated, and a very high success rate is achieved. The ureteroscopic treatment of renal calculi is a very practical technique that can be used as primary therapy in selected patients.

TYPES AND USES OF URETEROSCOPES

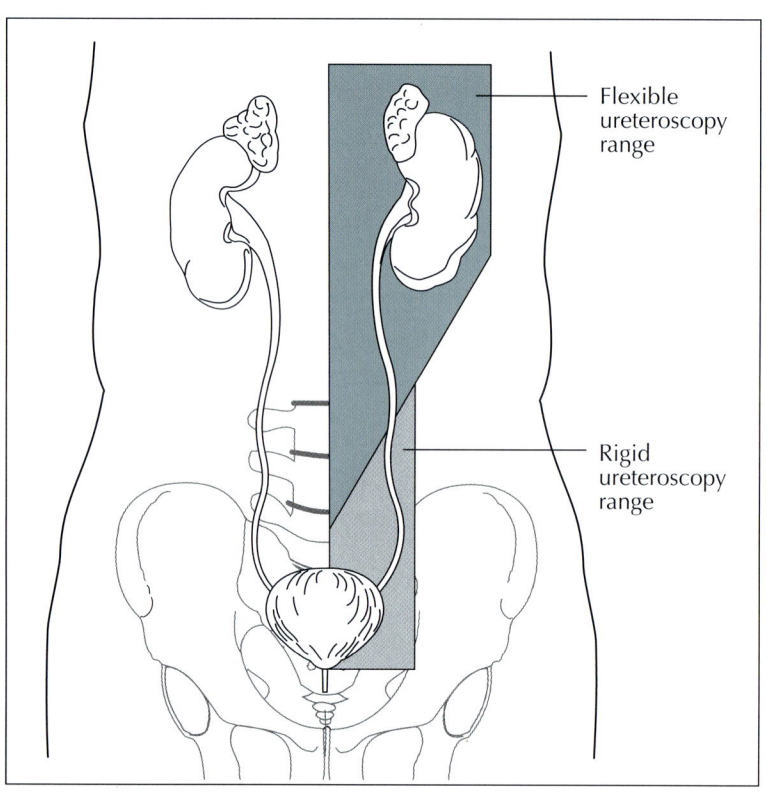

▶ **FIGURE 10-1.** Ureteroscopes. The rigid and flexible ureteroscopes are complementary instruments, each with its optimal area of access within the ureter and intrarenal collecting system [13]. The small-diameter rigid ureteroscopes can be placed under direct vision, usually without prior dilation. The rigid ureteroscopes can be expected to reach to the lower margin of the bony pelvis in any patient regardless of body configuration or sex. This rigid instrument can often be passed further, to the mid- or even proximal ureter or even into the renal pelvis, particularly in thin women. Because it is usually easier to manipulate and work through a rigid endoscope, it is the instrument of choice if it will reach the selected point in the ureter easily. It is more difficult to pass a rigid ureteroscope above the iliac vessels, however, and in this case the flexible ureteroscope is preferentially used. The optimal area for the flexible ureteroscope is the mid and proximal ureter, as well as the intrarenal collecting system.

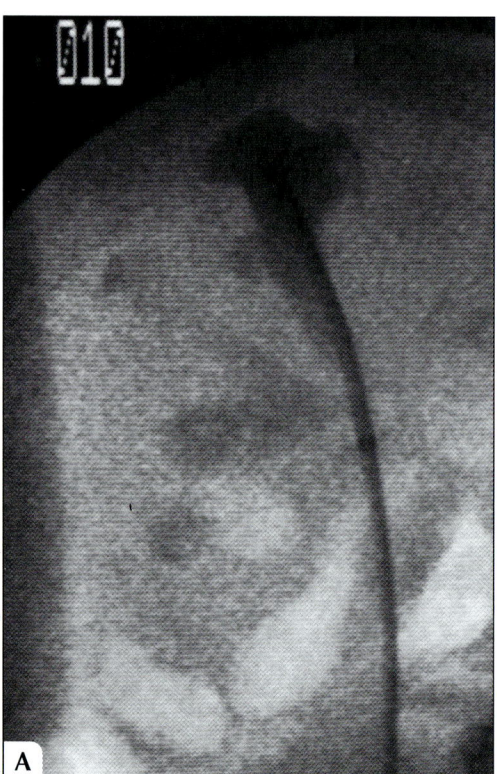

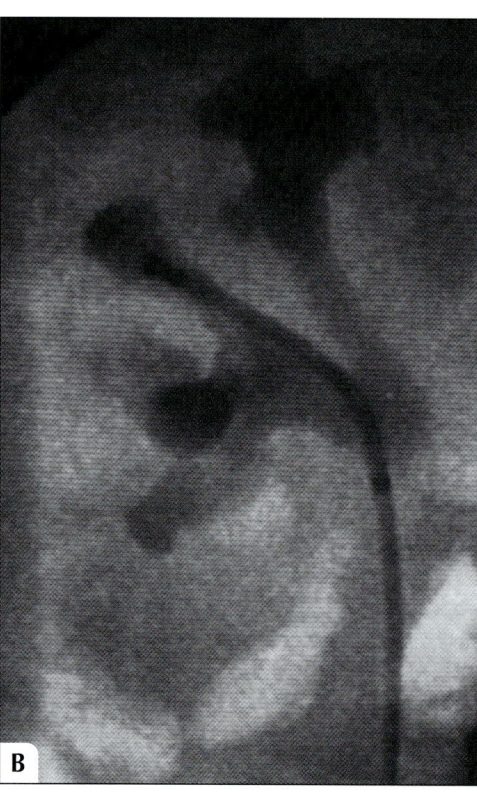

▶ **FIGURE 10-2.** Use of the flexible ureteroscope. Within the kidney, the flexible ureteroscope can be used to access the entire collecting system in more than 90% of patients (**A** to **D**).

(*Continued on next page*)

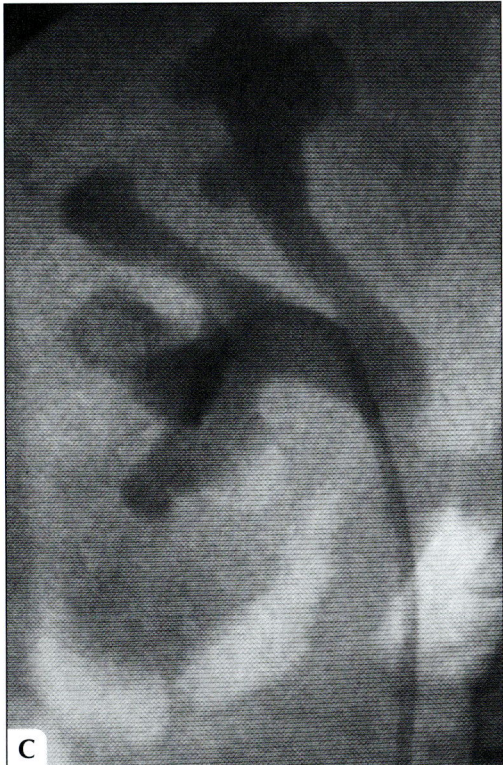

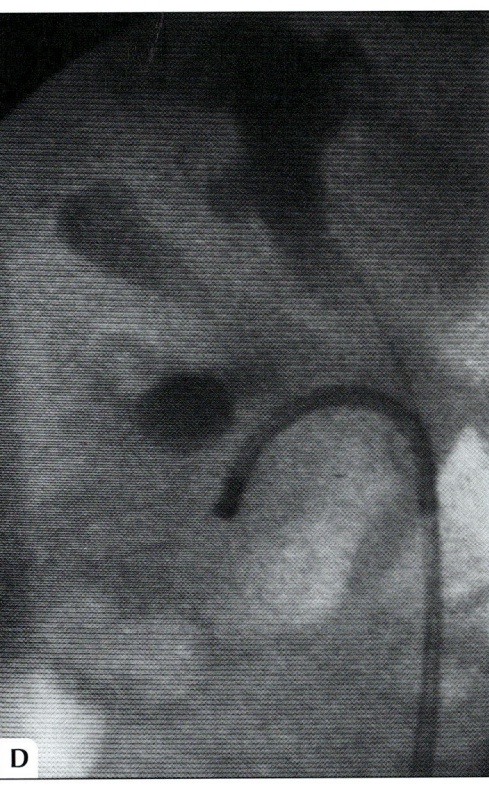

▶ **FIGURE 10-2.** (*Continued*) It is always more difficult to reach the lower infundibula, however (*panel D*). The position can be followed fluoroscopically. When any working instrument is present within the channel, deflection will be limited [14]. The extent of this loss of deflection is related to the specific working instruments. Stiffer devices, such as larger retrieval instruments or larger-diameter laser fibers, limit deflection more than small, more flexible devices.

POSITIONING

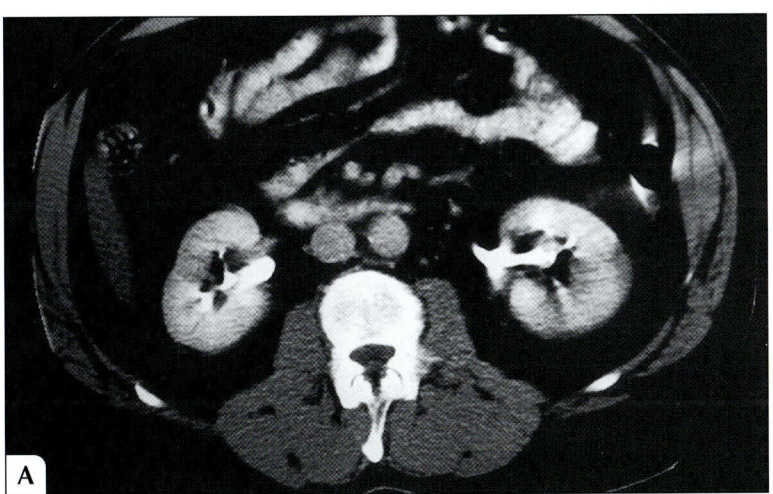

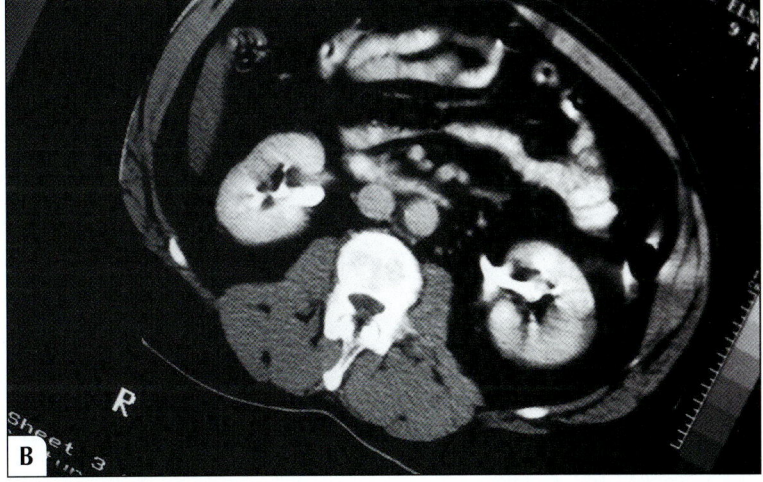

▶ **FIGURE 10-3.** Position of a posterior infundibulum with the patient in two positions. The patient can be positioned to increase the chance of a calculus remaining within the renal pelvis or even passing to the upper infundibulum. The proper positioning minimizes the chance of a calculus falling into a lower infundibulum that is more difficult to access. Because the posterior infundibula pass quite steeply posteriorly and the anterior infundibula are more lateral, elevation of the ipsilateral flank can render the anterior infundibula more truly anterior and the posterior more nearly lateral. These CT scans of the kidney with contrast in the collecting system demonstrate the position of a posterior infundibulum with the patient in the supine position (**A**) and also when the flank is elevated 30° (**B**).

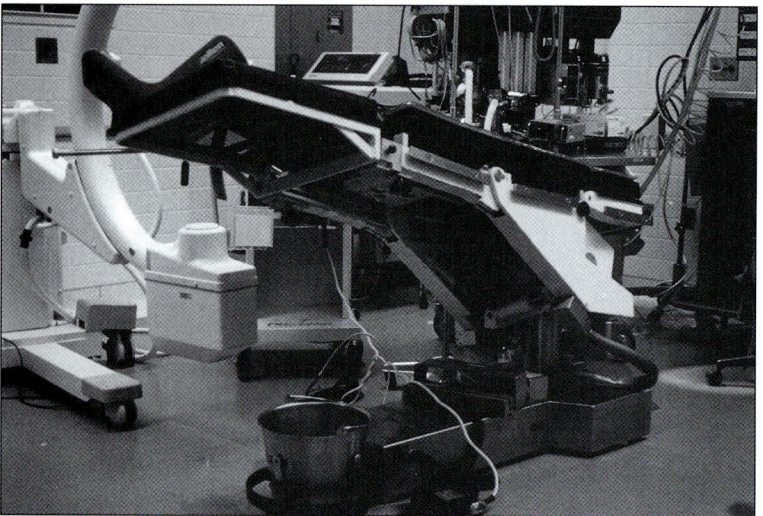

▶ **FIGURE 10-4.** Position of machinery. Placing the patient in the Trendelenburg position will render the renal pelvis or the upper infundibula more dependent. Therefore, a stone or fragments within the renal pelvis are more likely to remain in the pelvis or even to pass into the upper infundibulum in a patient in the Trendelenburg position with the ipsilateral flank elevated than in a patient who is lying flat. In comparison, the reverse Trendelenburg position (previously used for ureteral stones) would tend to encourage a stone or fragment to fall into the lower infundibulum, where it is less accessible to the flexible ureteroscope.

STONE RETRIEVAL

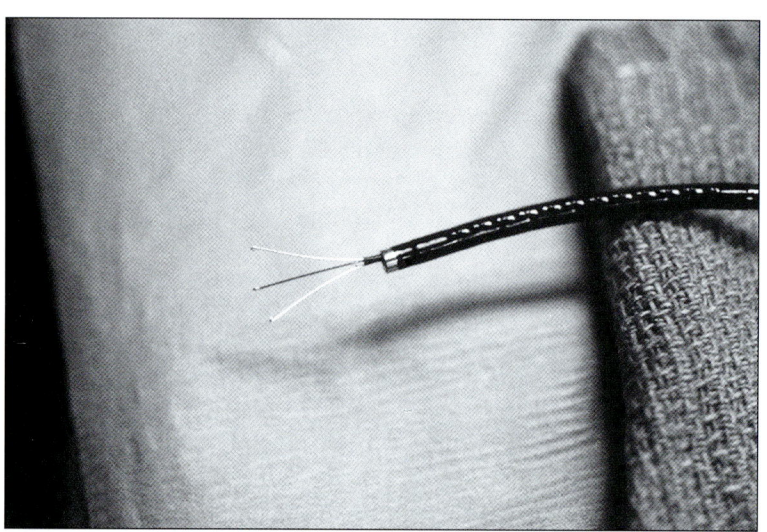

▶ **FIGURE 10-5.** (*See* Color Plate) A wire-pronged grasper for stone retrieval. Retrieval of the calculus within the kidney is the most effective technique to remove the entire stone. It can be performed only when the stone is small enough to pass through the ureter. Because the flexible ureteroscopes contain a single channel, only one working device can be placed through the channel and still leave adequate room for irrigation. Therefore, a device that can reversibly grasp the calculus is preferred. A wire-pronged grasper (*ie*, the three-pronged grasper) is most effective. It offers a compromise between firmly holding the calculus and being able to release it.

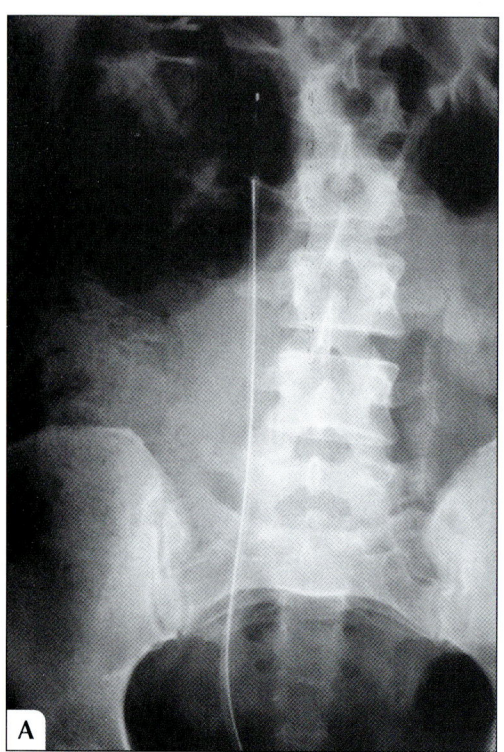
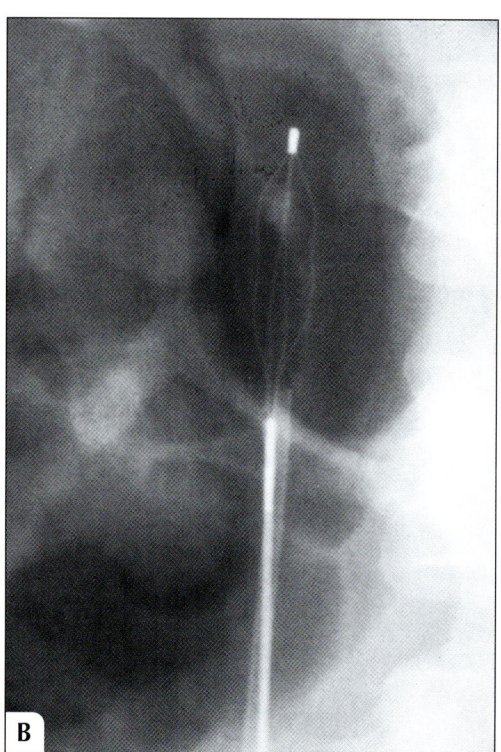

A

B

▶ **FIGURE 10-6.** The use of a basket for stone retrieval (**A** and **B**). Some authors have recommended the use of a basket within the kidney for retrieval of stones. The risk with this device is that the stone being withdrawn may become lodged in the ureter. In this situation, the handle must be removed to allow removal of the ureteroscope, which can then be placed into the ureter again beside the shaft of the basket to fragment the stone within the basket.

Comparison of Endoscopic Lithotriptors

	Effective Fragmentation	Safety	Stone removal	Cost
EHL	+++	+	0	+
Ultrasound	++	+++	++++	+
Impact	++++	+++	0	+
Lasers				
Pulsed dye	++	+++	0	++++
Holmium	++++	++	++	+++

▶ **FIGURE 10-7.** Comparison of endoscopic lithotriptors. Calculi that are too large to be removed intact through the ureter must be fragmented within the kidney for removal. There are several devices that can be placed through the channel of the flexible ureteroscope to break calculi. The major instruments for this purpose are the electrohydraulic lithotriptor (EHL) [15,16], the pulsed dye laser [17,18], and the holmium yttrium-aluminum-garnet (YAG) laser [10,11,19].

The electrohydraulic lithotriptor has been used widely throughout the urinary tract. Probes as small as 1.6 to 1.9 F are available. These limit deflection of the flexible ureteroscope very little. The fragmentation effect produced with a bubble formed at the tip of the probe during activation is predominantly directed parallel to the device from the tip [16]. There is some lateral scattering of energy that can affect the urothelium. It can also be used for fragmentation of calculi, particularly in the lower pole when direct contact with the laser fiber or the electrohydraulic lithotriptor probe is impossible. During fragmentation, no volume of stone is removed; fragments are formed that must either be removed or allowed to pass. It remains an effective device for endoscopic lithotripsy.

The pulsed dye laser was the first practical laser for endoscopic lithotripsy [17]. It is a very safe device that has minimal effect on tissue but can fragment most calculi. It is not effective against cystine stones, however, and is less effective against very hard, dense stones such as calcium oxalate monohydrate or brushite. This laser can also be used through a small 200-μm fiber. Its limitations are practical considerations in that it is expensive to operate and can be used only for calculi. Its limited effectiveness is also a negative factor.

The most effective and efficient endoscopic lithotriptor for use in the flexible ureteroscope, particularly within the kidney, is the holmium YAG laser [10,11,19,20]. This device fragments a urinary calculus and removes the volume of the calculus during the fragmentation. Small particles of stone are released into the irrigant and washed from the kidney. A large volume of the stone is removed during fragmentation with the holmium laser. Numerous small pieces also remain and must be broken into fragments small enough to pass or be withdrawn through the ureter. This is the most difficult and tedious part of the procedure but is extremely important to its success. The holmium laser is delivered through a bare fiber, and any energy is absorbed within 0.4 mm of water. Therefore, the fiber must touch the surface of the calculus to be effective. Various fibers are available with a 365-μm or 200-μm core and are most effective for ureteroscopic lithotripsy. The smaller fiber limits deflection of the flexible ureteroscope by only a few degrees, whereas the larger fiber limits deflection to approximately 90°.

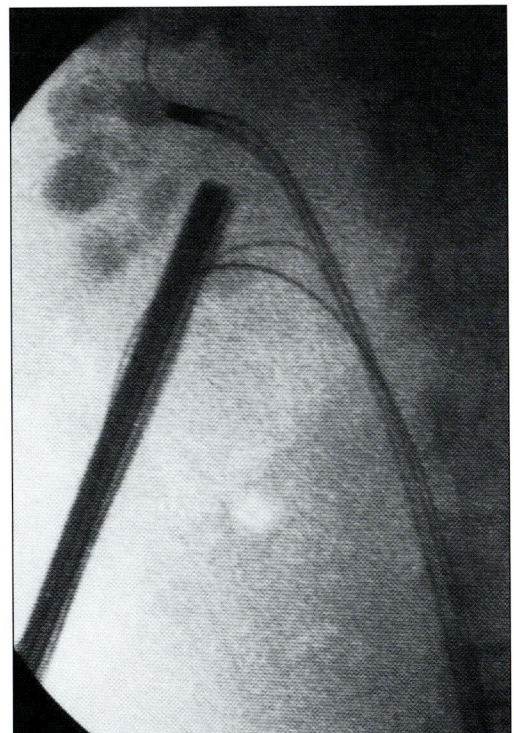

▶ **FIGURE 10-8.** Ureteroscopy. This technique can be used with other techniques for treatment of calculi. Simultaneous percutaneous nephrostolithotomy and ureteroscopic lithotripsy can be very effective in combining the major benefits of each approach [21,22]. Percutaneous nephrostolithotomy allows removal of a large volume of calculus, particularly that accessible to a rigid endoscope and the ultrasonic lithotriptor. The flexible ureteroscope can be used to access portions of the intrarenal collecting system that are inaccessible or accessible only with difficulty through a percutaneous tract. Some areas can be approached better from a different angle. For example, infundibula parallel and adjacent to the percutaneous nephrostomy tract may be very difficult to reach through that tract, whereas they may be quite accessible to a flexible ureteroscope passed through the ureter.

Simultaneous ureteroscopy and shock-wave lithotripsy (SWL) can be performed on some lithotriptor tables. The ureteroscope can be used to determine the effect of shock-wave lithotripsy and the extent of fragmentation and then to fragment the stone should SWL be unsuccessful. This combined technique has produced a nearly 100% success rate in treating renal stones in one series.

Ureteroscopic Treatment of Renal Calculi

	Percent
Overall success	89
Stone free	77
Asymptomatic fragments (< 3 mm)	12
Simultaneous ureteral calculi	56

▶ **FIGURE 10-9.** Ureteroscopic treatment of renal calculi. This treatment has been very successful. In a series of 100 patients with renal calculi treated with ureteroscopy, Fabrizio *et al.* [6] found an overall success rate of 89%. This included the 77% of patients who had complete clearance of their renal calculi after ureteroscopic treatment within 3 months and another 12% who had asymptomatic fragments less than 3 mm in diameter remaining. Some of these patients (56%) also had ureteral calculi treated simultaneously, and all those stones were removed at the same time. Many of the renal calculi were actually incidental stones noted at the time of treatment of the ureteral stones. Of the targeted renal stones, however, 98% were removed or fragmented.

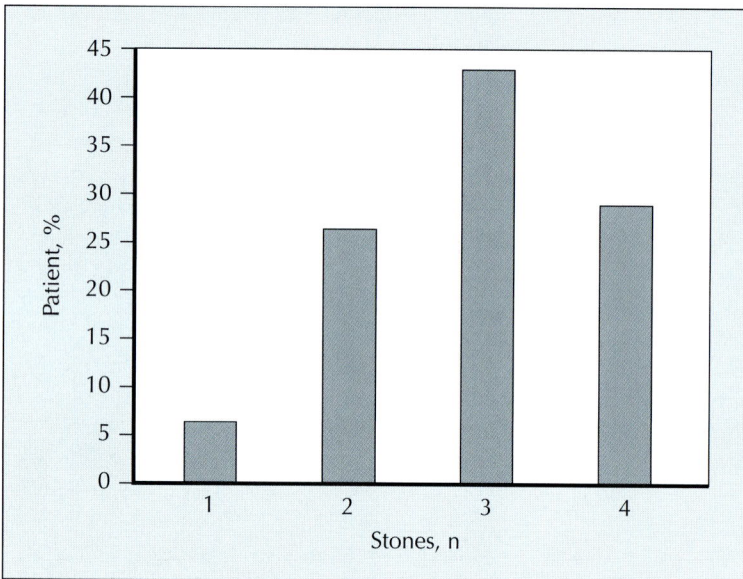

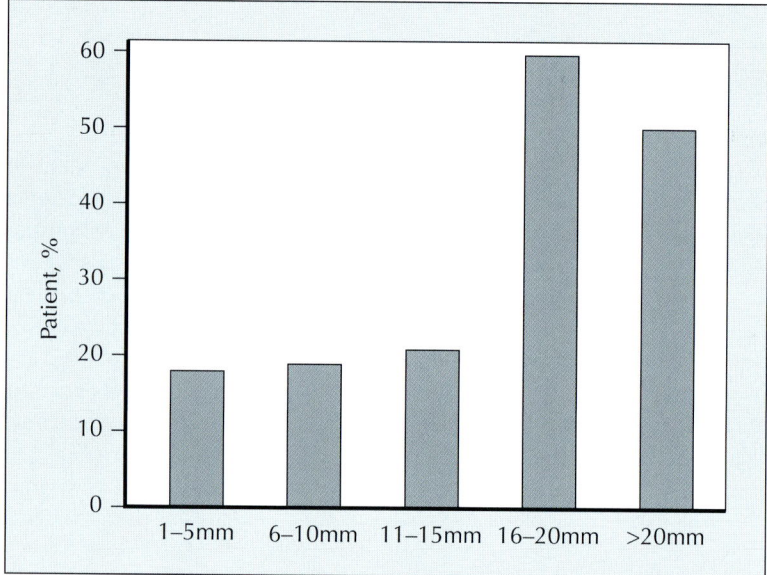

▶ **FIGURE 10-10.** Residual calculi versus original number of renal calculi. The success of treatment was related to the number of renal stones present and also to their size. When there was a single renal stone, only 6% had residual calculi. This rate of residual stones increased to 42% when there were three stones present, however, and there was a residual rate of more than 25% for both two and four or more stones. (*From* Fabrizio [6].)

▶ **FIGURE 10-11.** Residual calculi versus original renal calculi size. The residual stone rate was similar at less than 20% for stones 5 to 15 mm in diameter. The rate increased from 50% to 60% for stones 16 mm and more in diameter, however. (*From* Fabrizio [6].)

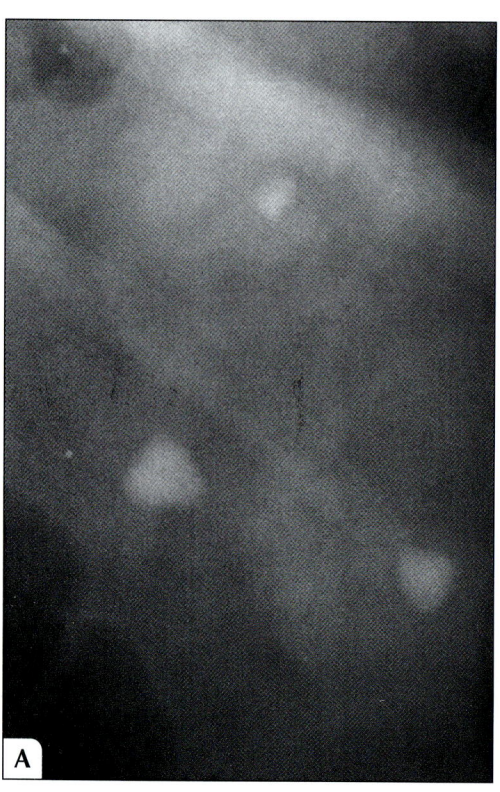

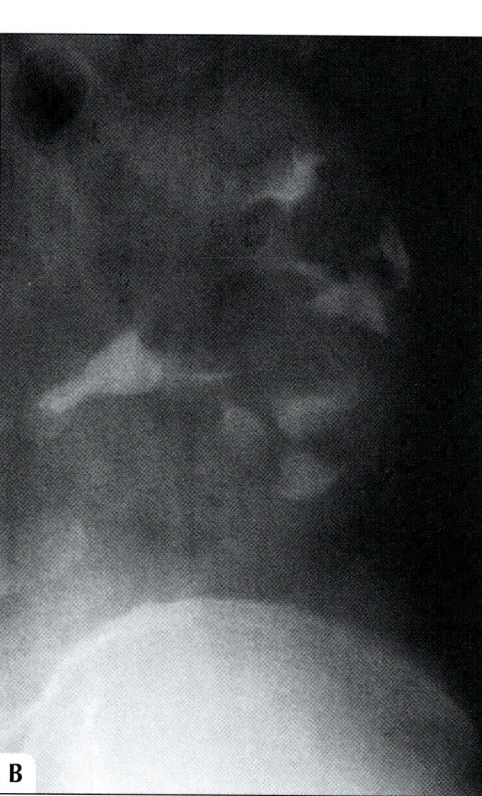

▶ **FIGURE 10-12.** Use of ureteroscopic laser lithotripsy for large stones. Even larger volumes of stone (≥ 2 cm in largest dimension), can be successfully treated with ureteroscopic laser lithotripsy [23,24]. **A,** One of the first patients treated this way was a 350-lb man with three renal stones. **B,** A film from the excretory urogram demonstrates the three calculi located in the renal pelvis and the upper and lower calyces. Any percutaneous access would allow a rigid endoscope to reach only two of the stones, necessitating a flexible endoscopic approach to the remaining stone. Therefore, the patient was treated with flexible ureteroscopic holmium laser lithotripsy. Each calculus could be reached and fragmented effectively.

(*Continued on next page*)

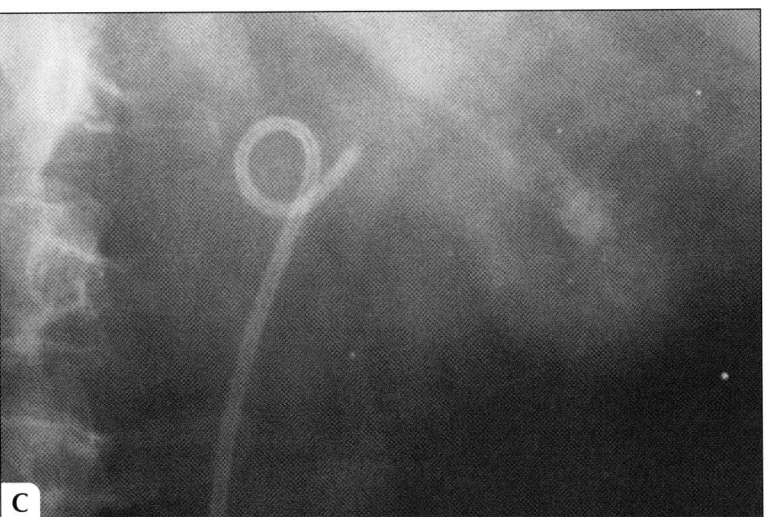

▶ **FIGURE 10-12.** (*Continued*) **C,** After surgery there were several small fragments in the lower pole only. These fragments subsequently cleared. The results in this patient demonstrate the potential for effective therapy in patients with a large stone burden.

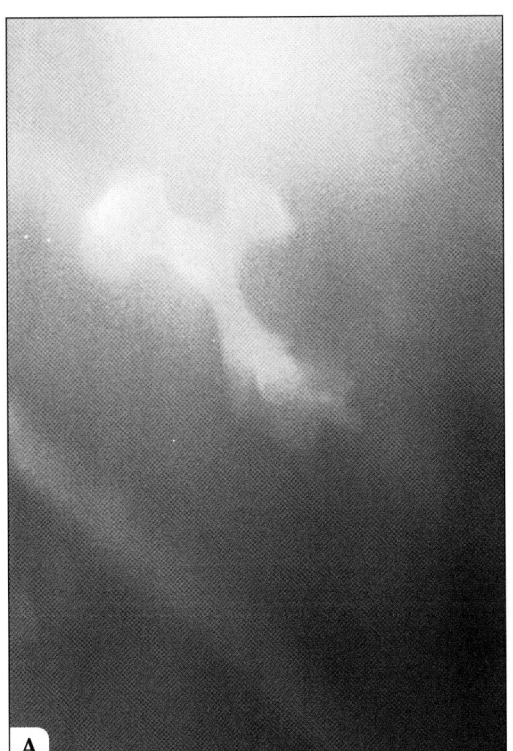

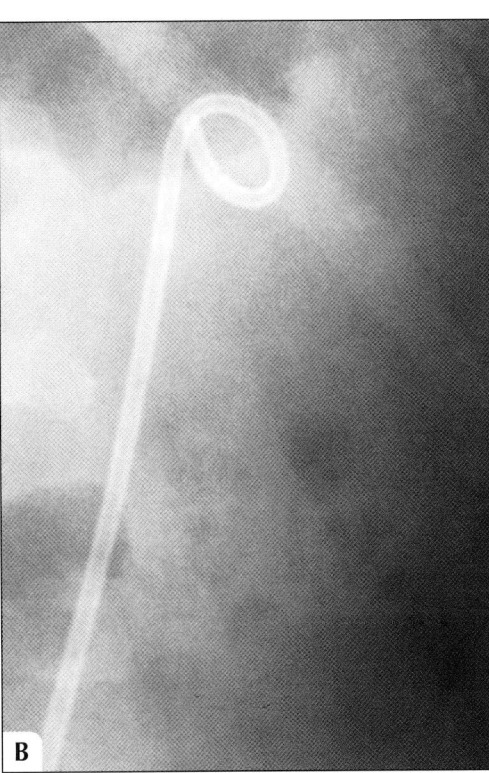

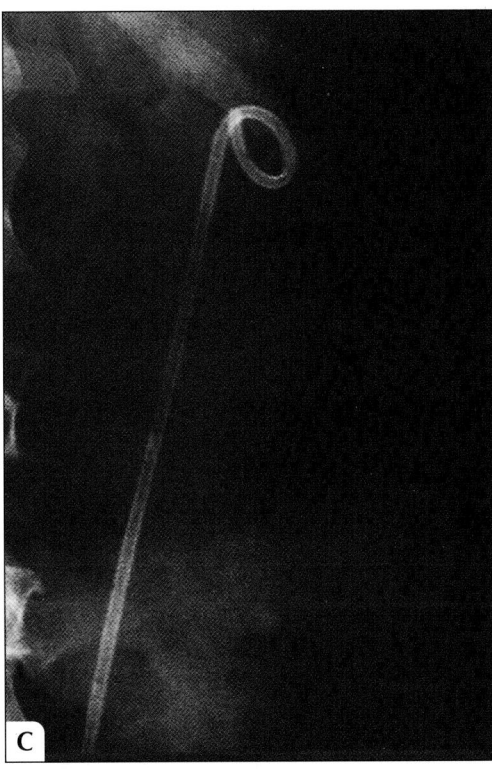

▶ **FIGURE 10-13.** Ureteroscopic laser lithotripsy for difficult cases. **A,** A 33-year-old woman evaluated for microscopic hematuria was found to have a 50 x 15 mm branched calculus in the left upper pole. The entire upper pole of the kidney was located above the 12th rib, and a portion of it was above the 11th rib. Because of the patient's size (*ie,* 275 lbs), and the location of the stone, it was believed that direct access to the calculus with percutaneous nephrostomy would be difficult. Shock wave lithotripsy was not considered a good choice because of the high failure rate for a stone of this size. The patient was offered ureteroscopic laser lithotripsy. The advan-

tages of this procedure are the possibility of a single procedure as an outpatient without the need for a nephrostomy or hospitalization and the higher failure rate associated with shock wave lithotripsy. The stone was treated with a 7.5-F flexible ureteroscope using the holmium laser. A total of 16.8 kJ of energy was used for stone fragmentation. **B,** At the completion of the procedure, a kidney, ureter, and bladder film demonstrated scattered small fragments of stone in the upper pole. **C,** Six days later, there were multiple fragments in the lower pole. The stent was removed at that time, and the remaining fragments have subsequently cleared.

ADVANTAGES OF URETEROSCOPIC APPROACH

Indications for Ureteroscopic Treatment of Renal Calculi

Failed ESWL
Obesity
Medical conditions precluding ESWL or PCN
Simultaneous ureteral calculi
Advantages of lithotomy position

▶ **FIGURE 10-14.** Indications for ureteroscopic treatment of renal calculi. There are several advantages of ureteroscopic laser lithotripsy for certain patients. It has been applied to patients with special indications, including those in whom extracorporeal shock wave lithotripsy (ESWL) has failed, the obese patient, and those with medical indications such as severe pulmonary disease. Others who have refused the percutaneous nephroscopic approach have also been treated successfully with ureteroscopic laser lithotripsy.

There are also specific advantages of the ureteroscopic approach, including the ability to place the patient in the lithotomy position for therapy. In addition, there is no need for a percutaneous nephrostomy tract. The calculi can be treated with a high success rate with holmium laser lithotripsy in a single procedure. The remaining options are to use other endoscopic lithotriptors available (*ie*, the electrohydraulic lithotriptor (EHL), or the pulsed dye laser). The endoscopic procedure can be combined with ESWL when necessary. PCN—percutaneous nephrostomy.

REFERENCES

1. Drach GW, Dretler SP, Fair WR, *et al.*: Report of the United States cooperative study of extracorporeal shock wave lithotripsy. *J Urol* 1986,135:1127–1133.

2. LeRoy AJ, Segura JW, Williams HJ, Jr., Patterson DE: Percutaneous renal calculus removal in an extracorporeal shock wave lithotripsy practice. *J Urol* 1987, 138:703–706.

3. Segura JW, Patterson DE, LeRoy AJ, *et al.*: Percutaneous removal of kidney stones: review of 1,000 cases. *J Urol* 1985,134:1077–1081.

4. Lam HS, Lingeman JE, Barron M, *et al.*: Staghorn calculi: analysis of treatment results between initial percutaneous nephrostolithotomy and extracorporeal shock wave lithotripsy monotherapy with reference to surface area. *J Urol* 1992, 147:1219–1225.

5. Fuchs A, Fuchs G: Retrograde intrarenal surgery for calculus disease: new minimally invasive treatment approach. *J Endourol* 1990, 4:337–345.

6. Fabrizio MD, Behari A, Bagley DH: Ureteroscopic management of intrarenal calculi. *J Urol* 1998, 159:1139–1143.

7. Abdel-Razzak OM, Bagley DH: The 6.9 F semi-rigid ureteroscope in clinical use. *Urology* 1993, 41:45–48

8. Grasso M, Bagley DH: A 7.5 F actively deflectable, flexible ureteroscope: a new plateau in both diagnostic and therapeutic upper urinary tract endoscopy. *Urology* 1994, 43:435–441.

9. Johnson DE, Cromeens DM, Price RE: Use of the holmium: YAG laser in urology. *Lasers Surg Med* 1992, 12:353–363.

10. Denstedt JD, Razvi HA, Sales JL, Eberwein P: Preliminary experience with holmium: YAG laser lithotripsy. *J Endourol* 1995, 9:255–258.

11. Erhard MJ, Bagley DH: Urologic applications of the holmium laser: preliminary experience. *J Endourol* 1995, 9:383–386.

12. Erhard MJ, Salwen J, Bagley DH: Ureteroscopic removal of mid and proximal ureteral calculi. *J Urol* 1996, 155:38–42.

13. Bagley DH: Ureteroscopic stone retrieval: rigid versus flexible endoscopes. *Semin Urol* 1994, 12:32–38.

14. Poon M, Beaghler M, Baldwin D: Flexible endoscope deflectability: changes using a variety of working instruments and laser fibers. *J Endourol* 1997, 11:247–249.

15. Reuter HJ, Kern E: Electronic lithotripsy of ureteral calculi. *J Urol* 1973, 110:181–183.

16. Vorrenther R: New tip design and shock wave pattern of electrohydraulic probes for endoureteral lithotripsy. *J Endourol* 1993, 7:35–43.

17. Dretler SP, Watson G, Parrish JA, Murray S: Pulsed dye laser fragmentation of ureteral calculi: initial clinical experience. *J Urol* 1987, 137:386–386.

18. Grasso M, Shalaby MA, El-Akkad MA, Bagley DH: Techniques in endoscopic lithotripsy using the pulsed dye laser. *Urology* 1991, 37:138–144.

19. Bagley DH, Erhard MJ: Use of the holmium laser in the upper urinary tract. *Tech Urol* 1995, 1:25–30.

20. Grasso M: Experience with the holmium laser as an endoscopic lithotrite. *Urology* 1996, 48:199–206.

21. Grasso M, Nord RG, Bagley DH: Prone split leg and flank roll positioning: simultaneous antegrade and retrograde access to the upper urinary tract. *J Endourol* 1993, 7:307–310.

22. Nord RG, Goodman AC, Bagley DH: Prone split leg position for simultaneous retrograde ureteroscopic and percutaneous nephroscopic procedures. *J Endourol* 1991, 5:13–16.

23. Grasso M, Conlin M, Bagley DH: Retrograde ureteropyeloscopic treatment of large upper urinary tract (≥ 2 cm) and minor staghorn calculi. *J Urol* 1998, 160:346–351.

24. Poon M, Beaghler M: Ureterorenoscopy treatment of large upper urinary tract calculi. [abstract P2-15]. *J Endourol* 1997, 11(suppl 1):S97.

Incisional Surgery for Renal Stones

Silas Pettersson

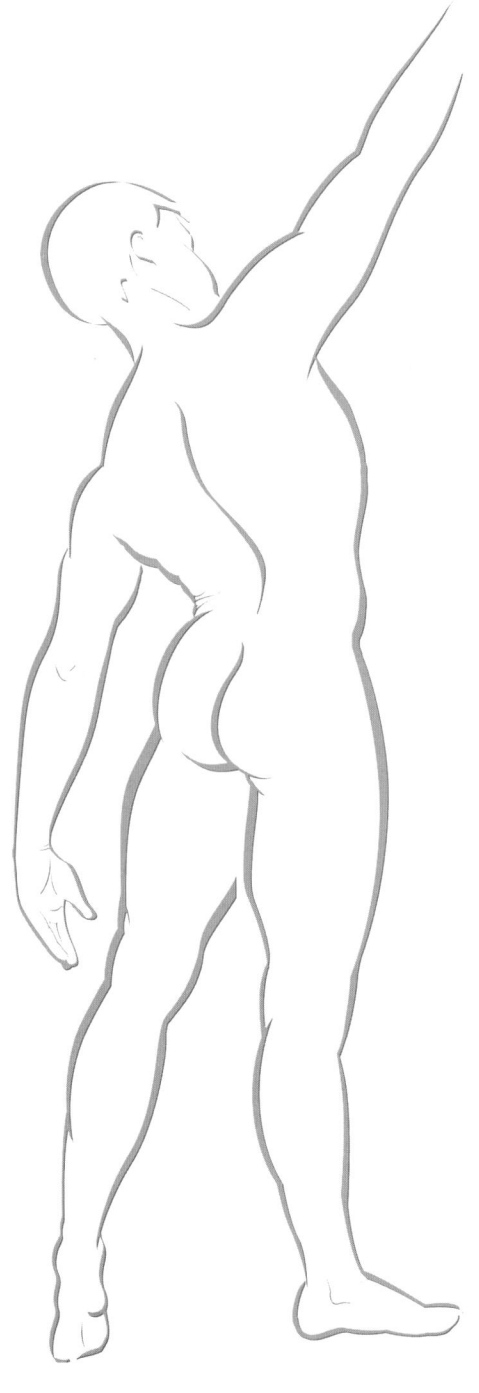

The first planned nephrectomy is usually attributed to Simon (1870) [1], the first nephrolithotomy to Morris (1880) [2], and the first pyelolithotomy to Czerny (1890) [3]. The latter used a longitudinal incision on the posterior surface of the pelvis. The length of the incision was limited on one side by the retropyelic artery and the renal parenchyma, and on the other side by the pyeloureteral junction. Because of these limitations and the previous descriptions by Hyrtl [4] and Brödel [5] of a relatively avascular plane on the lateral border of the kidney, urologists decided to use a bivalve nephrotomy for the removal of large stones. The frequent shortcomings of the above-described techniques (with a nephrectomy rate as high as 40% [6]) resulted in a resigned attitude regarding patients with complex stones like staghorn calculi, even though the urologist was well aware that these staghorn calculi eventually resulted in destruction of the kidney and a risk of septic complications [7]. Due to the limited access to the intrarenal collecting system from the pelvis in patients with large and more complex stones, a prolongation of the incision into the inferior calyx was suggested, incising the lower pole of the kidney [8]. Those enlarged pyelotomies, however, were soon abandoned because they often led to sectioning of the retropyelic vessels and, as a consequence, loss of renal parenchyma.

Based on the anatomic description by Henle [9] of the renal sinus and the fibrous diaphragm that secures the entrance to the sinus (as described by Disse [10]), Gil-Vernet introduced a new way to access the intrasinusal portion of the collecting system for pyelotomy and pyelofundibulotomy in 1965 [11]. Using this approach, damage to the parenchyma or its vessels could be avoided regardless of the extent of peripelvic sclerous reaction.

The atrophy that frequently resulted from a transparenchymal approach to a stone was simultaneously addressed in two different ways by separate groups. One was the anatrophic nephrotomy (ana-atrophic as opposed to atrophic) [12]; the other was the use of radial paravascular multiple nephrotomies [6,13]. Prerequisites for good results included ischemic hypothermia, introduced in renal surgery by Semb [14], and techniques of contact radiography [15].

INDICATIONS

Indications for Incisional Stone Surgery

Stones associated with anatomic abnormality requiring open operative
   intervention (*eg*, ureteropelvic junction obstruction, infundibular
   stenosis, calyceal diverticulum)
Complex stone burden for which only multiple percutaneous or extra-
   corporeal shock-wave procedures could render the patient stone
   free, as compared with a single open surgical procedure
Failure of previous extracorporeal shock wave lithotripsy or percuta-
   neous nephrostolithotomy
Ablative surgery of a nonfunctional stone-bearing kidney
Stones in morbidly obese patients
Comorbid medical disease
Patient preference

▶ FIGURE 11-1. Indications for surgery. The introduction of percutaneous and extracorporeal shock wave technologies dramatically changed the surgical management of renal stones. Today, less than 5% of patients are treated with open surgical techniques [16–19]. Although the basic indications for surgical treatment of stones have remained the same, the indications for an open operative intervention are relative, and the technique represents a reasonable alternative in only a limited number of patients.

PREOPERATIVE WORKUP

Preoperative Workup

Radiologic workup
   In anteroposterior and oblique projections (mandatory)
   Plain films (compulsory immediately prior to open surgery)
   Retrograde pyelography including rotational views (strongly recommended)
   Renal aortography (when anomalous arterial supply is anticipated)
Laboratory workup
   Serum creatinine/urea determination (mandatory)
   Total and separate glomerular filtration rate determination (strongly recommended in patients
      without normal contralateral kidney)
   Consultation with nephrologist (compulsory in severely depressed renal function)
   Urine culture (mandatory)
   Coagulation studies (mandatory before major surgery)
   Metabolic screening (strongly desirable)
Preparation of patient
   Hydration before surgery (strongly recommended)
   Antibiotics according to sensitivity testing (mandatory)
   Pulmonary embolus prophylaxis (mandatory)
   Kidney protective agents (according to the routines of the department)
   Marking kidney to be operated on (mandatory)

▶ FIGURE 11-2. Workup and preparation before surgery. Preoperative workup and preparation for open stone surgery differs in several respects from the workup required before minimally invasive stone procedures. A three-dimensional radiologic workup is desired for proper patient selection and to plan the type of intervention. An intravenous urogram (IVU), including tomography, is compulsory to demonstrate the number, size, and position of the stones; the configuration of the collecting system; and the outflow conditions. An IVU also provides information on the contralateral kidney. More detailed topographic information is obtained from retrograde pyelography, including anteroposterior, oblique, and lateral projections. A plain radiograph of the kidney and urinary tract is of utmost importance immediately before open surgery because the treatment strategy cannot be changed as easily once open surgery has begun; this is also true for large staghorn calculi.

A rough estimate of renal function is important to obtain. In patients with bilateral stone disease, a nonhealthy contralateral kidney, or stones in a solitary kidney, glomerular filtration rate plus computed isotope renography is warranted. If the renal function is severely impaired, estimations of serum electrolyte and bicarbonate levels are also of importance. In patients with severely depressed renal function, the patient should be informed that postoperative dialysis may be necessary.

Screening for urinary tract infections should always be undertaken before surgery so that the results of sensitivity testing are available a couple of days before surgery. Generalized coagulopathy should be ruled out by determining the platelet count, prothrombin time, bleeding time, and activated partial thromboplastin time. Metabolic screening with determination of the cause of the stones permits postoperative guidance and medical treatment, which are as important as the surgery itself in patients with urinary calculous disease.

Hydration is important if a period of vascular arrest is planned. It is achieved preferably by giving 1500 mL of lactated Ringer's solution by rapid infusion before induction of anesthesia [20]. Prophylaxis against pulmonary embolism should always be provided to this group of patients because the position during surgery impedes venous return; intermittent positive-pressure ventilation is required, and the intervention is usually fairly long. Minidose heparin (5000 U given subcutaneously 2 hours before surgery and then every 8 hours following surgery) is a common recommendation alone or in combination with antiembolic elastic stockings [21].

Antibiotic therapy should be started at least 48 hours before surgery. Prophylactic antibiotic therapy is provided according to departmental routine. As in all surgery on paired organs, it is of utmost importance to make sure that the correct kidney is operated on. It should therefore be a rule that the surgeon himself marks the appropriate side with a waterproof fiber-tipped pen after having checked with the patient, the records, and the radiographic films.

Useful Incisions for Open Stone Surgery

The classic loin incision with excision of the anterior portion of the 12th rib provides good access to the renal parenchyma and the posterior surface of the renal pelvis for nephro- or pyelolithotomy. The access to the upper pole is sometimes not optimal [22].

The supra 12 incision permits good access to the pelvis and the parenchyma [23]. As an alternative, a supra 11 incision may be used when required for lesions in the upper pole or in kidneys situated highly.

The posterior vertical lumbotomy incision is recommended for pyelolithotomy, pyeloplasty, and high ureteric stones [11]. It is associated with an easier recovery than flank incisions [24].

▶ **FIGURE 11-3.** Types of incisions. More than 40 types of incisions for approaching the kidney have been described. For incisional renal stone surgery, there are three well-established options. A flank incision below the 12th rib is often too low for renal stone surgery and should be avoided. Abdominal and thoracoabdominal incisions are mainly used for radical nephrectomy for tumors but may also be of value for stones when severe fibrosis is anticipated. These incisions give an excellent direct exposure to the renal pedicle and the kidney, but the access to the renal pelvis is less direct.

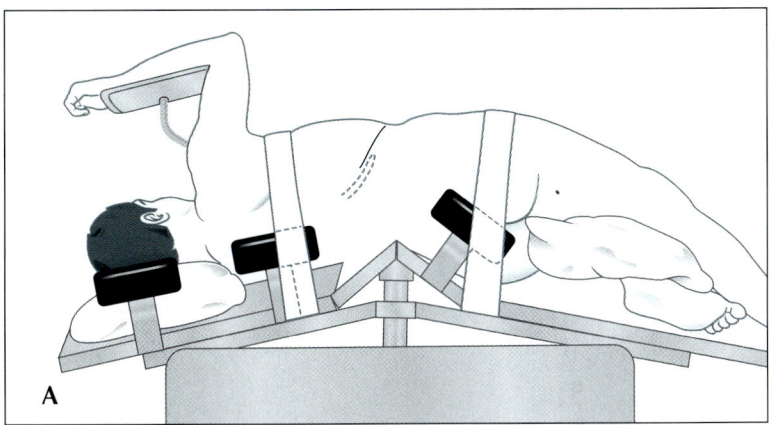

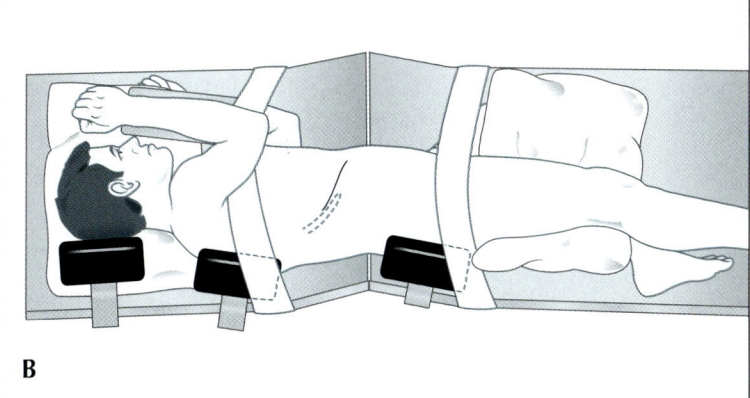

▶ **FIGURE 11-4.** Patient positioning (**A** and **B**) for classic loin incision (see Fig. 11-5) and supracostal (see Fig. 11-6) approach. For both approaches, the patient is placed in the lateral position with a vertical back, close to the edge of the operating table. The midlumbar spine should be placed at the level of the table break. The lower leg is flexed at a right angle and the upper leg is kept straight. The upper arm is supported in an arm rest. A pillow is placed between the knees, and a pad is placed under the axilla of the dependent arm to prevent compression of vessels and nerves. The table is then broken, but not so much that the lumbar spine begins to flex laterally. Breaking that is too pronounced may result in

hypotension as a result of decreased venous return from compression of the inferior vena cava and decreased aeration of the lung on the dependent side. A jackknife position that is too pronounced may also result in postoperative back pain, particularly in elderly patients. The position of the patient on the operating table is stabilized using T-piece table attachments in the sacral and upper thoracic regions and behind the neck. Straps are attached to the table for safety reasons and to avoid twisting of the trunk, which may render proper wound closure difficult [21]. Zinc oxide plaster may also be used to secure the patient to the table but may cause troublesome skin reactions in sensitive patients.

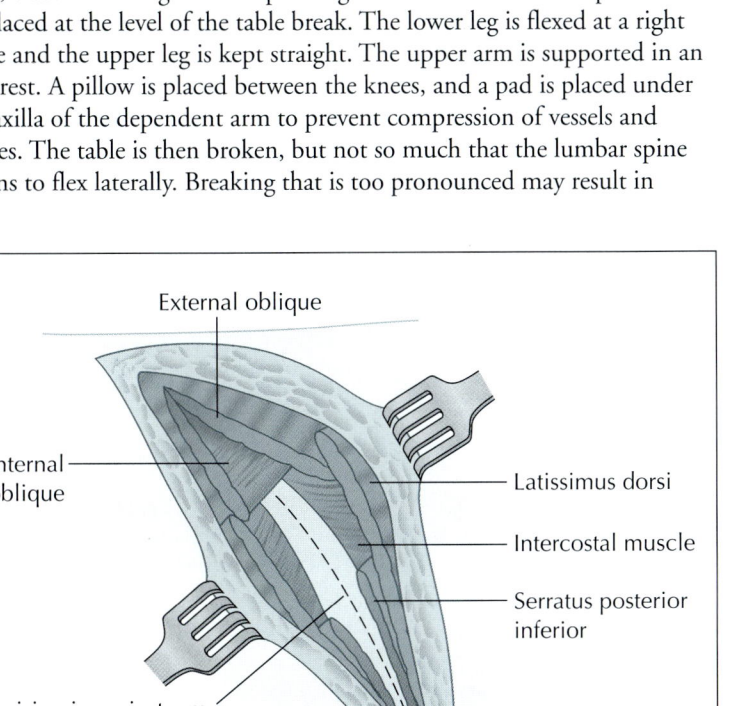

▶ **FIGURE 11-5.** Classic loin incision. With the decreasing frequency of open stone surgery and, consequenctly, less training for the young urologist, it is important that the incision be easy to learn, safe to practice, and applicable in difficult situations. The classic loin incision with excision of the 12th (occasionally the 11th) rib fulfills these criteria [22].

A, Skin incision. Before the skin is incised, scratches are made in the skin straight across the intended incision. The skin incision is made over the 12th rib, through the subcutaneous fat, down to the muscles. The latissimus dorsi and the underlying serratus posterior inferior muscles are incised, and the incision is continued 2 to 3 inches into the external oblique in line with the rib. The periosteum on the upper surface of the rib is incised via diathermy.

(Continued on next page)

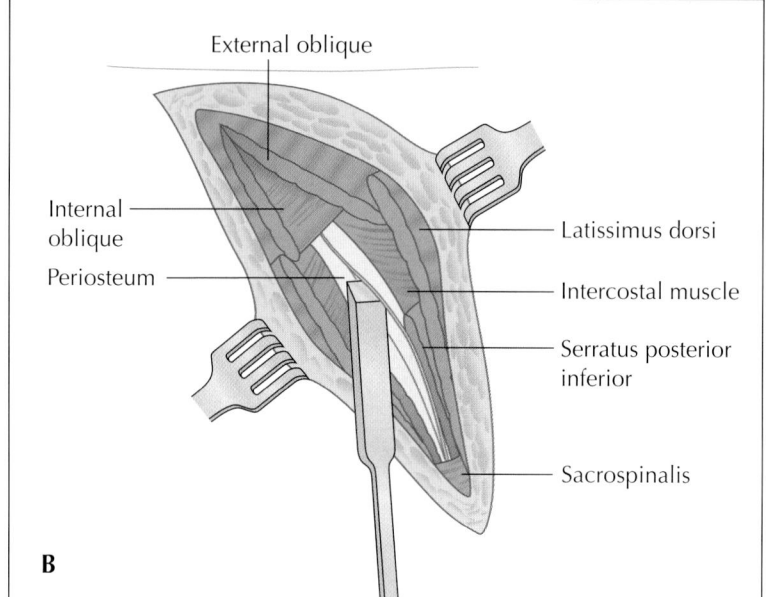

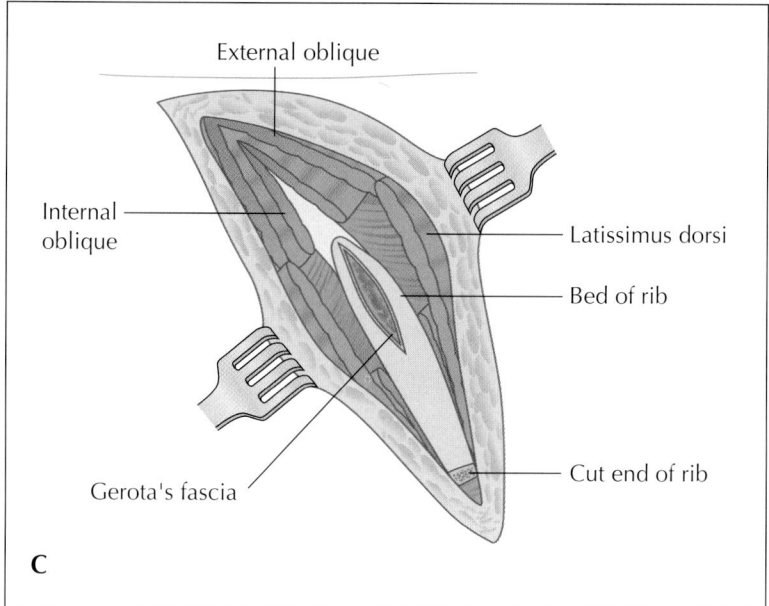

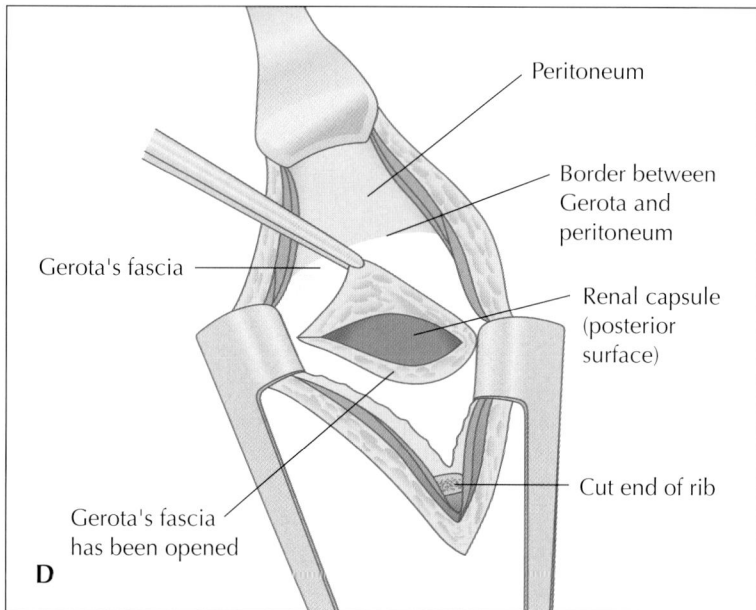

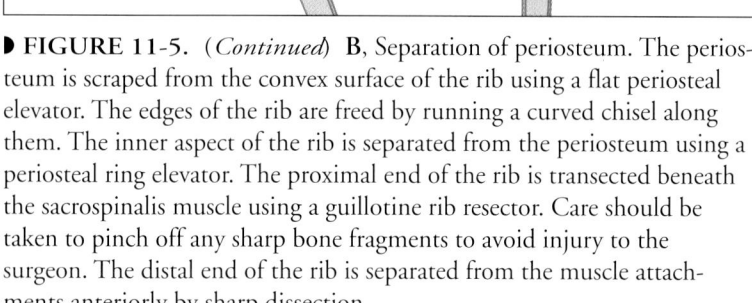

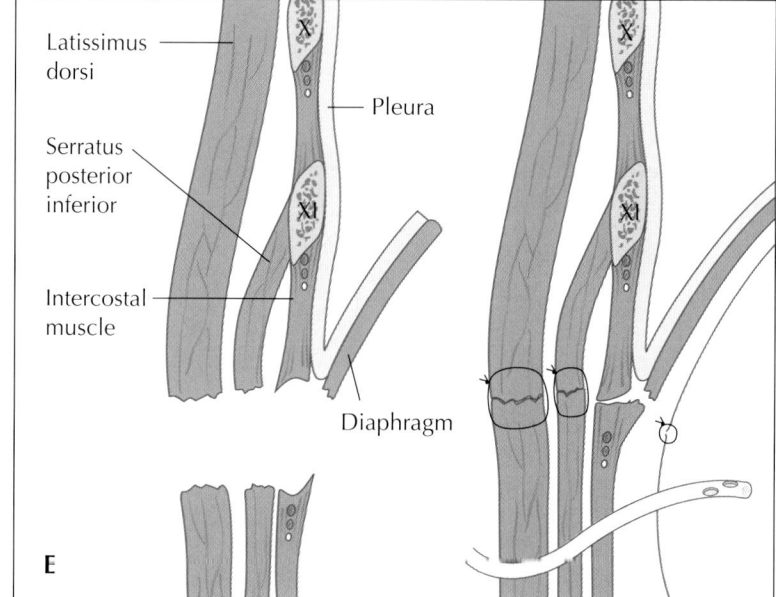

▶ **FIGURE 11-5.** (*Continued*) **B,** Separation of periosteum. The periosteum is scraped from the convex surface of the rib using a flat periosteal elevator. The edges of the rib are freed by running a curved chisel along them. The inner aspect of the rib is separated from the periosteum using a periosteal ring elevator. The proximal end of the rib is transected beneath the sacrospinalis muscle using a guillotine rib resector. Care should be taken to pinch off any sharp bone fragments to avoid injury to the surgeon. The distal end of the rib is separated from the muscle attachments anteriorly by sharp dissection.

C, Incising the internal oblique muscle with diathermy. By incising this muscle, the incision is continued a few inches anteriorly. The anterior part of the periosteal bed is incised entering the retroperitoneal space. A finger is then inserted into the perinephric space behind the posterior periosteal bed, which is incised to expose Gerota's fascia. The insertion of the diaphragm to the inner aspect of the periosteum and fascia is usually divided. To protect the pleura, it is gently pushed away with a finger. The transverse fascia and muscle are incised using a scalpel. There are vessels joining the 11th and 12th intercostal bundles that often bleed. Care should be taken not to injure the underlying peritoneum, which is swept forward with a finger. If the incision is made in the line of the rib, the subcostal neurovascular bundle, which runs between the internal oblique and transversus muscles, is not injured. The bundle is usually palpable.

D, Introduction of self-retaining retractor. A longitudinal incision is made in the posterior aspect of Gerota's fascia to avoid injury to the peritoneum. The posterior renal capsule is cleared from the perinephric fat. The dissection of the perinephric fat may be easy or cumbersome depending on the amount of pronounced sclerosis secondary to previous surgery or inflammation. The extent of mobilization depends on the planned procedure.

E, Closure of the wound. Before closing the wound, 0.5% bupivacaine is injected around the 11th and 12th intercostal nerves posterior to the incision. A drain is placed near the posterior surface of the kidney and brought out through a separate stab wound. Gerota's fascia is closed using a few interrupted resorbable sutures. The kidney rest is lowered, and the table is returned to its zero position. The initial scratches on the skin should be checked to avoid twisting when the wound is closed. The incision is closed in separate layers using interrupted resorbable sutures. Great care should be taken not to include the intercostal nerves in the sutures. The anterior layer of the periosteum may be sutured, but it is not recommended. Desensitization below the wound is a common sequela.

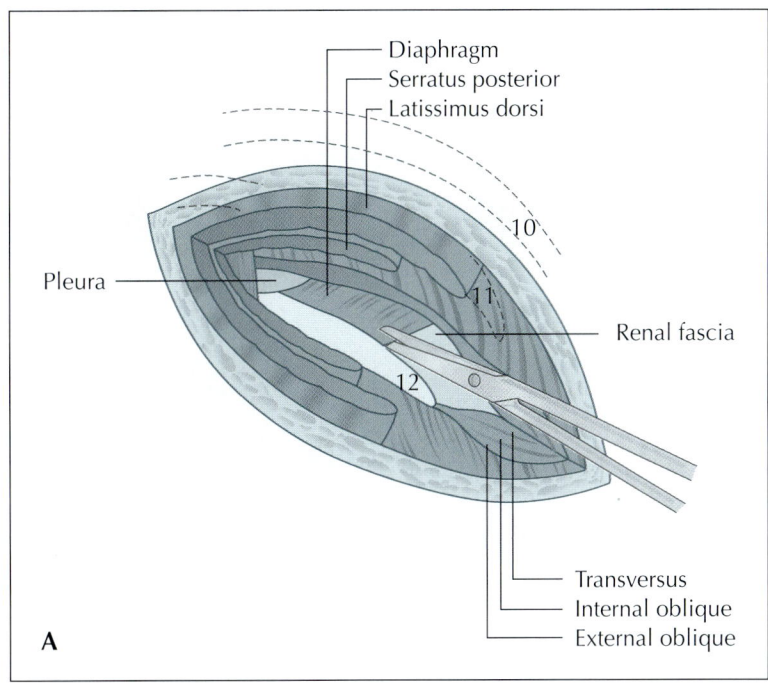

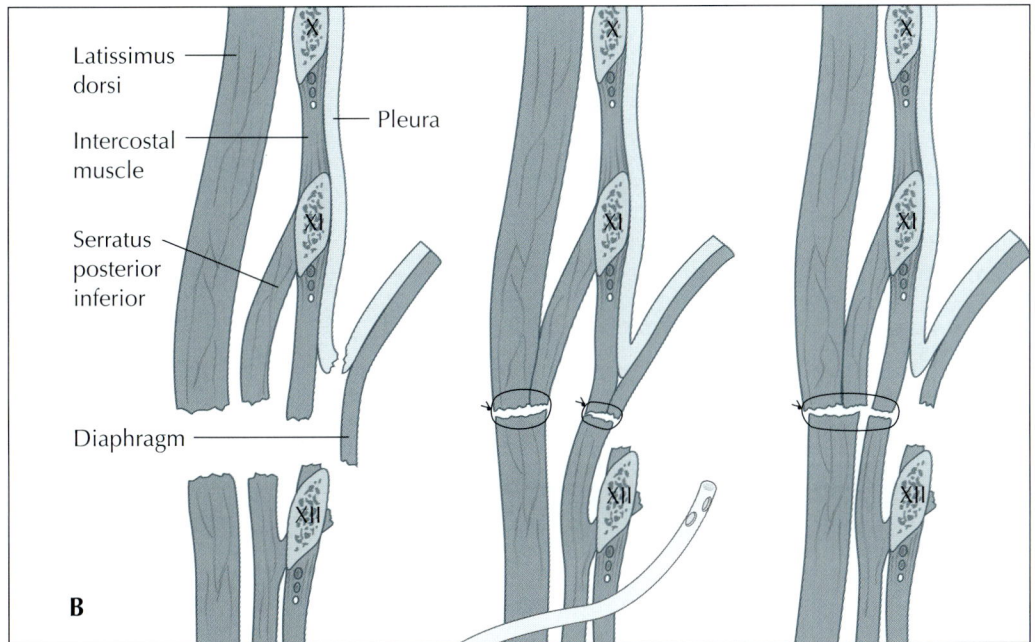

C. Risk of Lesion of the Pleura	
Type of Incision	*Percentage*
Supra 12th	15
Supra 11th	70

▶ **FIGURE 11-6.** The supracostal approach. The patient is placed in the lateral jackknife position. **A,** Incision is made using diathermy. The incision is parallel to the upper margin of the 12th rib through the latissimus dorsi and serratus posterior muscles, and it extends into the external and internal oblique muscles in the line of the rib [25]. The length of the incision depends on the extent of the procedure. For complete mobilization of the kidney, including intraoperative radiologic evaluation, the incision should start three fingers lateral to the dorsal spines. The transverse muscle, which mixes with the thoracolumbar fascia, is incised with the scalpel. Again, it is important to protect the peritoneum by sweeping it off the abdominal wall before the muscle is incised. The intercostal muscles are divided in a proximal direction along the upper margin of the rib; then the insertion of the diaphragm is divided. Care should be taken to protect the pleura by sweeping it away with a finger [23]. The dissection of the rib may proceed up to the vertebral column behind the erector spinae muscles, which are incised or retracted. To permit mobilization of the 12th rib, the costovertebral ligament is divided, and the crus of the diaphragm is elevated. The lower rib may now be swung down, resting on the quad-

ratus lumborum and psoas muscles. After the introduction of a self-retaining retractor, an excellent view of Gerota's fascia is obtained.

B, Closing the incision in two layers. The detached diaphragm is sutured, together with the upper edge of the intercostal muscle to the lower edge of the divided serratus posterior muscle external to the rib below. The latissimus dorsi and serratus muscles above are sutured to the edge of the latissimus dorsi below. Alternatively, the upper edges of the latissimus, serratus, and intercostal muscles are sutured to the lower edges of the latissimus and serratus muscles in one layer. The diaphragm and lower edge of the intercostal muscle are not sutured.

C, Lesion of the pleura. A lesion of the pleura is usually diagnosed during surgery by the detection of air escaping through the lesion. The rent is closed together with the diaphragm after expansion of the lung by positive-pressure ventilation before the sutures are tied. Sufficient closure can be checked by filling the wound with saline. A chest radiograph should always be obtained postoperatively when a lesion of the pleura is suspected or has been repaired. (Panel C *Adapted from* Barry and Hodges [25].)

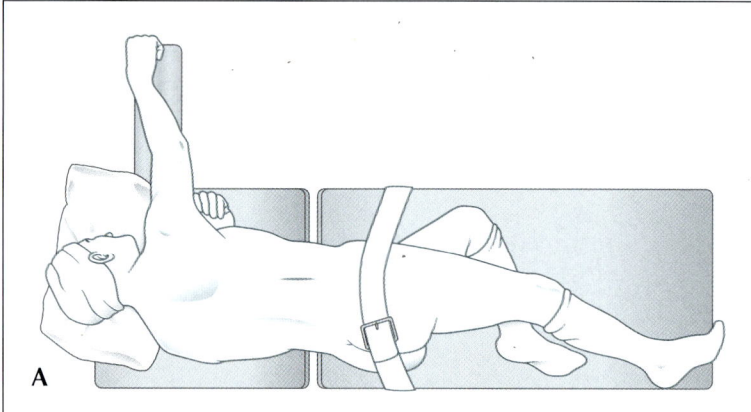

FIGURE 11-7. The dorsal lumbotomy. As popularized by Gil-Vernet in 1965, the dorsal lumbotomy was a slight modification of Simon's original incision for the first nephrectomy. According to Gil-Vernet, the dorsal lumbotomy has advantages over the oblique lumbotomy because 1) it avoids sectioning of any muscular fibers or nerves, and 2) it reaches the pelvis and the upper ureter from a posterior direction, which is direct and perpendicular to the pelvis and does not require mobilization of the kidney [11,24].

A, Unilateral procedure. The patient is placed in a half-lateral, half-prone position with the dependent leg flexed as in the classic loin position and with pillows between the knees and under the axilla. The table is slightly broken, extending the lumbar region. A sandbag is placed between the abdomen and the table to push the kidney posteriorly. For bilateral nephrectomy, the patient is placed in a prone position with support under the sternum and in the pubic region to avoid compression of the abdomen, which might interfere with respiration and venous return. The table is also broken in this position to improve access to the kidney.

B, Vertical incision along the lateral margin of the sacrospinalis muscle. The incision is made from the border of the 12th rib to 1 to 2 inches from the iliac bone. The lumbodorsal fascia is incised lateral to the sacrospinalis and quadratus lumborum muscles. These muscles are retracted medially until the transversalis fascia is exposed. The latter is transected longitudinally, after which Gerota's fascia is identified and incised longitudinally.

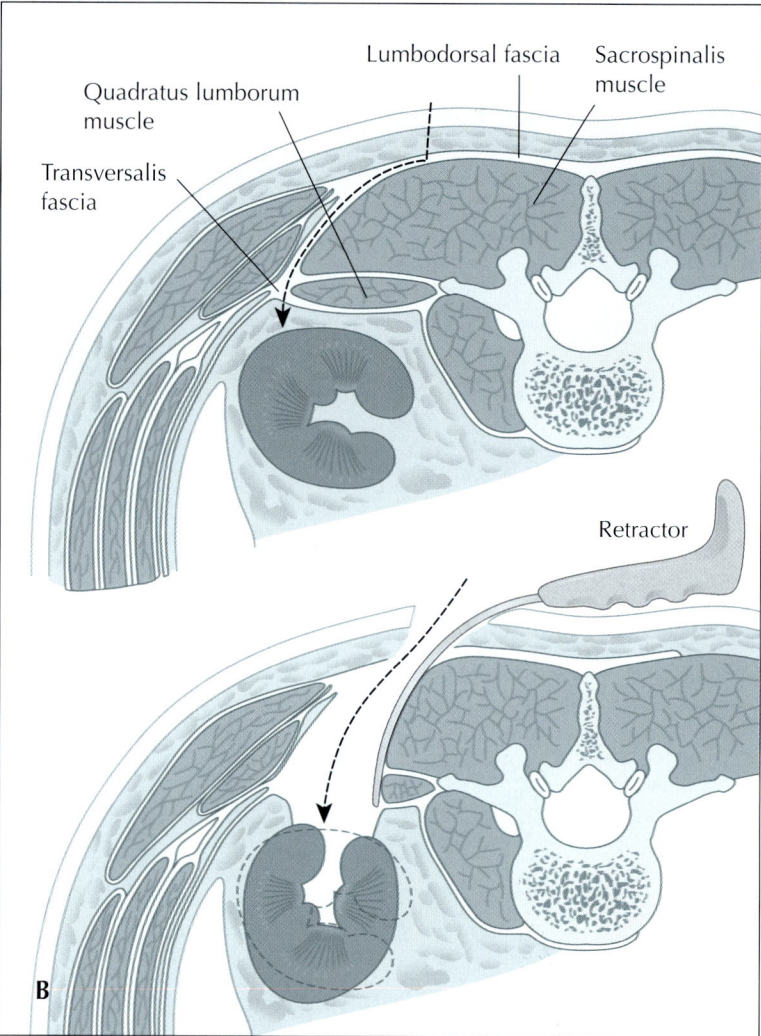

The incision is sufficient for pyelolithotomy and extended pyelolithotomy, for upper ureterolithotomy, and for pyeloplasty. The incision may also be used for the removal of small kidneys. The incision is closed in two layers: the transversalis fascia and the lumbodorsal fascia, respectively.

PYELOLITHOTOMY

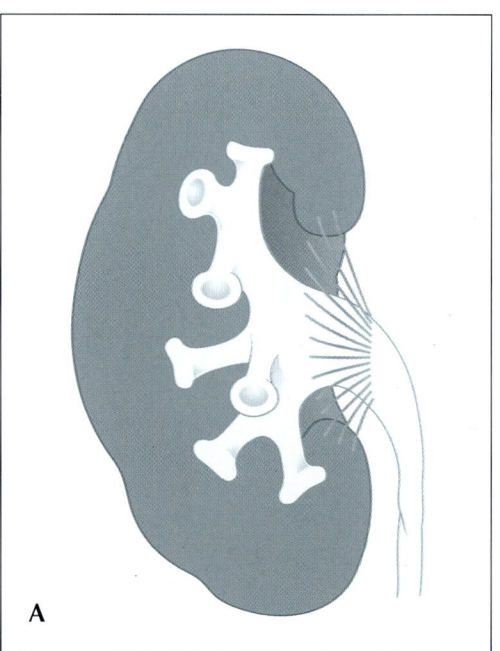

FIGURE 11-8. Approaching the renal sinus (**A**). To approach the renal sinus one must keep in mind that the renal fibrous capsule sends fibers to the renal pelvis and the pedicle. These fibers form a diaphragm that closes the renal sinus together with its contents of blood vessels, lymphatics, and the intrarenal collecting system, all embedded in fatty tissues [10,11]. Another fact to consider is that a thin sheet of fibers from the capsule reflects the posterior edge of the kidney, covering the inside of the parenchymatous lip. In this way it becomes stabilized, permitting a retractor to be placed around it.

(Continued on next page)

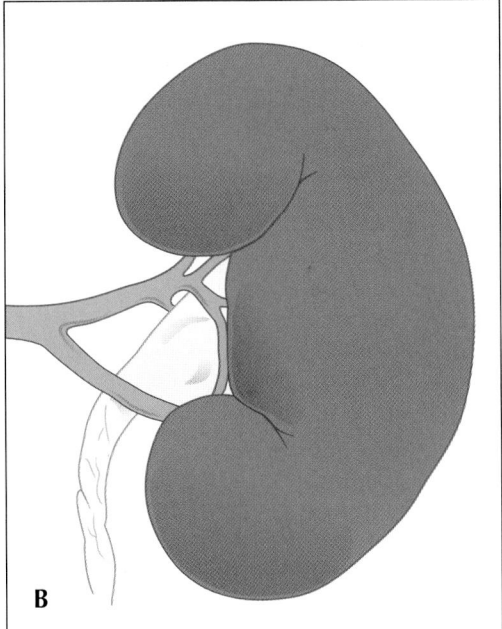

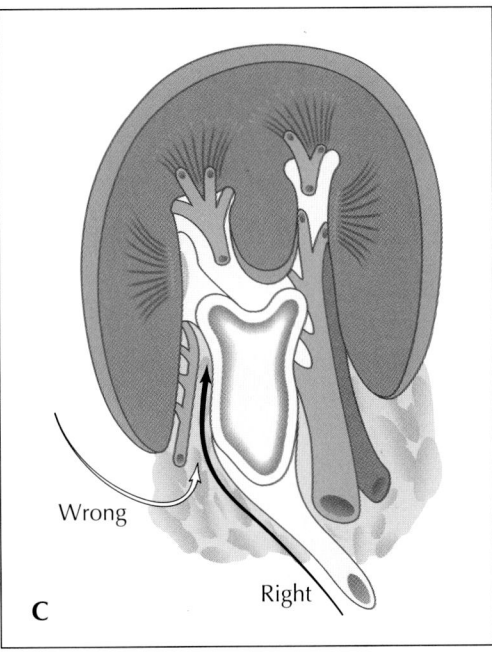

the sinus close to the parenchyma, where it is well protected. Less often, it runs slightly outside along the edge of the posterior lip, where it is prone to injury.

C, Dissection of the sinus. As long as the dissection of the sinus follows the adventitia of the posterior ureteropelvic wall, the risk of damage to the parenchyma or vessels is very low. The sinus should never be approached from the posterior renal surface around the posterior lip into the sinus; the risk of damage to the posterior artery in this instance is overwhelming. Once the sinus has been opened, a retractor or two may be placed. The posterior half of the kidney may now be firmly lifted up, causing the organ to turn and displaying the pelvis and the posterior aspect of the calyces. There is a risk that the retractors may compress the retropyelic vessels, impairing their circulation. Impaired circulation is usually signaled by the posterior surface of the kidney turning cyanotic, which indicates that the tension on the retractors must be diminished.

▶ **FIGURE 11-8.** (*Continued*) **B,** Position of the retropyelic artery. This artery supplies the posterior segment of the kidney. The retropyelic artery is a branch of the main renal artery and runs across the superior edge of the pelvis to the posterior area of the sinus. Usually, the artery proceeds inside

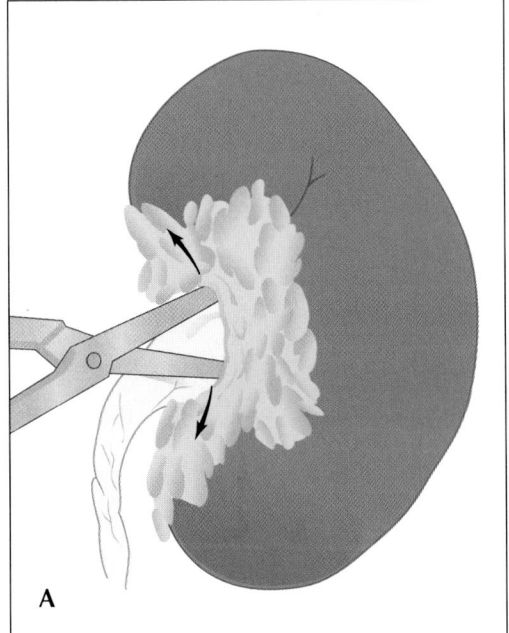

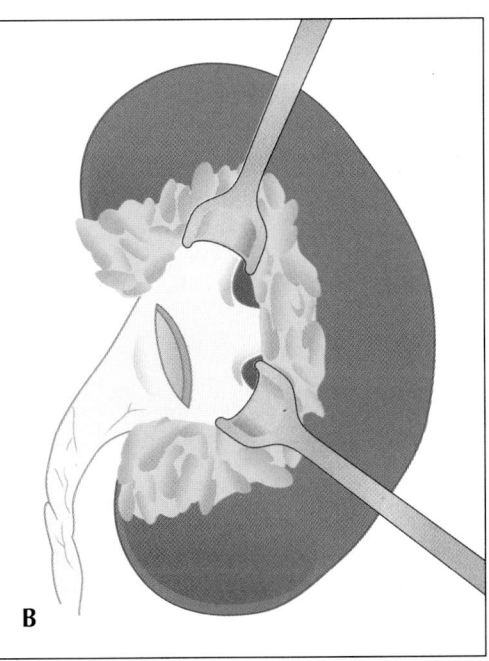

previously and there is no major sclerous reaction, a plane can easily be found between the adventitia of the pelvis and the capsular diaphragm by blind dissection. A pair of curved scissors is introduced and spread underneath the diaphragm in close contact with the adventitia. When the plane between the adventitia and the fibrous capsule is obliterated because of severe sclerosis, another plane can be obtained between the adventitia and the muscular wall of the pelvis [11].

B, The exposed renal pelvis is incised parallel to the parenchyma. A blunt retractor or two can now be introduced easily, and the posterior surface of the pelvis is displayed. To avoid cutting the spiral-shaped muscle fibers of the pelvis (which would interfere with its peristalsis) and to lower the risk of tearing the UPJ, a transverse incision parallel to the parenchyma should be made instead of a vertical one [11]. The incision is made against the stone. Preferably a hooked blade is used first, followed by an angulated pair of scissors. Avoid stay sutures, which may tear the pelvis. The stone is removed with a forceps and the pelvis is then irrigated with saline. Before closure, an infant feeding tube is passed to the bladder to confirm that the passage is clear.

▶ **FIGURE 11-9.** The simple pyelolithotomy. **A,** Exposing the lower pole of the kidney. The lower pole of the kidney is exposed after Gerota's fascia has been incised. For a simple pyelotomy, there is no need to mobilize the entire kidney. The proximal ureter is identified medial to the lower pole, and a sling is passed around it. Watch out for a lower segment artery from the aorta. Using blunt dissection, the ureter is followed in a proximal direction along its posterior wall between the fat and the ureteral adventitia until the ureteropelvic junction (UPJ) and the capsular diaphragm have been exposed [11]. If the patient has not been operated on

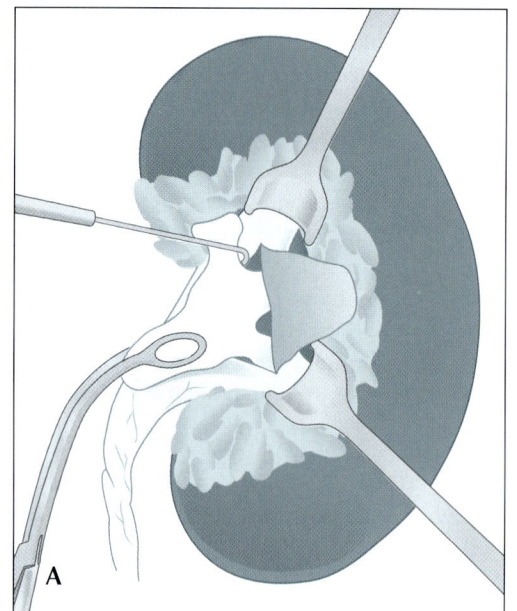

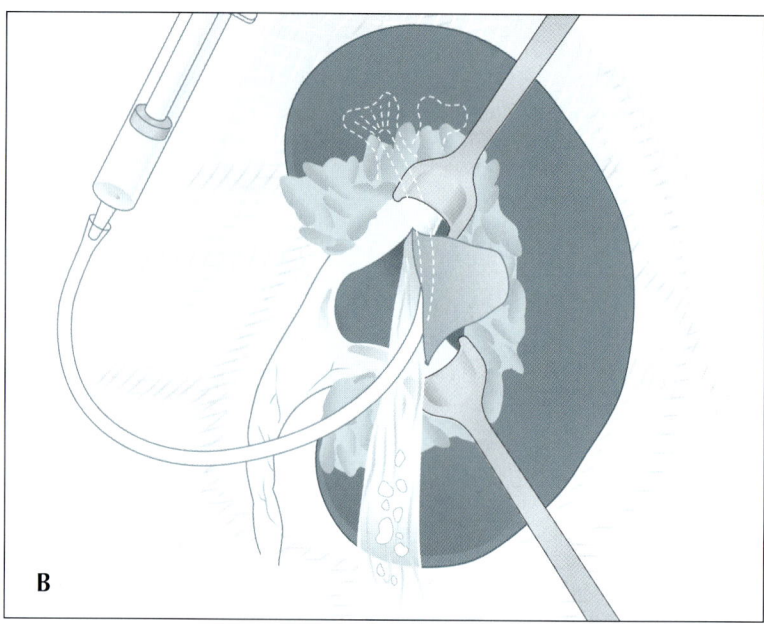

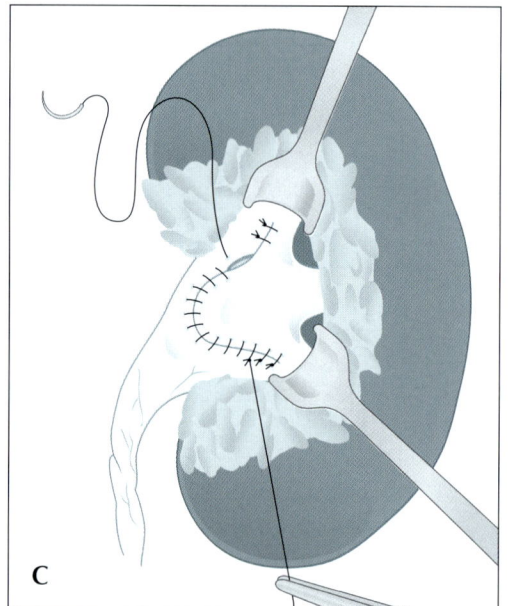

D. Results and Complications of Extended Pyelolithotomy for Staghorn Stones*

	Patients, n
Mortality	0
Hemorrhage	0
Wound infection	0
Persistent fistula	0
	Kidneys, n
Complete removal	42
Incomplete removal	12
Dust left behind	5
Fragments left behind	7

*Total number of patients, 45; total number of kidneys, 54.

▶ **FIGURE 11-10.** Extended pyelolithotomy. **A,** Blunt dissection. The pelvis and the infundibula of the main calyces are exposed by dissection. Dissection can usually be performed without any bleeding. A curved or u-shaped incision is made using angulated scissors. The extent of the incision should be adapted to the shape, size, and position of the stone. Sometimes it is extended onto one or more stone-bearing infundibula. The pelvic portion of the stone is first turned out through the incision. After the affected infundibula are incised longitudinally, shorter caliceal extensions are then mobilized. The branches are mobilized one by one. The entire stone can often be removed by gentle rotation along its axis; the goal should be to remove the stone in one piece. For larger stones with multiple extensions, this may not always be possible, and the stone may have to be divided under direct vision using a special stone-cutter or a robust pair of scissors.

B, Residual stones retrieved from the calyces. Residual stones can be retrieved by using a variety of fine stone forceps of different shapes or by flushing with saline. During flushing, the area around the opened pelvis should be protected with gauze to prevent stone fragments from being spread throughout the wound. Intraoperative pyeloscopy is often of great value in localizing residual stones [26]. Peripheral stones too large to extract through the infundibulum are removed using radial nephrotomies. Before the pelvis is closed, contact radiography should always be performed to confirm complete stone removal [15,27,28].

C, Closing the incision. The incision in the renal pelvis is closed, preferably using interrupted or running sutures of 4-0 or 5-0 polyglycolic acid or chromic catgut. A watertight closure should be the goal. Because of limited access, the most extreme parts of the infundibular incisions may be difficult to close and may have to be left open. Before the pelvis is closed, the patency of the ureter down to the bladder is checked using a ureteric catheter. When poor drainage is feared, an internal ureteric splint is left in place. Postoperative leakage is rare because the pelvic incision is covered by perihilar fat and the posterior lip.

D, Results and complications of extended pyelolithotomy for staghorn stones. In a review of 54 kidneys in 45 patients operated on for staghorn calculi using extended pyelolithotomy, excellent results were reported with regard to postoperative morbidity, blood loss, and stone clearance [29]. In an experimental study in dogs, the extended sinus approach was not associated with any functional or parenchymal loss [30]. (Panel D *Adapted from* Singh *et al.* [29].)

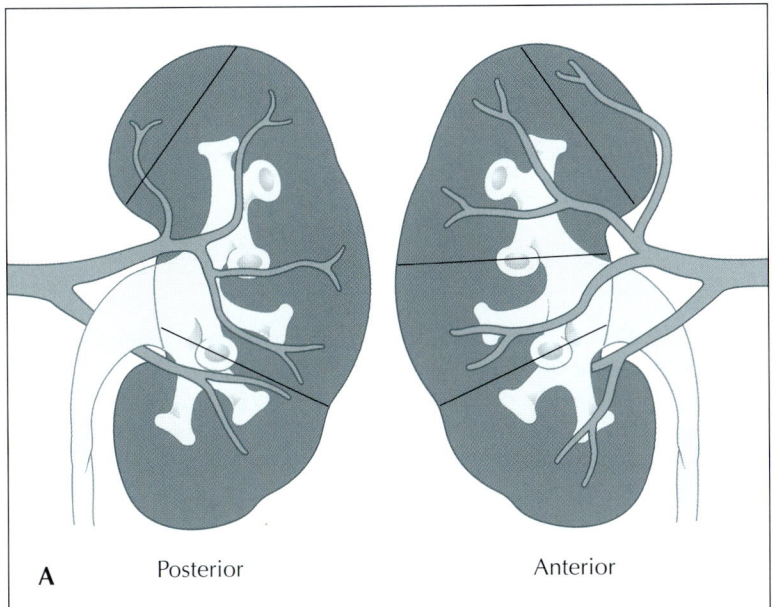

A | Posterior | Anterior

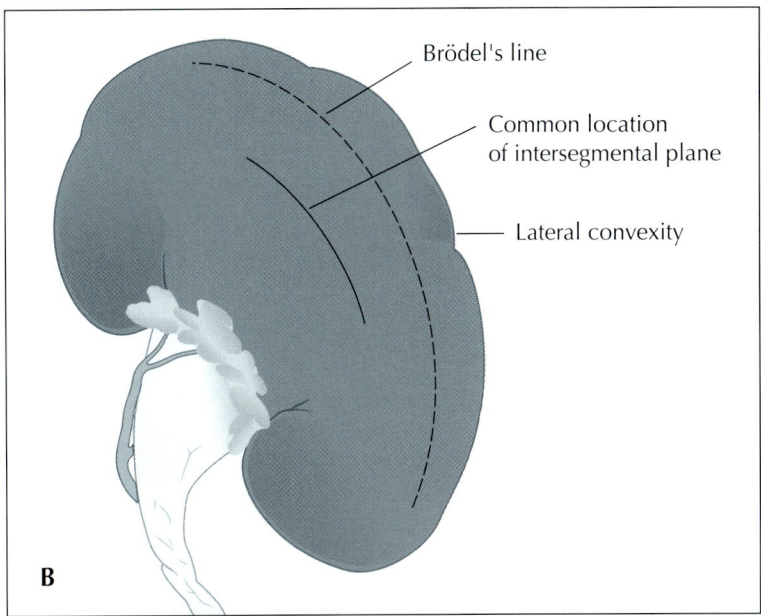

Brödel's line

Common location of intersegmental plane

Lateral convexity

B

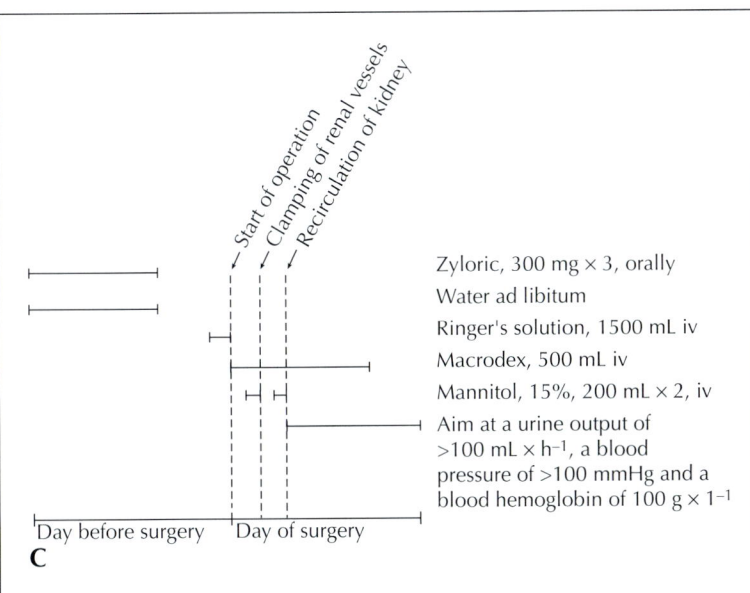

Start of operation
Clamping of renal vessels
Recirculation of kidney

Zyloric, 300 mg × 3, orally

Water ad libitum

Ringer's solution, 1500 mL iv

Macrodex, 500 mL iv

Mannitol, 15%, 200 mL × 2, iv

Aim at a urine output of >100 mL × h^{-1}, a blood pressure of >100 mmHg and a blood hemoglobin of 100 g × 1^{-1}

Day before surgery | Day of surgery

C

▶ **FIGURE 11-11.** Nephrolithotomy requires two basic skills. The first skill is proficient knowledge of the vascular anatomy and the parenchymal segments corresponding to different arteries [5,6,31]. The second skill is that the surgeon should be familiar with current renal preservation techniques. Another prerequisite is performance of good routines for intraoperative contact roentgenography.

A, Vascular supply to the five renal segments. To understand the structure of the kidney it is important to remember that during embryologic development multiple separate reniculi, each with its own papilla, medulla, cortex, and blood supply, fuse to form a kidney. Within the kidney there are venous and lymphatic collaterals between the reniculi. This is in contrast to the renal arteries, which are so-called end arteries (*ie*, circulation in one artery cannot replace circulation in a neighboring artery). The reniculi are usually grouped into five segments: a posterior, an apical, a lower, and two

anterior (upper and middle) segments. Each segment is supplied by its own artery [5,6,31]. The boundary between two neighboring segments is a relatively avascular zone that has been exploited in surgery.

B, Location of common intersegmented incision. The anterior and posterior segments do not, as a rule, meet on the lateral convex border of the kidney but on the posterior half, approximately two thirds of the way from the lateral convexity. The posterior renal artery is usually the first big branch from the main renal artery and is astride the upper edge of the renal pelvis on its way to the posterior segment of the kidney. The avascular line between the anterior and posterior segments thus differs from the original one described by Brödel [5,6,31].

C, Renal preservation. Renal preservation starts the day before surgery by ensuring that the patient is well hydrated with salt-containing solutions at the time of surgery, which counteracts activation of the renin-angiotensin system [32–34]. The routine of giving 1500 mL by slow infusion overnight can usually be replaced by rapid infusion a couple of hours before surgery [35]. Based on animal experiments, we routinely give the patient allopurinol, 300 mg three times daily, the day before surgery to prevent the formation of some of the noxious free radicals at recirculation [36]. The most important part of the renal preservation program is kidney hypothermia, which decreases cellular metabolic activity [37], including the consumption of high-energy phosphates. The easiest and most efficient technique for cooling the kidney is to pack it in slush ice. To prevent the spread of ice in the wound, the kidney and the ice are included in a plastic bag opened at the bottom and tied around the pedicle. It is important to let the kidney cool for a minimum of 10 minutes before surgery starts because a core temperature of 10° C to 20° C is the goal [38]. Another cornerstone in renal preservation is mannitol (15%), which is given both before clamping the artery (200 mL) and before recirculation (another 200 mL). Mannitol increases the renal capillary blood flow, prevents intracellular edema, induces an osmotic diuretic effect (which flushes the renal tubules), and serves as a scavenger of free radicals [39,40].

(Continued on next page)

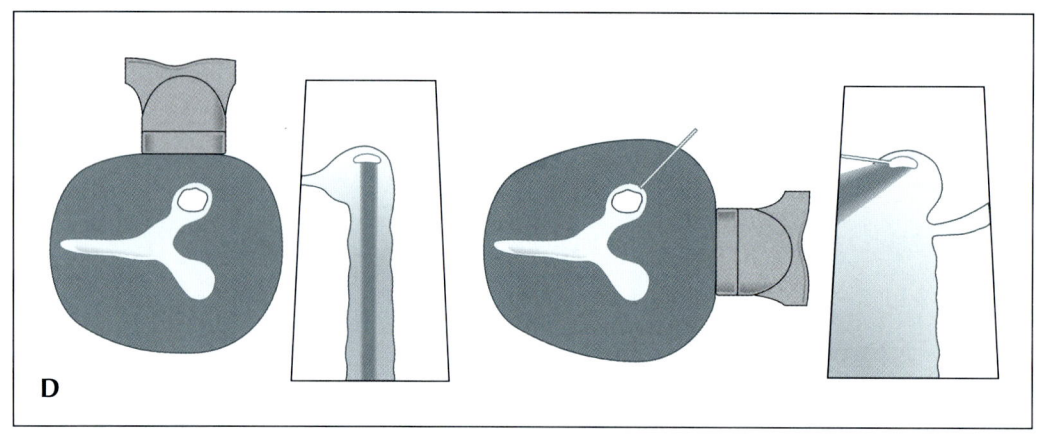

D

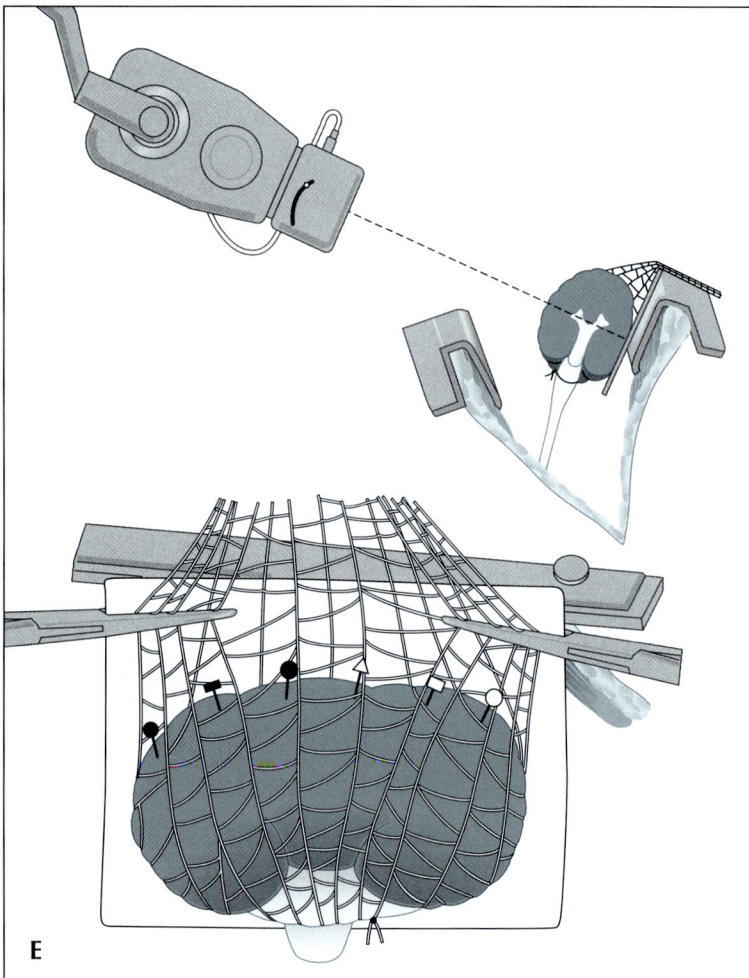

E

▶ **FIGURE 11-11.** (*Continued*) **D,** Control of residual stones. For complex stones, for which most open surgical procedures are done today, intraoperative control of residual stones is as important as the surgery itself. Intraoperative pyeloscopy may be of great help in localizing residual stones, but it does not guarantee complete inspection of the whole collecting system or provide any documentation of the end result [26,41,42]. Intraoperative ultrasonography has the same limitations as pyeloscopy. It may be useful in the localization of residual stones, but it is difficult to use in assessing the result at the end of a surgical intervention [42,43]. Fluoroscopy using a C-arm may be considered a useful tool in the localization of residual stones. It has poor resolution, however, partly due to interposition of soft tissue, and is difficult to maneuver in a surgical field. Long exposure times are also associated with high radiation doses [44].

E, Intraoperative radiography. Existence of a facility that can provide good-quality intraoperative radiography is a prerequisite before open renal stone surgery. A portable radiograph unit is available in most departments. Special kidney surgery films are not commercially available, but a pack of mammography films and an intensifying screen in a sterile plastic bag or glove may be used [27]. The radiologic technician must be thoroughly familiar with organ radiography. After complete mobilization, the kidney is supported in a sling or a net. The exposures are made at precise right angles to the film, which is placed in direct contact with the kidney in the wound. Anteroposterior and oblique exposures are usually obtained. To provide reference points for the localization of the stones, various-shaped needles may be used to indicate the stones. The first film is exposed before an incision is made in the kidney. A final roentgenogram is made to check complete removal of all fragments before repair of the kidney is started.

A technique of three-dimensional intraoperative contact radiography that does not require total mobilization of the kidney has been developed [28]. The technique, however, is cumbersome and requires special films and carriers that may be difficult to obtain.

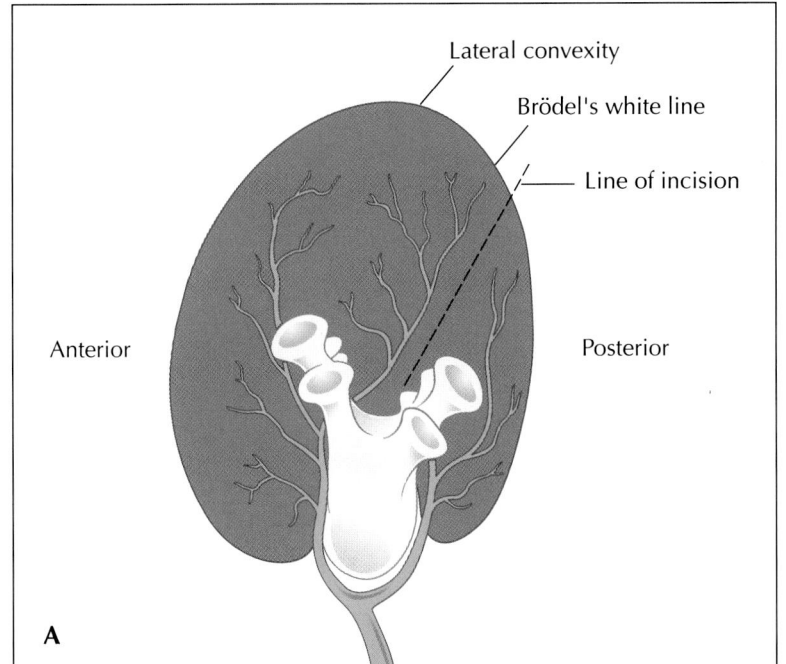

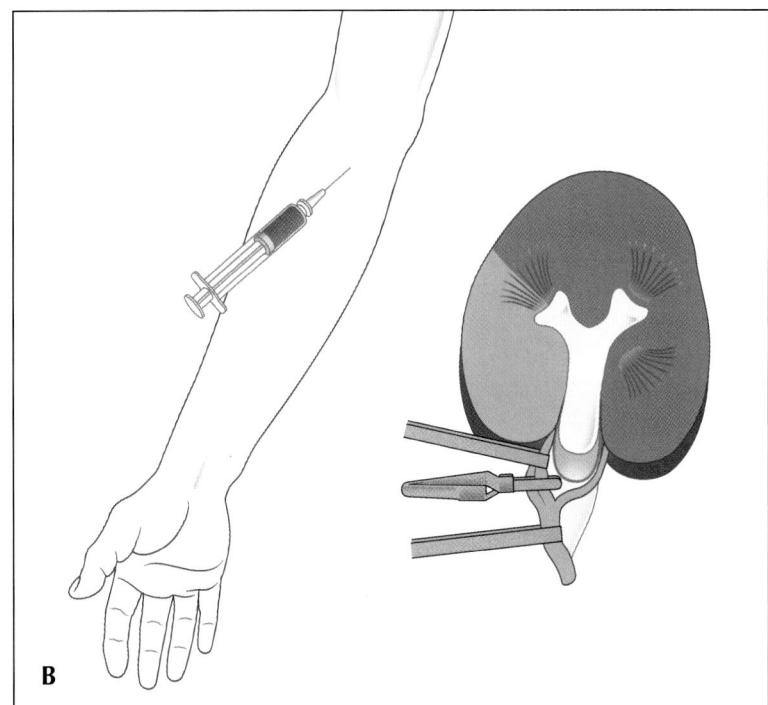

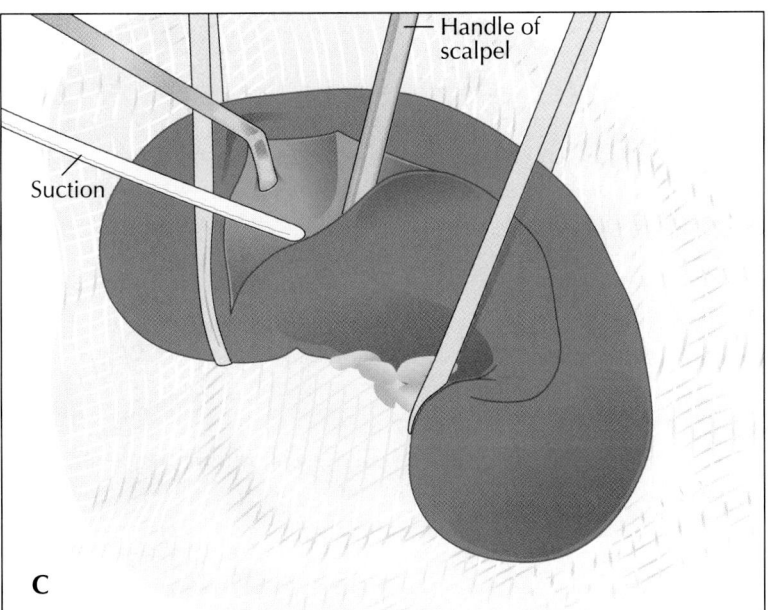

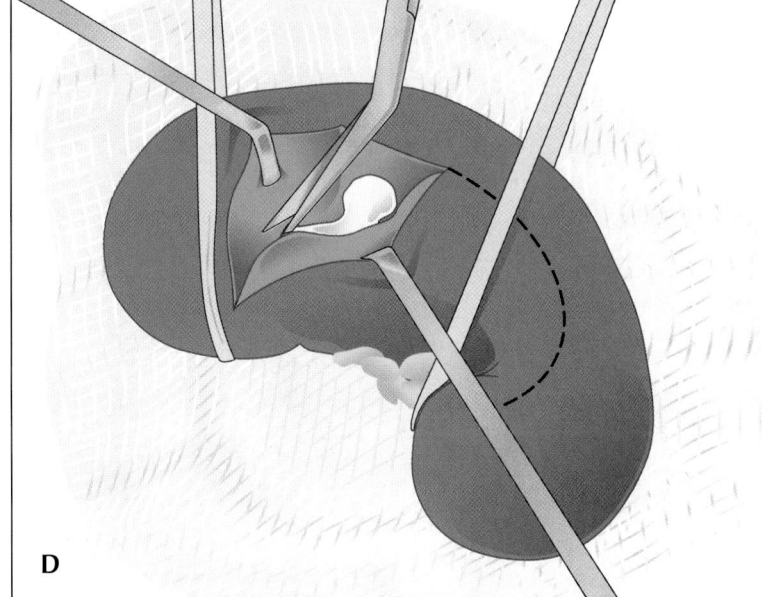

▶ **FIGURE 11-12.** Anatrophic nephrolithotomy. In contrast to previously described procedures for removal of stones via the collecting system, the anatrophic nephrolithotomy by definition is performed in a relatively avascular plane to avoid secondary atrophy [12,45].

A, Line chosen for the incision is the plane between the anterior and the posterior segments. This line is approximately 0.5 to 1 cm posterior to Brödel's white line, which is about 2 cm behind the lateral convexity of the kidney.

B, The "avascular" line must be mapped for each kidney. The kidney is mobilized and suspended in a sling or in a net. The main renal artery and the posterior segment artery are carefully dissected. Mannitol is given, and an atraumatic rubber-shed bulldog clamp is put on the posterior artery. Approximately 10 to 20 mL of methylene blue is injected intravenously or into the aorta proximal to the renal arteries to visualize the boundary between the posterior segment and the rest of the kidney. The avascular

line is indicated on the capsule by using methylene blue or simply by diathermy. The bulldog clamp is transferred to the main renal artery, and the kidney is cooled (see Fig. 11-11C).

C, An incision is made along the line of demarcation through the renal capsule. Blunt dissection, using the handle of the scalpel, is made down through the parenchyma, which is split, not cut. The correct dissection plane is between the posterior and anterior arterial segments just anterior to the posterior calyces and infundibula down to the renal pelvis.

D, The exposed pelvis is opened. The stone is not removed until the nephrotomy is completed. It is important that as few branches of the stone as possible are fractured. The branches should be carefully retracted, displacing calyceal mucosa or incising stenotic infundibula, so as not to damage the collecting system. Before the kidney is reconstructed, another contact film should be taken to ensure that the kidney is stone-free.

(*Continued on next page*)

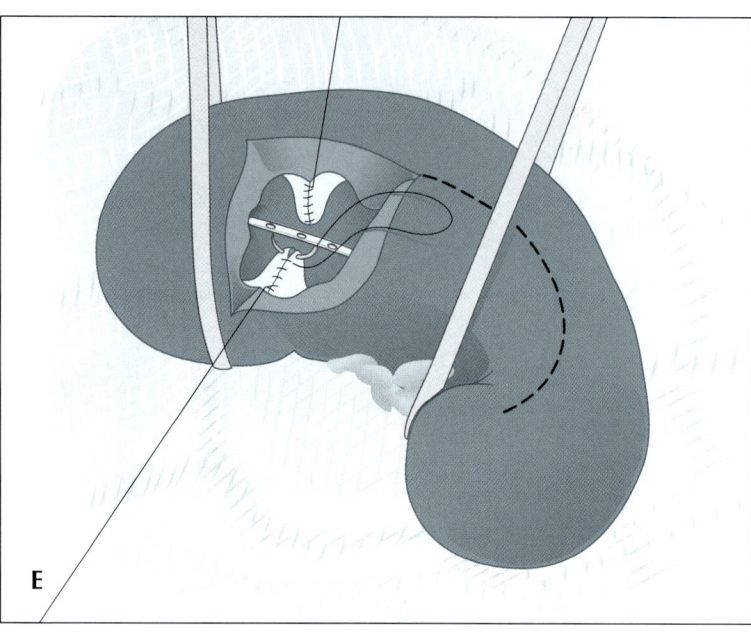

E

▶ **FIGURE 11-12.** (*Continued*) E, Reconstructing the collecting system. The collecting system is reconstructed by suturing adjacent infundibula to each other. Peripelvic fat should not be included in the closure. The collecting system is finally closed with running 4-0 chromic sutures. Any cross-cut small arteries and venous bleeding spots are suture-ligated using 5-0 chromic catgut sutures. The renal capsule is closed using a running 4-0 resorbable suture. After another infusion of mannitol, the vascular clamp is removed. A stent is left from the renal pelvis down to the bladder. Bleeding from the incision may be stopped by gentle pressure. If the bleeding continues, supplementary 2-0 catgut mattress sutures may be placed for compression. If the bleeding does not stop despite these measures, the capsular incision may have to be opened after the artery is reclamped and local hypothermia is again applied. Not until the bleeding is controlled are Gerota's fascia and the incision closed. Wrapping the kidney with omentum contributes to resorption of infected material postoperatively and facilitates future re-exploration [46]. Drains should always be placed.

F, Results and complications. Anatophic nephrolithotomy often requires an operation time of more than 5 hours in a hyperextended lateral position, which often implies considerable postoperative morbidity, particularly involving the lungs. It should be considered a major surgical intervention. The impact on renal function is usually low. The true surgical complications include postoperative hemorrhage, urinary drainage, acute tubular necrosis, and vascular injury. The urinary leakage can usually be handled by stent placement, and rarely by open surgery. In patients with major bleeding, selective renal angiography should be performed to localize the bleeding spot, which then may be closed by embolization or open surgery. In a series of 44 patients with bilateral staghorn calculi in whom anatrophic nephrolithotomy was performed, all patients were stone-free at the end of the intervention, and there were no postoperative deaths [45]. In an experimental study of canine kidneys, anatrophic intersegmental nephrotomy was associated with a 30% decrease in function and a significant parenchymal loss [30]. (Panel E *Adapted from* Resnick and Boyce [45].)

F. Results and Complications of Anatrophic Nephrolithotomy in 44 Patients with Bilateral Staghorn Calculi

Complications	Incidents, n
Mortality	0
Urinary drainage	1
Prolonged ileus	2
Hemorrhage	7
Atelectasis	10
Residual stones	0

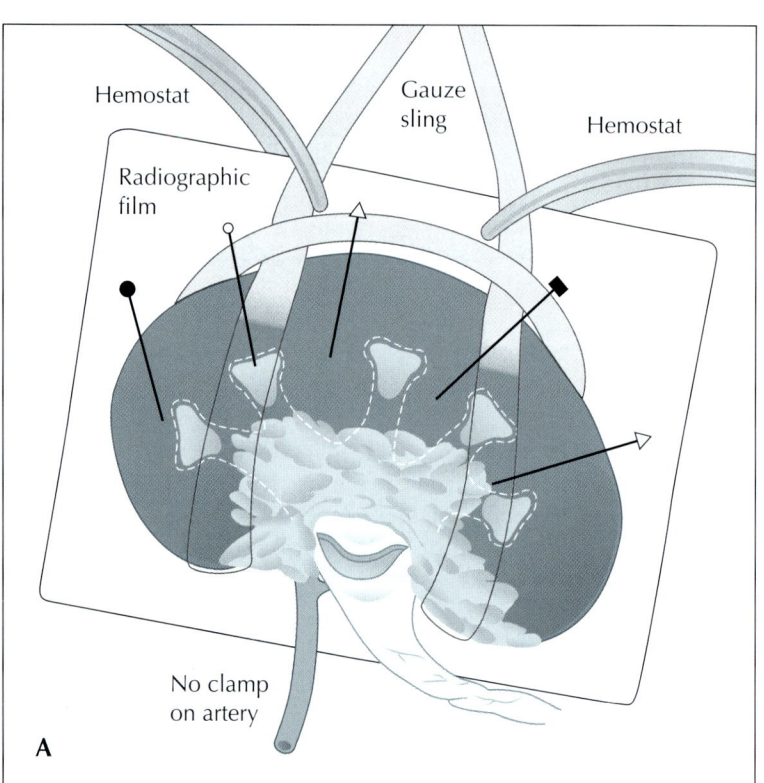

Hemostat · Gauze sling · Hemostat · Radiographic film · No clamp on artery

A

▶ **FIGURE 11-13.** Radial paravascular multiple nephrolithotomy. A, Perioperative contact radiography. Based on the radial arrangement of the intrarenal arteries, a technique of paravascular nephrotomy was developed by Wickham [6,13]. To avoid major intrarenal vessels, the radial incisions should be made peripherally on the posterior surface as far away from the hilus as possible, aiming at the bottom of the calyx. More than 60% of all calyces can be approached in this way [6]. The procedure requires a flank incision with good access to the kidney, which has to be completely mobilized. For complex staghorn calculi, the procedure should start with an extended pyelolithotomy to remove the bulk of the stones. When peripheral residual stones not obtainable through the collecting system have been demonstrated on contact radiographic films, clamping of the renal artery and preservation of the parenchyma are instituted as described in Figure 11-11C. It is sometimes possible to palpate stones in dilated calyces through the parenchyma. When the artery has been clamped, the kidney shrinks in size and becomes floppy. Most large stones can then be palpated. When the parenchyma is thick, small retained stones may be localized on contact radiographic films by using marking needles as reference points or by means of intraoperative ultrasound [15,42].

(Continued on next page)

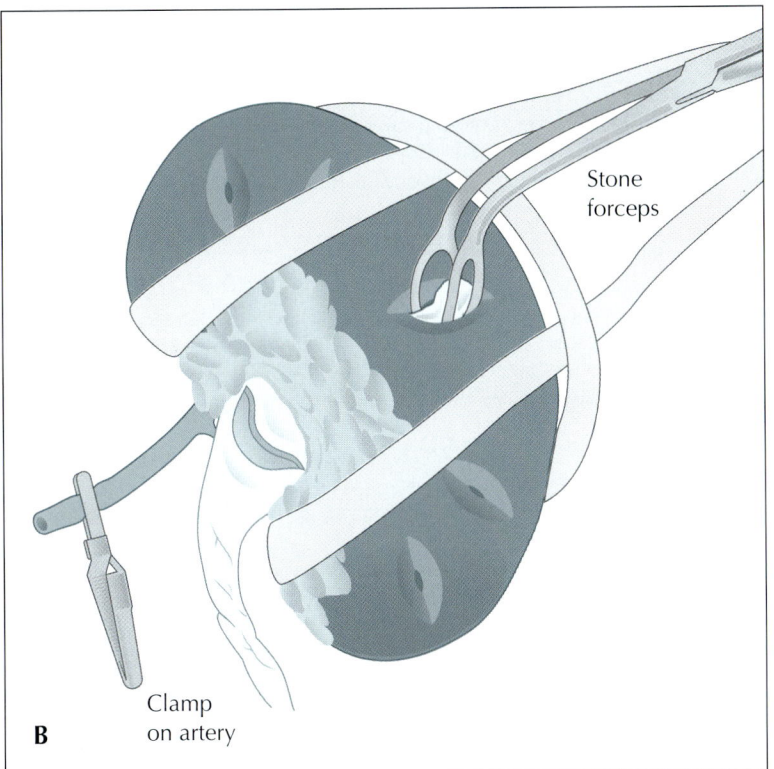

B

Stone forceps

Clamp on artery

▶ **FIGURE 11-13.** (*Continued*) B, Radial paravascular multiple nephrolithotomies. Larger vessels can be localized and avoided by using a Doppler probe [42,43]. The position of a stone can often be confirmed using a number 1 hypodermic needle. After contact with the stone, a radial incision (0.5 to 1.0 cm) is made in the capsule. By blunt dissection, the needle is followed down to the stone. When complete stone removal has been documented, the incisions are closed using interrupted 4-0 chromic catgut sutures in the capsule. A nephrostomy tube is recommended, and a drain is placed. Omentum may be used to wrap the kidney [46].

C. Results and Complications in 250 Patients Undergoing Multiple Nephrotomies for Stones

Stone free rate	86%
Nephrectomy	
For hemorrhage	3
For infection	3
Blood replacement	
< 500 mL	69%
> 1000 mL	9%
Renal function	
Mean preoperative creatinine	142 mmol/L
Mean follow-up creatinine	143 mmol/L
Urine fistula	—

C, Results and complications in 250 patients operated on with multiple nephrolithostomies. Of 250 patients operated on for complex stones using multiple paravascular nephrotomies, 86% were primarily cleared of calculi. Most of the residual calcifications were intraparenchymal [6]. Six kidneys had to be removed. Blood replacement was less than one unit in the majority of cases. Postoperative fistula formation was not a problem. Renal function as estimated from serum creatinine levels remained stable. In an experimental study in dog kidneys, radial paravascular nephrotomies were followed by a 20% decrease in function but no significant parenchymal loss [30]. (Panel C *Adapted from* Wickham [6].)

REFERENCES

1. Simon G: Exstirpation einer Niere am Menschen [German]. *Dtsch Klin* 1870, 22:137.

2. Morris H: A case of nephrolithotomy; or the extraction of a calculus from an undilated kidney. *Trans Clin Soc Lond* 1881, 14:30–44.

3. Czerny HE: Ueber Nierenexstirpation beitr 2 [German]. *Klin Chir* 1890, 6:485.

4. Hyrtl J: Handbuch der Topographischen Anatomie und Ihre Praktisch Medizinisch [German]. *Chirurgischen Awendugen* 1882, 1:834.

5. Brödel M: The intrinsic blood vessels of the kidney and their significance in nephrotomy. *Johns Hopkins Hosp Bull* 1901, 12:10–13.

6. Wickham JEA: The radial paravascular multiple nephrotomy. In *Intrarenal Surgery*. Edited by Wickham JEA. New York: Churchill Livingstone; 1984:1–29, 166–176.

7. Singh M, Chapman R, Tresidder GC, *et al.*: The fate of the unoperated staghorn calculus. *Br J Urol* 1973, 45:581–585.

8. Turner Warwick RT: Lower pole pyelo-calycotomy, retrograde partial nephrectomy, and uretero-calycostomy. *Br J Urol* 1965, 37:673–677.

9. Henle J: *Handbuch der Systematischen Anatomie des Menschen*. Göttingen: Braunschweig; 1862.

10. Disse JSG: In *Anatomie van den Mensch*. Edited by Groeve JG. Rotterdam: 1891.

11. Gil-Vernet J: New surgical concepts in removing renal calculi. *Urol Int* 1965, 20:255–288.

12. Smith M, Boyce W: Anatrophic nephrotomy and plastic calyrrhaphy. *Trans Am Assoc Genitourin Surg* 1967, 59:18–24.

13. Wickham JA, Coe N, Ward JP: 100 cases of nephrolithotomy under hypothermia. *J Urol* 1974, 112:702–705.

14. Semb C: Partial resection of the kidney: anatomical, physiological and clinical aspects. *Ann R Coll Surg Engl* 1956, 19:137–155.

15. Boyce WH: The localization of intrarenal calculi during surgery. *J Urol* 1977, 18:152–157.

16. Segura JW, Preminger GM, Assimor DG, *et al.*: Nephrolithiasis clinical guidelines panel summary report on the management of staghorn calculi. *J Urol* 1994, 151:1648–1651.

17. Paik ML, Wainstein MA, Spirnak JP, *et al.*: Current indications for open stone surgery in the treatment of renal and ureteral calculi. *J Urol* 1998, 159:374–379.

18. Assimos DG, Boyce WH, Harrison LH, *et al.*: The role of open stone surgery since extracorporeal shock wave lithotripsy. *J Urol* 1989, 142:263–267.

19. Kane CJ, Bolton DM, Stoller ML, *et al.*: Current indications for open stone surgery in an endourology center. *Urology* 1995, 45: 218–221.

20. Streem SB, Novick AC, Hodge E, *et al.*: Preoperative hospitalization to hydrate living kidney donors can be omitted without sacrificing graft function. *J Urol* 1993, 150:1779–1781.

21. Samuel JR, McLeskey CH: Anaesthesia for intra-renal surgery. In *Intrarenal Surgery*. Edited by Wickham JEA. Edinburgh: Churchill Livingstone; 1984.

22. Hess E: Resection of the rib in renal operations. *J Urol* 1939, 42:943–956.

23. Turner Warwick RT: The supracostal approach to the renal area. *Br J Urol* 1965, 37:671–672.

24. Gardiner RA, Naunton-Morgan TC, Whitfield HN, *et al.*: The modified lumbotomy versus the oblique loin incision for renal surgery. *Br J Urol* 1979, 51:256–259.

25. Barry JM, Hodges CV: The supracostal approach to the kidney and adrenal. *J Urol* 1975, 114:666–669.

26. Zingg EZ, Futterlib A: Nephroscope in stone surgery. *Br J Urol* 1980, 52:333–337.

27. Marberger M, Hruby W: Intraoperative radiology: the film. In *Intrarenal Surgery*. Edited by Wickham JEA. Edinburgh: Churchill Livingstone; 1984:307–315.

28. Gil-Vernet J, Culla A: Advances in intraoperative renal radiography: 3-dimensional radiography of the kidney. *J Urol* 1981, 125:614–619.

29. Singh M, Tresidder GC, Blandy J: The long-term results of removal of staghorn calculi by extended pyelolithotomy without cooling or renal artery occlusion. *Br J Urol* 1971, 43:658–664.

30. Fitzpatrick JM, Sleight MW, Braack A, *et al.*: Intrarenal access: effects on renal function and morphology. *Br J Urol* 1980, 52:409–414.

31. Graves FT: The anatomy of the intrarenal arteries and its application to segmental resection of the kidney. *Br J Urol* 1954, 42:132–139.

32. Pettersson S: Renal preservation in extracorporeal surgery. In *Renal Preservation.* Edited by Marberger M, Dreikorn K. Baltimore: Williams & Wilkins; 1983:139–142.

33. Pettersson S: Bench surgery and renal autotransplantation for calculi. In *Renal Tract Stone.* Edited by Wickham JEA, Colin BA. Edinburgh: Churchill Livingstone; 1990:501–516.

34. McDougal WS: Renal perfusion/reperfusion injuries. *J Urol* 1988, 140:1325–1330.

35. Streem SB, Novick AC, Hodge E, *et al.*: Preoperative hospitalization to hydrate living kidney donors can be omitted without sacrificing graft function. *J Urol* 1993, 150:1779–1781.

36. Hansson R, Johansson S, Jonsson O, *et al.*: Effects of free radical scavengers on renal circulation after ischemia in the rabbit. *J Clin Sci* 1986, 71:245–251.

37. Fuhrman FA, Field J: The reversibility of the inhibition of rat brain and kidney metabolism by cold. *Am J Physiol* 1943, 139:193–196.

38. Ward JP: Determination of the optimum temperature for regional renal hypothermia during temporary renal ischaemia. *Br J Urol* 1975, 47:17–24.

39. Nosowsky EE, Kaufman JJ: The protective action of mannitol in renal artery occlusion. *J Urol* 1963, 89:295–299.

40. Freeman AB, Crapo JD: Biology of disease, free radicals and tissue injury. *Lab Invest* 1982, 47:412–426.

41. Makato M, Yoshio I, Toyohie M: Operative nephroscopy with fiberoptic scope: preliminary report. *J Urol* 1978, 119:166–168.

42. Alken P: Radial nephrolithotomy under ultrasound and Doppler probe control; Intraoperative radiology; Intra-operative pyeloscopy. In *Urolithiasis: Therapy, Prevention. Encyclopedia of Urology*, vol 17. Edited by Schneider HJ. Berlin: Springer; 1986:140–180.

43. Lytton B: Intraoperative ultrasound for nephrolithotomy. *J Urol* 1983, 130:213–217.

44. Rubenstein MA, Norris DM, Chun LS: Intraoperative localization of renal calculi using the Polarex 2 C-arm image intensifier. *J Urol* 1979, 121:562–563.

45. Resnick MI, Boyce WH: Bilateral staghorn calculi: patient evaluation and management. *J Urol* 1980, 123:338–341.

46. Turner Warwick R: The use of the omental pedicle graft in urinary tract reconstruction. *J Urol* 1976, 116:340–347.

Medical Therapy for Urolithiasis

Villis R. Marshall

Integral to our attempts to understand the cause of urolithiasis has been the desire to apply that knowledge to develop a therapy that will bring about stone dissolution. The stability of calcium oxalate in urine has made this little more than a dream. However some success has been achieved, particularly with uric acid stones. Unfortunately, such stones represent only a relatively small proportion of the total stone incidence. Therefore, medical therapy appears to have two practical means of influencing urolithiasis: primary prevention and the prevention of recurrence. This chapter explores how these options can be applied and examines the evidence available to support the effectiveness of medical therapy.

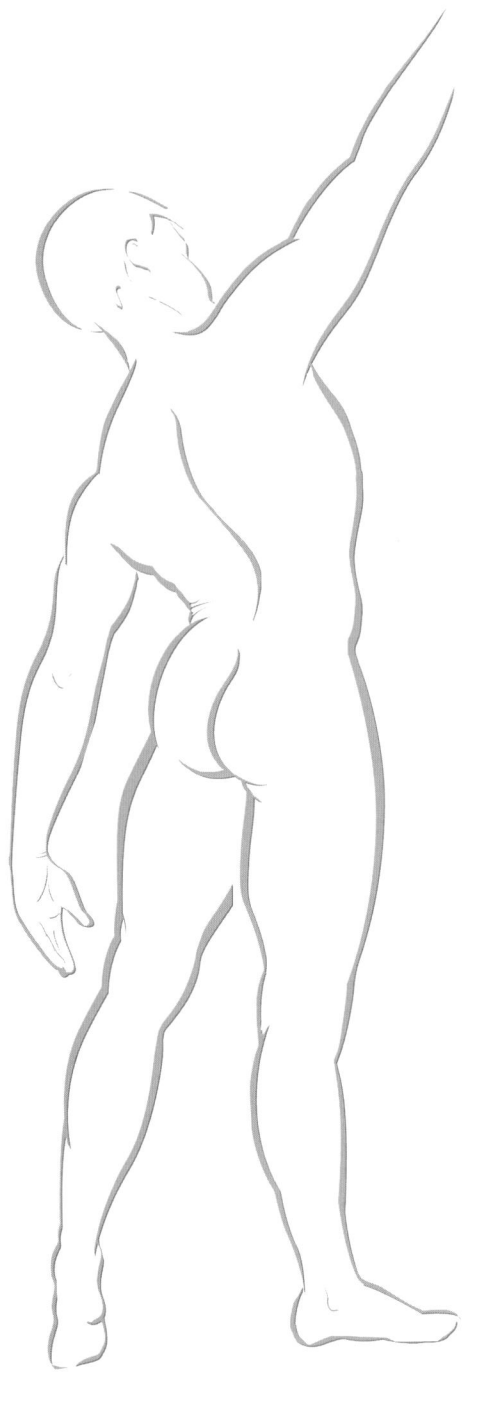

Types of Urinary Stones

Calcium oxalate, calcium phosphate
Uric acid
Struvite
Cystine
Dihidroxyadenine
Xanthine
Triamterene
Silicate

▶ **FIGURE 12-1.** The stone types identified in humans. The latter two, triamterine and silicate, are extraordinarily rare; these are iatrogenic stones, and avoidance of triamterine and silicate in antacid preparations should ensure that these stones no longer occur. Unfortunately, primary prevention of the more common stone types is by no means as simple. The initial step in the formation of any stone is the formation of crystals of the stone-forming substance. Thus, for crystals to occur, the urine needs to become supersaturated with a particular salt. Although it is acknowledged that crystallization is only one step in the chain that results in stone formation, this appears to be the initial critical step. If crystallization could be prevented, stone formation would not take place. It does not, however, mean that other strategies that may result in prevention of crystal aggregation may not be an extremely effective means of preventing stone formation.

PRIMARY PREVENTION OF CALCIUM OXALATE STONES

The Key Determinants of Calcium Oxalate Stone Prevention

Fluid output
Diet

▶ **FIGURE 12-2.** Prevention of calcium oxalate stones. It would appear that maintaining a high fluid intake and, hence, fluid output coupled with an appropriate diet is the best means of preventing calcium oxalate stone formation. Although this appears to be sound advice, there is little published evidence to show that a high fluid intake is associated with low rates of stone occurrence. The work of Blacklock [1] is frequently cited. In that study, he reported that stone formation dropped by 86% in British sailors when the average urine output was increased from 800 to 1200 mL. Note that a 1200-mL output did not entirely prevent stone formation, however, and it would seem necessary for the urine output to exceed this volume consistently for prevention of stone formation. Even with a high 24-hour urine output, the urine may still become supersaturated with calcium oxalate, particularly at night or after meals. As indicated, it seems that 1.2 L probably represents an underestimation of the output needed. On the basis of epidemiologic studies [2], an output of more than 2 L per day appears to be the minimum requirement to prevent stone formation.

Dietary Factors Capable of Increasing the Risk of Calcium Oxalate Lithiasis

High sodium intake
High-protein diet
High calcium intake

▶ **FIGURE 12-3.** Possible risk-increasing factors for developing calcium oxalate lithiasis. High sodium intake, high protein intake, and high-calcium diet have all been proposed to be risk factors for the formation of calcium oxalate stones.

Proposed Mechanisms of Action of Sodium

Causes increase in urinary calcium excretion
Causes reduction in urinary citrate excretion
Causes increased saturation of sodium urate

▶ **FIGURE 12-4.** Possible sodium mechanisms of action. It has been postulated that because high sodium intake has these documented abilities, lowering the sodium intake may reduce stone recurrence rates. However, a large epidemiologic study was unable to demonstrate a significant correlation between sodium intake and stone incidence [3]. Thus, a low-sodium diet does not appear to be beneficial.

Proposed Mechanisms of Action of Protein

Increases urinary calcium excretion
Reduces urinary pH
Reduces urinary citrate excretion
Increases uric acid excretion

FIGURE 12-5. The mechanism of action of protein determined from the metabolic studies of Breslau *et al.* [4] and Fellström *et al.* [5]. Epidemiologic studies have failed to establish an association between calcium oxalate stone formation and the protein content of the diet [6–8]. Therefore, on theoretical grounds, it remains attractive to suggest that a low-protein diet will be protective, but more careful epidemiologic or case-controlled studies are necessary before a causative effect can be established with certainty.

•• HIGH CALCIUM INTAKE ••

Dietary Calcium and Stone Formation

Low dietary calcium levels may reduce the binding of oxalate in the gut resulting in increased absorption of oxalate
Oxalate is more important in determining urinary calcium oxalate saturation than calcium

FIGURE 12-6. Dietary calcium and oxalate in stone formation. The observation by Flocks [9] that a high level of urinary calcium excretion was a common finding in patients with calcium oxalate stones has helped spawn the idea that lowering calcium intake would be beneficial in reducing stone formation. However, our belief that this is a valuable approach has been challenged by recent epidemiologic studies. Curhan *et al.* [3] found that subjects on a high-calcium diet had a lower incidence of stones than those who had a low consumption of calcium. The question then is how we can reconcile this observation with the theoretical aspects of calcium oxalate crystallization. This somewhat paradoxical situation is due to the fact that if calcium is reduced in the diet, less oxalate is bound to calcium in the gut. As a result, enteric oxalate absorption is increased. Because oxalate is more important in determining the urinary saturation of calcium oxalate than calcium, it has the potential to increase crystal formation. Thus, lowering calcium levels in the diet is not protective unless the level of oxalate is also lowered. Perhaps the best approach to calcium restriction is summarized by Coe *et al.* [10]: "...Physicians should drop dietary calcium restriction from their list of preventive and therapeutic measures for patients who are at risk for formation of calcium oxalate stones." Thus, one of the bastions of stone prevention, namely a low-calcium diet, seems destined for the dustbin of history.

PREVENTION OF CALCIUM OXALATE STONE RECURRENCE

Risk Factors for Stone Recurrence

Urinary volume
Urinary calcium excretion
Urinary oxalate excretion
Urinary urate excretion
Urinary citrate excretion
pH
Inhibitors

FIGURE 12-7. Risk factors for stone recurrence. As previously discussed, there is very good theoretical evidence to suggest that maintaining adequate hydration is helpful in preventing stone recurrence. At present, there is sparse evidence from randomized trials to support this concept in clinical practice, with only one report published recently [11]. Although a "stone clinic effect" is well recognized [12], and some studies have shown that patients who maintain an increased fluid intake have a low stone occurrence rate, the lack of randomized trials still places this in the "good idea basket." Also, the lack of randomized trials [13] makes it very difficult to advise patients effectively in clinical practice regarding what output they should maintain and over what period of time to achieve a beneficial effect. One important question regarding who needs to undergo preventive measures, needs to be answered. This question is particularly pertinent because recurrence rates quoted range from 5% to 15% [13,14]. Also, the other question that has to be addressed is whether a lifetime of treatment justifies the prevention of a single recurrence. The stone may pass spontaneously or could be dealt with by a relatively noninvasive modality, such as extracorporeal shock wave lithotripsy. To try to resolve this dilemma, attempts have been made to define risk factors for recurrence. The ones that have been most frequently chosen are shown in this figure. Considerable confusion has arisen because— despite many studies over many years by many workers in the field—it has not been possible to get consistent results. Although one group of researchers has found a significant change in a particular parameter in stone-formers, almost equivalent numbers of researchers have been unable to repeat their findings [15]. The other important practical fact is that there is no convincing evidence that patients with abnormal values have higher recurrence rates than stone-formers whose levels of a particular parameter fall within the normal range [16]. Thus, it is still difficult to determine who should have medical treatment, particularly after the first stone episode. It seems that in light of our inability to predict with surety those at high risk of recurrence, the timing of the introduction of therapy may best be determined by the natural history of the disease in a given patient. One other piece of information that may be of value in deciding whether early treatment is appropriate is the observation that the size of the initial stone appears to predict the likely size of future recurrences [17]. Because the size of the stone is usually an important indicator of the need for surgical intervention, patients who may have a greater potential to require surgical intervention could be offered preventive treatment sooner rather than later.

Factors That Influence the Supersaturation of Urine With Calcium Oxalate

Concentration of calcium
Concentration of oxalate
Concentration of urate
Concentration of citrate
Concentration of inhibitors
Concentration of promoters
pH

▶ **FIGURE 12-8.** Tailoring therapy to correct a particular abnormality. From this figure, it is evident that the metastable limit for and supersaturation of calcium oxalate in the urine can be influenced by many factors. These factors are all interdependent. The most important seems to be oxalate, although unfortunately its output in the urine seems to be the parameter that is least easily influenced. The practical aspect of the interdependence of these agents is the observation that even if a particular parameter is not abnormal, it does not mean that lowering the concentration will not have a beneficial effect on calcium oxalate stone recurrence. It is interesting to note that a number of studies found that the risk of recurrence was reduced whether or not the patients initially had high or normal calcium levels when agents that had the capacity to lower calcium excretion were used in randomized trials [18–20]. Therefore, there is doubt whether there is value in trying to tailor therapy to correct a particular abnormality.

Potential Mode of Action of Thiazides in Preventing Stone Recurrence

Thiazides augment calcium absorption in the distal tubule
Extracellular volume depletion as a result of thiazide administration
  leads to enhanced calcium absorption
Possible direct effect of calcium reabsorption from the gut
Possible reduction in urinary oxalate excretion
Thiazides improve the urinary inhibitory activity by increasing the
  excretion of zinc and magnesium

Documented Side Effects of Thiazide Diuretics

Fatigue
Impotence
Malaise
Constipation
Metabolic disorders
  Hypocalcemia
  Hypouricuria
  Metabolic alkalosis

Agents Used to Reduce Recurrence in Calcium Oxalate Stone-Formers

Thiazides
Orthophosphate
Sodium cellulase phosphate
Potassium citrate
Magnesium
Allopurinol

▶ **FIGURE 12-9.** Agents most frequently used to try to prevent stone recurrence. To date, thiazides have probably been the most widely used; in the view of Coe *et al.* [10], they are the best in the prevention of stone recurrence. In this era of greater emphasis on evidence-based medicine, the value of any of these agents must be challenged because of the paucity of randomized trials. In the case of diuretic therapy for the prevention of stones, Menon *et al.* [21] were able to find seven randomized trials up to 1998. Interestingly enough, even in those randomized trials, four did not find a significant difference in stone recurrence rates. Unfortunately, all the trials can be criticized because of poor stratification, the inability to be certain of the dropout rates, and the small numbers of participants. All but one trial had fewer than 100 participants, and the total number in the seven studies was just over 500 subjects. It is, in many ways, quite surprising that so few patients have been subjected to randomized trials, given that millions of people have been treated with lithotripsy over the last decade!

▶ **FIGURE 12-10.** The role of thiazides in preventing stone recurrence. The need for long-term randomized trials of thiazides is further reinforced by the finding that in patients with absorptive hypercalciuria [22], the hypocalciuric effect was not maintained at 5 years, but if the patients had renal hypercaliuria, the reduction was maintained. In both studies, however, the number of subjects involved was small (12 and 10, respectively). This aspect of the long-term effect of thiazides needs further evaluation and highlights the importance of careful classification of patients before they are entered into randomized trials. The need to assess carefully the potential value of thiazides before commencing treatment is particularly important because of the significant number of adverse side effects associated with them. It has been reported that 30% to 50% of patients may cease treatment as a consequence of these effects [23].

▶ **FIGURE 12-11.** Documented side effects of thiazides that highlight why many patients will stop taking these agents.

•• ORTHOPHOSPHATE IN THE PREVENTION OF •• CALCIUM OXALATE STONE RECURRENCE

Mode of Action of Orthophosphate in Preventing Stones

Reduces serum 1,25-(OH)2 D levels
Decreases calcium excretion
Increases pyrophosphate and citrate excretion
(both inhibitors of crystallization)

▶ **FIGURE 12-12.** Possible mechanisms by which orthophosphate may influence calcium oxalate stone formation. Although some uncontrolled studies have shown a reduction in stone formation, a randomized trial [24], albeit with a small number of subjects (71) and follow-up of less than 3 years, was unable to show a significant reduction in stone recurrence rates. Therefore, the value of this agent has yet to be proven, although it would certainly seem that further studies are justified. The major side effect is diarrhea.

•• SODIUM CELLULOSE PHOSPHATE IN THE PREVENTION •• OF CALCIUM OXALATE STONE RECURRENCE

Actions of Cellulose Phosphate

Strong binder of calcium in the gut
Increases the excretion of oxalate
(potentially negative effect)

▶ **FIGURE 12-13.** Actions of cellulose phosphate. A number of studies have shown that cellulose phosphate is active in reducing stone formation, but it has not been subjected to appropriate randomized trials. This agent also has the potential to cause both hypomagnesemia and hyperoxaluria. This outcome is likely to promote stone formation and therefore offset the beneficial effect of reducing the calcium level. A practical problem associated with its use is that patients need to take 10 to 15 grams a day with meals, and patient compliance is therefore likely to be low. Although there are some advantages associated with this agent, it has not achieved wide usage, and it seems unlikely to find an ongoing place in the medical management of calcium oxalate urolithiasis.

•• POTASSIUM CITRATE IN THE PREVENTION •• OF CALCIUM OXALATE STONES

Mode of Action of Potassium Citrate

An inhibitor of calcium oxalate crystal aggregation
Complexes with calcium to form a soluble calcium citrate salt
May increase the renal absorption of calcium

▶ **FIGURE 12-14.** Use of citrate. In recent years, there has been an increase in the use of citrate to reduce stone recurrence. This increase was supported by the observation that hypocitruria was found quite frequently in stone-formers, although this has not been by any means a universal finding [15]. Again, there is a paucity of randomized trials (only four studies currently identified) [25–28]. These studies do not all show a significant improvement; the number of subjects in the studies is relatively small, and follow-up is short. Nevertheless, the results do appear promising. Further studies are needed before citrate be unequivocally recommended as an effective preventive agent. The major side effect is gastrointestinal disturbance. Because of this somewhat lower side-effect profile, it may be a better alternative than thiazide for the prevention of recurrence.

Mechanisms by Which Urate May Promote Calcium Oxalate Lithiasis

Epitaxial nucleation
Neutralization of urinary inhibitors such as glycosaminoglycans
Salting out calcium oxalate by urate

▶ **FIGURE 12-15.** Role of urate in calcium oxalate lithiasis. Since the work of Yu and Gutman [29], there has been considerable interest in the mechanism by which urate may promote calcium oxalate lithiasis. As can be seen from this figure, both epitaxial nucleation of calcium oxalate crystallization by urate and the reduction in the activity of urinary inhibitors have been proposed as the mechanism for this effect of allopurinol, but neither mechanism has been demonstrated to occur under physiologic conditions. More recent studies [30,31] have indicated that salting out is the most likely explanation for this phenomenon, and it would seem that the other proposed mechanisms should now be rejected. A number of studies have shown a reduction in stone recurrence, but there has been a paucity of randomized trials (five studies have been identified), again with variable outcomes [20,32–35]. Uncertainty still remains regarding 1) the effectiveness of allopurinol in the prevention of calcium oxalate stone recurrence and 2) which abnormal urinary findings will predict a beneficial response to therapy.

•• OXALATE IN THE PREVENTION OF STONE FORMATION ••

Methods of Reducing Oxalate Expression

Diet
Vitamin C reduction
Pyridoxine supplements
Magnesium supplements

▶ **FIGURE 12-16.** Lowering oxalate excretion. Many of the treatments investigated to date have been based on real or presumed differences in the excretion of a number of substances between stone-formers and non–stone-formers, but little attention has been paid to lowering the amount of oxalate. On theoretical grounds, because of the important physicochemical properties of oxalate in this process, it would seem that greater attention needs to be given to lowering oxalate levels. One of the major problems has been finding an agent that can effectively achieve this goal. This figure indicates a number of strategies by which the urinary oxalate level may be reduced. Although all these steps can be used to try to lower oxalate levels, to date no randomized trials have been attempted to quantify the beneficial effect. However, it would certainly appear to be a fertile area for further research.

MAGNESIUM AND PREVENTION OF STONES

Mode of Action

Increased mode of action of magnesium supplements
Increased magnesium excretion with a resultant inhibitory effect on crystal aggregation
Reduction in tubular citrate reabsorption

▶ **FIGURE 12-17.** Possible mechanism by which magnesium supplementation may reduce urinary stone formation. Relatively few studies have been undertaken; however, two randomized trials [36,37] were unable to show a significant difference in recurrence rates between the treated and untreated individuals. Once again, the numbers involved in these studies were small, and both studies were lacking in detail regarding the stratification and randomization of the patients. Therefore, further studies are required before magnesium therapy can be discarded. In addition, intestinal side effects are a problem. Again, it seems unlikely that this form of therapy will attain prominence in the future, particularly since it has been almost a decade since the last significant trial was published.

PRIMARY PREVENTION OF URIC ACID STONES

Sources of Uric Acid

Diet (accounts for approximately 50% of uric acid production)
De novo synthesis
End-product of tissue breakdown

▶ **FIGURE 12-18.** Uric acid sources. As with other stone types, urate will be precipitated only if the solubility product is exceeded. Quite distinct from calcium oxalate, however, its solubility is markedly influenced by the urine pH as well as by its concentration. This figure indicates the potential sources of urate. Thus, in the primary prevention of uric acid stones, diet does have the potential to play a very important role. Fish, poultry, and red meats are significant sources of purines, which cause a high level of uric acid excretion. Fluid intake is also of considerable importance. It would seem that low fluid intake coupled with a high-purine diet leads to persistently acidic urine. Individuals who have gouty diathesis frequently have acidic urine; it may well be that the key factor in stone formation in this group is the acidity of the urine rather than the high level of urate.

URIC ACID STONE DISSOLUTION

Strategies for the Dissolution of Uric Acid Stones

Increase the pH level of urine to 6 to 6.5
Have the patient monitor urinary pH level
Reduce uric acid excretion by the use of allopurinol

▶ FIGURE 12-19. Dissolution of uric acid stones. Uric acid stones have the almost unique distinction of being able to be dissolved. This figure lists the strategies that are most frequently used to achieve this outcome. The urinary pH level can be best adjusted by the use of either potassium citrate or sodium bicarbonate. The usual dose of sodium citrate is 30 to 60 mEq/L in divided doses, and the usual dose of sodium bicarbonate is 650 mg three times a day. It is important whenever possible to get the patient to monitor the urinary pH level because the ideal level is around 6.5. Levels higher than 7 may predispose to calcium oxalate crystal and stone formation, although this may be more a theoretical than practical consideration.

PREVENTION OF URIC ACID STONE RECURRENCE

Indications for Allopurinol Therapy

Hyperuricemia
Recurrent uric acid lithiasis despite adequate dietary and alkalization measures
Chemotherapy for myeloproliferative disorders

▶ FIGURE 12-20. Indications for allopurinol therapy. The hallmark of treatment to prevent uric acid stone recurrence is a high fluid intake (more than 2 L in 24 hours) and a diet low in fish, poultry, and red meats. The other valuable addition is the alkalization of the urine. Allopurinol is well tolerated, and the major side effects are a rash and gastrointestinal symptoms.

STRUVITE STONES

Key Factors in Struvite Stone Formation

pH >7.2
Ammonia in the urine
Urease-producing bacteria

▶ FIGURE 12-21. Struvite stone formation. Struvite stones are relatively uncommon, accounting for fewer than 5% of stones in most series. Control of infection coupled with adequate hydration is the key to preventing recurrence of these stones. The choice of antibiotics depends on the antibiotic sensitivity of the infecting organism. The control of infection will be compromised in the presence of residual stones or fragments. The ability of infecting organisms to produce urease is important; although it may not be possible to eradicate the infection completely, a valuable adjunct is to try to inhibit the urease produced by the bacteria. To this end, acetohydroxyamine has been used. Three randomized trials have shown a benefit when this agent was used [38–40]. As can be seen in Figure 12-22, however, it has a very significant side-effect profile. Given this long list of side effects, it is not surprising that even though this agent has been beneficial in preventing stone growth or recurrence, significant numbers of patients had to be withdrawn from trials [39].

▶ FIGURE 12-22. Acetohydroxamic acid has a wide range of troublesome side effects.

Side Effects Attributed to Acetohydroxamic Acid

Tremor	Alopecia
Headache	Anemia
Nausea	Diarrhea
Hallucination	Palpitations

Inhibitors of Urease

Fluorofamide
Hydroxyurea
Hydrocarbomide
Hydroxamic acid

▶ **FIGURE 12-23.** Other known inhibitors of urease. Although these agents may be useful in the treatment of staghorn stones, little more than pilot studies have been undertaken with these agents to date, and thus their value is yet to be established.

CYSTINE STONES

Solubility of Cystine and pH

pH	Solubility, mg/L
5.0	300
7.0	400
	1000

▶ **FIGURE 12-24.** Influence of pH on the solubility of cystine. Cystine stones usually account for fewer than 1% of stones in most series. Consequently, the two most frequently used methods of preventing cystine stone recurrence are lowering its concentration and raising the pH of the urine. To maintain the concentration of cystine at a safe level requires a urinary output of at least 3 L per 24 hours. In many patients this is difficult to achieve, particularly since the volume almost invariably results in nocturia; compliance with this degree of hydration is often poor. The pH level needs to be higher than 7.5 to dissolve cystine crystals. This requires massive amounts of bicarbonate, up to 25 grams per day. If hydration and alkalization fail, then cystine-complexing agents can be used. The two that have been tried are D-penicillamine and a mercaptoproprionyl glycine. The dose of each needs to be titrated to try to reduce the concentration of cystine to less than 200 mg/L. In some instances, the dose required is not sustainable because of the adverse side effects. The major side effects are gastrointestinal and dermatologic.

MISCELLANEOUS STONES

Treatment of Dihydroxyadenine and Xanthine Stones

Allopurinol—Hydration
Xanthine—Hydration

▶ **FIGURE 12-25.** Treatment of these extremely rare types of stone. Once again, aggressive hydration is the best treatment. Allopurinol is useful for dihydroxyadenine stones.

REFERENCES

1. Blacklock NJ: The pattern of urolithiasis in the Royal Navy. In *Renal Stone Research Symposium*. Edited by Hodgkinson A, Nordin BEC. London: Churchill Ltd; 1969:33–47.

2. Harvey JA, Hill KD, Pak CYC: Similarity of urinary risk factors among stone-forming patients in five regions of the United States. *J Lithotr Stone Dis* 1990, 2:124.

3. Curhan GC, Willett WC, Rimm EB, *et al.*: A prospective study of dietary calcium and other nutrients and the risk of symptomatic kidney stones. *N Engl J Med* 1993, 328:833–838.

4. Breslau NA, Brinkley L, Hill KD, *et al.*: Relationship of animal protein-rich diet to kidney stone formation and calcium metabolism. *J Clin Endocrinol Metab* 1988, 65:140–146.

5. Fellström B, Danielson BG, Karlström B, *et al.*: Effects of high intake of dietary animal protein on mineral metabolism and urinary supersaturation of calcium oxalate in renal stone formers. *Br J Urol* 1984, 56:263–269.

6. Brockis JG, Vevitt AJ, Cruthers SM: The effects of vegetable and animal protein diets on calcium, urate and oxalate excretion. *Br J Urol* 1982, 54:590–593.

7. Power C: Diet and renal stones: a case-control study. In *Urinary Stone*. Edited by Ryall RL, Brockis JG, Marshall VR, Finlayson B. London: Churchill Livingstone, 1983:30–33.

8. Goldfarb S: Diet and nephrolithiasis. *Endocrinol Metab Clin North Am* 1994, 45:235–243.

9. Flocks RH: Calcium and phosphorus excretion in the urine of patients with renal or ureteral calculi. *JAMA* 1939, 113:1466–1471.

10. Coe FL, Parks JH, Favus MJ: Diet and calcium: the end of an era? *Ann Intern Med* 1997, 126:553–555.

11. Borghi L, Meschi T, Amato F, *et al.*: Urinary volume, water and recurrences in idiopathic calcium nephrolithiasis: a 5-year randomized prospective study. *J Urol* 1996, 155:839–843.

12. Hosking DH, Erickson SB, Van Den Berg CJ, *et al.*: The stone clinic effect in patients with idiopathic calcium urolithiasis. *J Urol* 1983, 130:1115–1118.

13. Strauss A, Coe FL, Deutsch L, *et al.*: Factors that predict relapse of calcium nephrolithiasis during treatment: a prospective study. *Am J Med* 1982, 72:17–24.

14. Joost J, Putz A: Calcium oxalate stone formers: five years later. In *Urolithiasis and Related Clinical Research*. Edited by Schwille PO, Smith LH, Robertson WG, Vahlensieck W. New York: Plenum Press; 1985:557–560.

15. Ryall RL, Marshall VR: The investigation and management of idiopathic urolithiasis. In *Renal Tract Stone: Metabolic Basis and Clinical Practice*. Edited by Wickham JEA, Buck AC. London: Churchill Livingstone; 1990: 307–331.

16. Parks JH, Coe FL: An increasing number of calcium oxalate stone events worsens treatment outcome. *Kidney Int* 1994, 45:1722–1730.

17. Blandy JP, Marshall VR: Size of renal calculi recurrence rate and follow-up. *Br J Urol* 1976, 45:525–530.

18. Ljunghall S, Backman U, Danielson BG, *et al.*: Epidemiology of renal stones in Sweden in a middle aged male population. *Acta Med Scand* 1975, 197:439–445.

19. Laerum E, Larsen S: Thiazide prophylaxis of urolithiasis: a double blind study in general practice. *Acta Med Scand* 1984, 215:383–389.

20. Smith MJV: Placebo vs allopurinol for renal calculi. *J Urol* 1977, 117:690–692.

21. Menon M, Parulkar BG, Drach GW: Urinary lithiasis: etiology, diagnosis and medical management. In *Campbell's Urology*. Edited by Walsh PC, Retik AB, Vaughan ED Jr, Wein AJ. Philadelphia: WB Saunders Co; 1998:2661–2733.

22. Preminger GM, Pak CYC: Eventual attenuation of hypocalciuric response to hydrochlorothiazide in absorptive hypercalciuria. *J Urol* 1987, 137:1104–1109.

23. Yendt ER, Guay GF, Garcia DA: The use of thiazides in the prevention of renal calculi. *Can Med Assoc J* 1970, 102:614–620.

24. Ettinger B: Recurrent nephrolithiasis: natural history and effect of phosphate therapy: a double blind controlled study. *Am J Med* 1976, 61:200–206.

25. Abdulhadi MH, Hall PM, Streem SB: Can citrate therapy prevent nephrolithiasis? *Urology* 1993, 41:221–224.

26. Barcelo P, Wuhl O, Servitage E, *et al.*: Randomized double-blind study of potassium citrate in idiopathic hypocitraturic calcium nephrolithiasis. *J Urol* 1993, 150:1761–1766.

27. Hofbauer J, Hobarth R, Szabo N, *et al.*: Alkali citrate prophylaxis in idiopathic recurrent calcium oxalate urolithiasis: a prospective randomized study. *Br J Urol* 1994, 73:362–365.

28. Ettinger B, Pak CYC, Citron JT, *et al.*: Randomized trial of potassium magnesium citrate in the prevention of recurrent calcium oxalate nephrolithiasis. In *Urolithiasis*. Edited by Pack CYC, Resnick MI, Preminger GM. Dallas: Millet The Printer Inc; 1996:437–439.

29. Yu T-F, Gutman AB: Uric acid nephrolithiasis in gout: predisposing factors. *Ann Intern Med* 1967, 67:1133–1148.

30. Grover PK, Ryall RL, Marshall VR: Effect of urate on calcium oxalate crystallization in human urine: evidence for a promotory role of hyperuricosuria in urolithiasis. *Clin Sci* 1990, 79:9–15.

31. Grover PK, Ryall RL, Marshall VR: Dissolved urate promotes calcium oxalate crystallization: epitaxy is not the cause. *Clin Sci* 1993, 85:303–307.

32. Wilson DR, Strauss Al, Manuel MA: Comparison of medical treatments for the prevention of recurrent calcium nephrolithiasis [abstract]. *Urol Res* 1984, 12:39–40.

33. Ettinger B, Citron JT, Tang A, *et al.*: Prophylaxis of calcium oxalate stones: clinical trials of allopurinol, magnesium hydroxide and chlorthalidone. In *Urolithiasis and Related Clinical Research*. Edited by Schwille PO, Smith LH, Robertson WG, Vahlensieck W. New York: Plenum Press; 1985:549–552.

34. Miano L, Petta S, Paradiso GG, *et al.*: A placebo controlled double-blind study of allopurinol in severe recurrent idiopathic renal lithiasis: preliminary results. In *Urolithiasis and Related Clinical Research*. Edited by Schwille PO, Smith LH, Robertson WG, Vahlensieck W. New York: Plenum Press; 1985:521–524.

35. Robertson WG, Peacock M, Selby PL: A multicenter trial to evaluate three treatments for recurrent idiopathic calcium stone disease: a preliminary report. In *Urolithiasis and Related Clinical Research*. Edited by Schwille PO, Smith LH, Robertson WG, Vahlensieck W. New York: Plenum Press; 1985:545–548.

36. Wilson DR, Strauss AL, Manuel MA: Comparison of medical treatments for the prevention of recurrent calcium nephrolithiasis [abstract]. *Urol Res* 1984, 12:39–40.

37. Ettinger B, Citron JT, Tang A, *et al.*: Prophylaxis of calcium oxalate stones: clinical trials of allopurinol, magnesium hydroxide and chlorthalidone. In *Urolithiasis and Related Clinical Research*. Edited by Schwille PO, Smith LH, Robertson WG, Vahlensieck W. New York: Plenum Press; 1985:549–552.

38. Williams JJ, Rodman JS, Peterson CM: A randomized double-blind study of acetohydroxamic acid in struvite nephrolithiasis. *N Engl J Med* 1984, 311:760–764.

39. Griffith DP, Khonsari F, Skurnick JH: Experimental and clinical trials of lithostat (acetohydroxamic acid-AHA). In *Inhibitors of Crystallization in Renal Lithiasis and Their Clinical Application*. Edited by Martelli A, Buli P, Marchesini B. Bologna, Italy: Acta Medica; 1988:228–235.

40. Gleeson MJ, Griffith DP: Infection stones. In *A Medical and Surgical Reference*. Edited by Resnick MI, Pak CYC. Philadelphia: WB Saunders Co; 1990:113–132.

Laparoscopic Nephrectomy

Hamdy El Kappany
Ibrahim Eraky
Mohamed A. Ghoneim

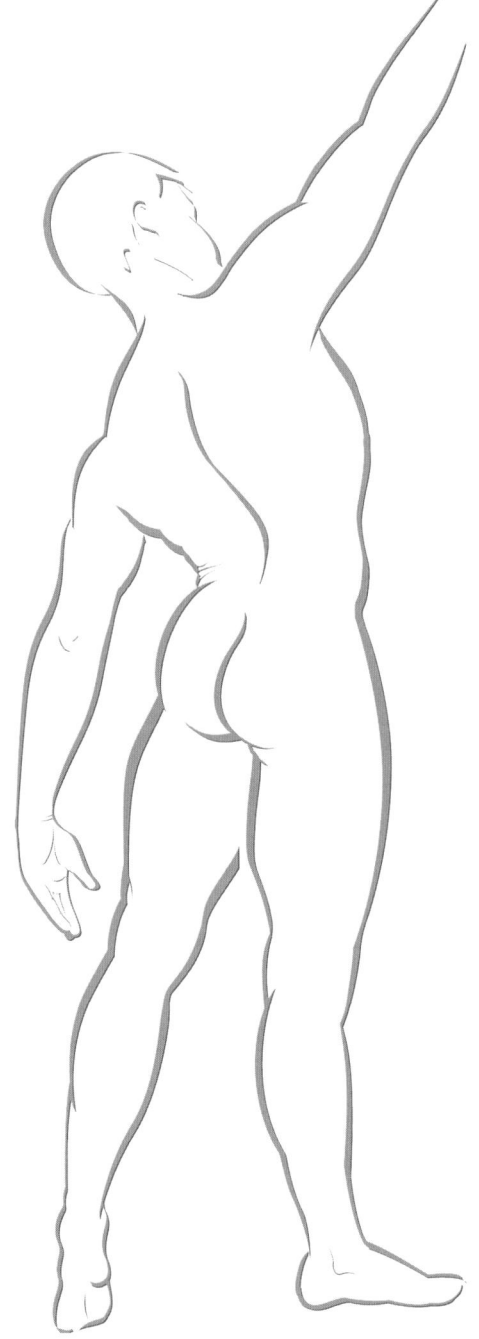

Laparoscopic nephrectomy became a reality when Clayman *et al.* [1,2] performed their first case through a transperitoneal approach after their extensive experimental studies using a pig animal model. They resolved the technical problem of the retrieval of the dissected kidney through a 10-mm port. This retrieval was achieved by designing a special bag for kidney entrapment and using an electrical tissue morcellator to fragment and aspirate the kidney inside the bag.

Initially, the procedure was restricted to patients with small, nonfunctioning kidneys having benign pathology [3,4]. As a result of refinement of laparoscopic instrumentation and the surgical experience gained with this technique, the scope of indications has progressively increased. Currently, the procedure is used for all types of benign renal disease: xanthogranulomatous pyelonephritis, polycystic kidney disease, native donor nephrectomy, and renal tumors [5–11].

Until a few years ago, most laparoscopic nephrectomies had been performed via the transperitoneal approach. In 1992, Gaur [12] introduced the retroperitoneal approach. A balloon was used for creation of the retroperitoneal space [12]. So far, more than 600 laparoscopic nephrectomies via the transperitoneal or retroperitoneal approach have been performed for benign disease in many medical centers worldwide. More than 200 cases have been performed in the Urology and Nephrology Center in Mansoura, Egypt [4,8,10,11]. Based on our experience there, we recommend the retroperitoneal approach for removal of small and average-sized kidneys and the transperitoneal approach for large kidneys and when dissection difficulties are expected, as in obese patients or when there is suspicion of severe perirenal adhesions.

For safe and proper handling of the ureter, kidney, and renal pedicle, a good understanding of the anatomy of the kidney region is important. Good positioning of the surgical ports is essential with proper use of suitable instruments.

The average operating time ranges from 55 minutes to 6 hours. However, the operating time decreased with the surgeons' increasing experience [5–8]. Laparoscopic nephrectomy has the advantage of a short hospital stay (3 to 6 days) and convalescence (1 to 2 weeks) with a marked decrease in the need for postoperative analgesics. In contrast to open nephrectomy with its inherent operative and postoperative complications [13–16], laparoscopic nephrectomy is associated with less surgical trauma (such as muscle-cutting incision); this allows rapid convalescence and early return to work. The total complication rate is about 12% to 15%; the major complication rate is about 3%. The conversion rate to open surgery due to difficulty of the procedure (elective) or major intraoperative complication (emergency) was 3% to 9% [8,17].

INDICATIONS AND CONTRAINDICATIONS

Indications for Laparoscopic Nephrectomy

Benign symptomatic nonfunctioning kidneys
  Hydronephrosis
  Chronic pyelonephritic kidneys
  End-stage renal disease
  Renal hypoplasias and dysplastic kidneys
Donor nephrectomy (?)
Malignant renal condition (?)

▶ **FIGURE 13-1.** Indications for laparoscopic nephrectomy. The most common indication for removal of the kidneys through a laparoscopic approach is nonfunction secondary to a benign cause. These cases include nonfunctioning kidneys (such as kidneys in hydronephrosis or chronic pyelonephritis with or without vesicoureteral reflux) associated with reno-vascular hypertension and small kidneys in patients with chronic renal failure [5–8]. The condition must be symptomatic to a degree that justifies this intervention, such as recurrent pain or urinary tract infection. Live-donor nephrectomy is feasible through this approach in both experimental work and the clinical setting [18,19]; however, most surgeons are still reluctant to adopt this approach in view of the high level of safety that must be ensured [8]. Some investigators reported the removal of malignant kidneys in select cases. To avoid the hazard of spread to trocar sites, morcellation is avoided, and the kidney is extracted through a small incision [11]. The safety of this approach is not guaranteed, however, and many reports of malignant spread in other abdominal tumors have been published [20]. Also, this approach is challenged by the recent trend toward conservative surgical management of small renal tumors [21].

Contraindications to Laparoscopic Nephrectomy

Uncorrected coagulopathy
Severe cardiopulmonary disease
Previous multiple abdominal operations
Previous renal surgery
Malignant renal conditions (?)

▶ **FIGURE 13-2.** Contraindications to laparoscopic nephrectomy. Bleeding tendency and severe cardiopulmonary conditions are contraindications to any surgical intervention. Previous multiple abdominal operations are a relative contraindication to the transperitoneal approach. It could be tried using Hasson's technique, but the retroperitoneal approach is better in these cases. Previous renal surgery is a contraindication because the kidney is always surrounded by a dense fibrous reaction, which cannot be safely handled with the available dissection techniques [8].

SURGICAL ANATOMY

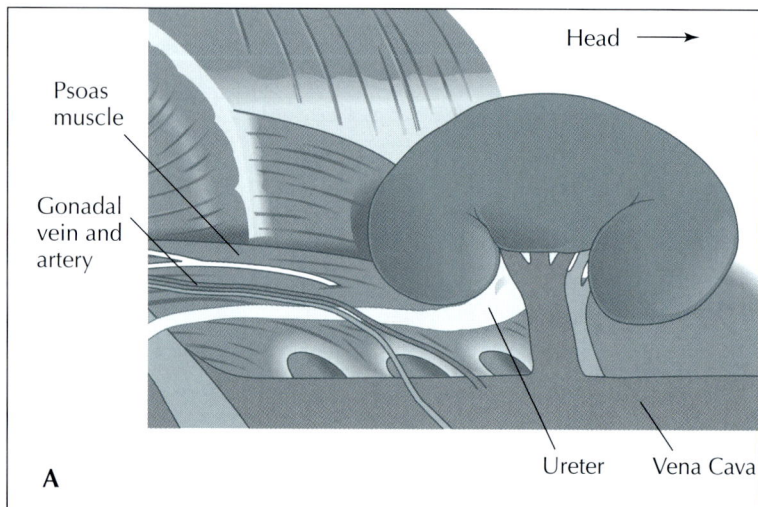

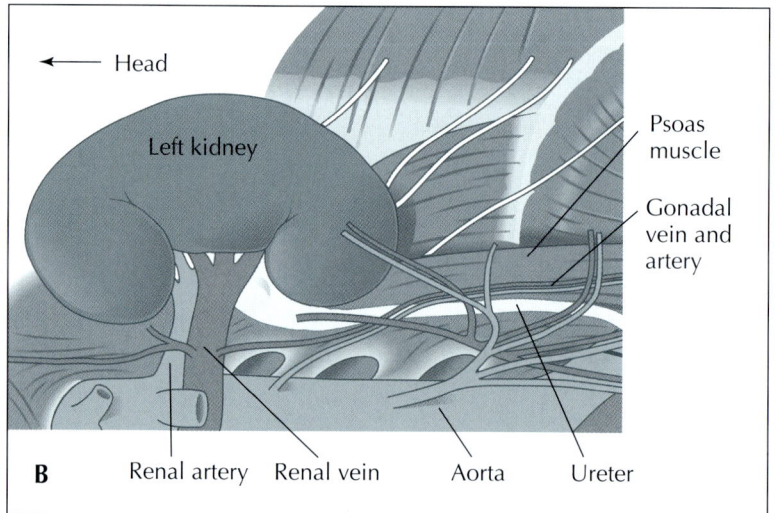

▶ **FIGURE 13-3.** Anatomy for the transperitoneal approach. The patient lies in the lumbar position. The surgeon stands on the abdominal side of the patient. The colon passes anterior to the kidney and ureter. The kidney becomes visible after reflection of the colon. The ureter passes anteromedial to the psoas major muscle until it reaches the renal hilum.

The identification and dissection of the ureter are facilitated by upward traction on the lower pole of the kidney. Proximal dissection of the ureter leads to the medial side of the renal pelvis, where the renal artery and vein can be safely dissected. The renal vein is anteroinferior to the renal artery. In some cases, exposure of the vena cava in right-sided nephrectomy allows better visualization of the renal vein (**A**), whereas on the left side the aorta is the landmark for the left renal artery (**B**). Exposure of the pedicle stump allows better and earlier control and avoids the need to deal with multiple branches and tributaries.

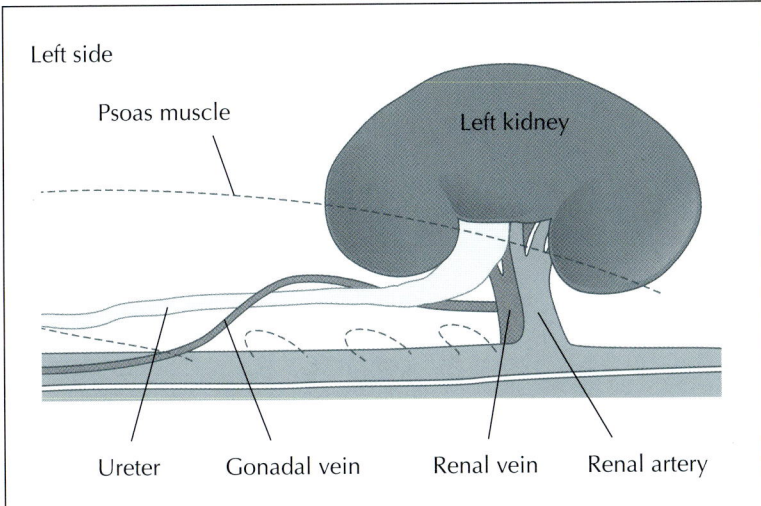

FIGURE 13-4. Anatomy for the retroperitoneal approach. The patient lies in the lumbar position. The surgeon stands on the dorsal side of the patient. The main landmark for orientation is the psoas muscle. A fibrous outer layer of Gerota's fascia is incised near the medial border of the psoas muscle to expose the perirenal fat. The ureter appears as a white band anteromedial to the psoas muscle, with its surrounding vascular supply. If it is followed up to the kidney with dissection of the perirenal fat, the renal pelvis will be exposed; here the renal artery appears first and is posterosuperior to the renal vein. The gonadal vessel appears clearly on the left side of this vein. On both right and left sides, gonadal veins appear medial to the ureter when they reach the renal hilum.

Preoperative Preparation

General anesthesia
Antibiotic prophylaxis
Urethral catheter
No need for ureteric catheter
No need for renal artery embolization

FIGURE 13-5. Preoperative preparation. The procedure is performed with the patient under general anesthesia using endotracheal intubation and good muscle relaxation. Acidosis due to CO_2 absorption is totally abolished with end-tidal CO_2 monitoring. Usually, prophylactic antibiotics are administered after fixation of the intravenous line. The urethral catheter is routinely fixed. Fixation of Ryle's tube is optimal. Familiarity with the surgical anatomy of the laparoscopic approach leads to easier identification of the ureter and control of the renal artery without fixation of the ureteric catheter or renal artery embolization.

TECHNIQUE OF TRANSPERITONEAL LAPAROSCOPIC NEPHRECTOMY

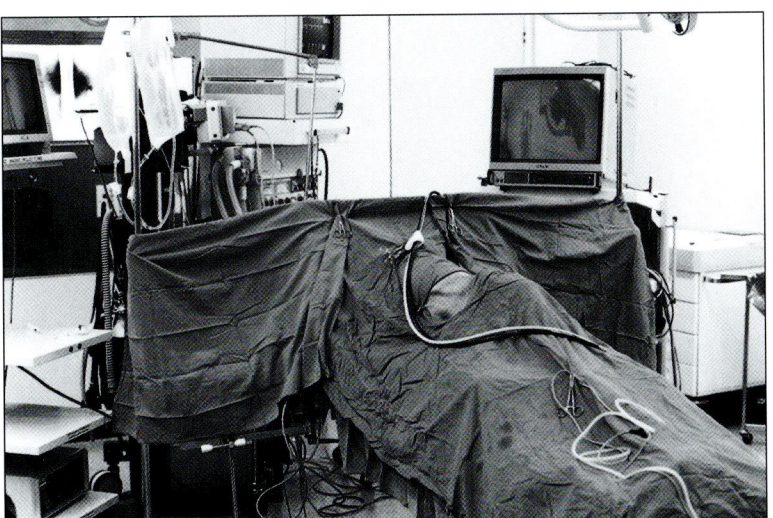

FIGURE 13-6. Patient positioning. The patient is put in a standard lumbar position. The surgeon stands on the abdominal side of the patient. Performing the operation in this position from the start avoids the need to reposition the patient after creation of a pneumoperitoneum in the supine position, as advocated by some surgeons [2]. This may play a role in shortening the operative time. It also facilitates the medial reflection of the colon by the effect of gravity just after incision of the posterior peritoneum. Also, if an open intervention is needed to deal with uncontrolled bleeding or a difficult dissection, a direct lumbar approach is feasible in a few minutes.

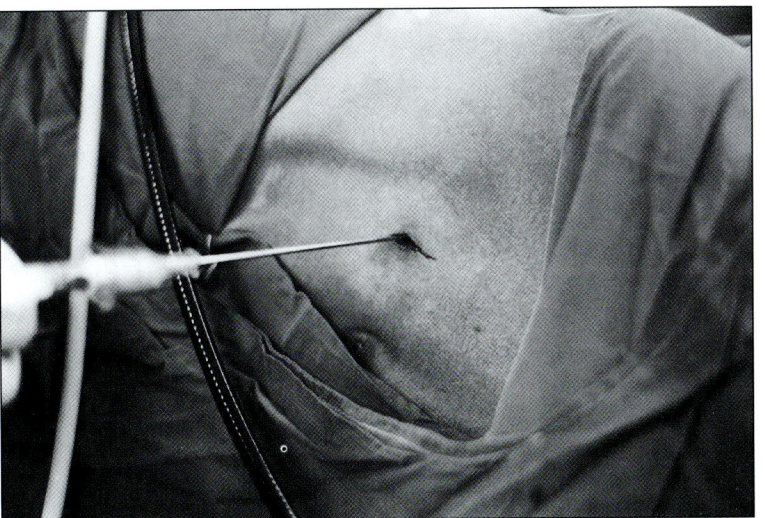

FIGURE 13-7. Creation of a pneumoperitoneum. The pneumoperitoneum is created using a Veress needle. The needle is introduced in a horizontal plane at the lateral border of the rectus muscle at the level of the umbilicus. The intraperitoneal position of the tip of the needle can be ensured by the visual and tactile verification of release of the needle spring, by the hanging drop test, and by easy injection of 2 mL of saline with failure of its retrieval on suctioning. Then CO_2 insufflation is started using slow filling at 1 L/min to avoid incidental air embolism until generalized resonance is achieved. The peritoneal cavity usually requires 3 to 6 L of CO_2 to be completely and safely inflated. In children, 1.5 to 3.0 L are required. Then the flow is increased to maintain intraperitoneal pressure at 15 mm Hg using an automatic insufflator.

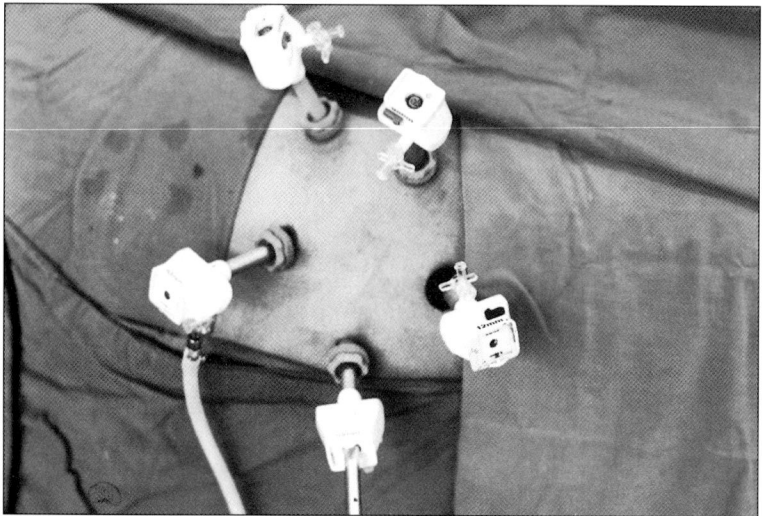
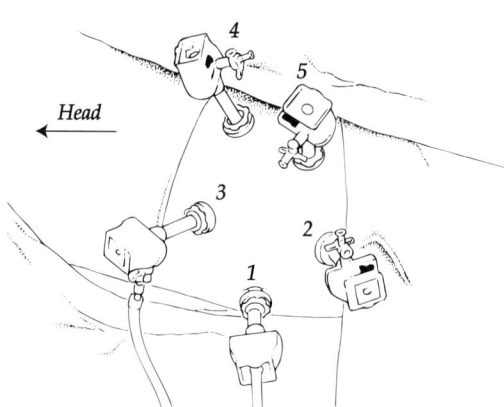

▶ **FIGURE 13-8.** Fixation of surgical ports. Four or five ports are used to accomplish this procedure. The first port (10 mm) is fixed at the site of the Veress needle. This port is used to introduce the laparoscope (10 mm, 0°). The whole procedure is visualized via two monitors at the head of the table using a high-quality charge-coupled device (CDD) camera connected to the laparoscope. Under endoscopic guidance, the second port (12 mm) is fixed midway between the first port and the anterior superior iliac spine. This port is used to introduce a dissecting electroscissors to control the renal vasculature, and the endoscopic pouch to entrap the kidney at the end of the operation. The third port (10 mm) is inserted below the costal margin at the midclavicular line and is used to introduce the Maryland forceps for tissue manipulation. The fourth port (10 mm) and the fifth port (5 or 10 mm) are inserted in the midaxillary line and are used for traction on tissues with the EndoBabcock (United States Surgical Corp., Norwalk, CT) or toothed forceps. Thorough inspection of the abdominal cavity is essential to exclude any inadvertent trauma, especially to the colon or blood vessels.

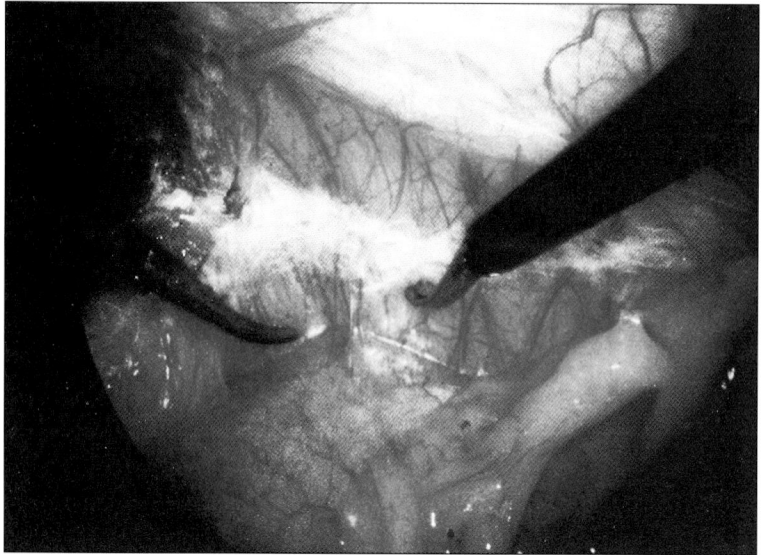
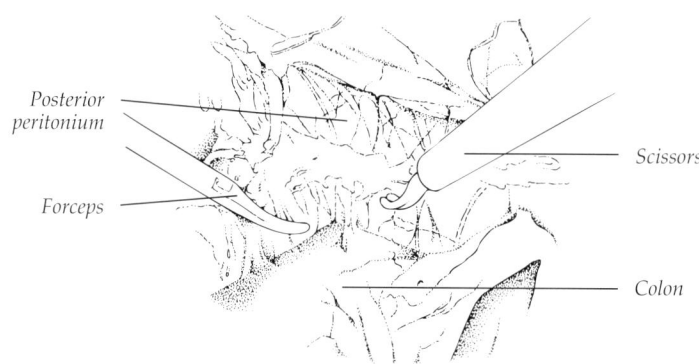

▶ **FIGURE 13-9.** (*See* Color Plate) Reflection of the colon. The peritoneum lateral to the colon (line of Toldt) is incised. This incision is performed using diathermy scissors and extends from the level of the iliac vessels distally to 10 cm above the colic flexures proximally. A safety distance (about 1 cm) lateral to the colon should be respected to avoid diathermy injury of the colon. By a combination of blunt and sharp dissection posterior to the colon, the colon becomes free from the posterior abdominal wall and is reflected medially under the effect of gravity.

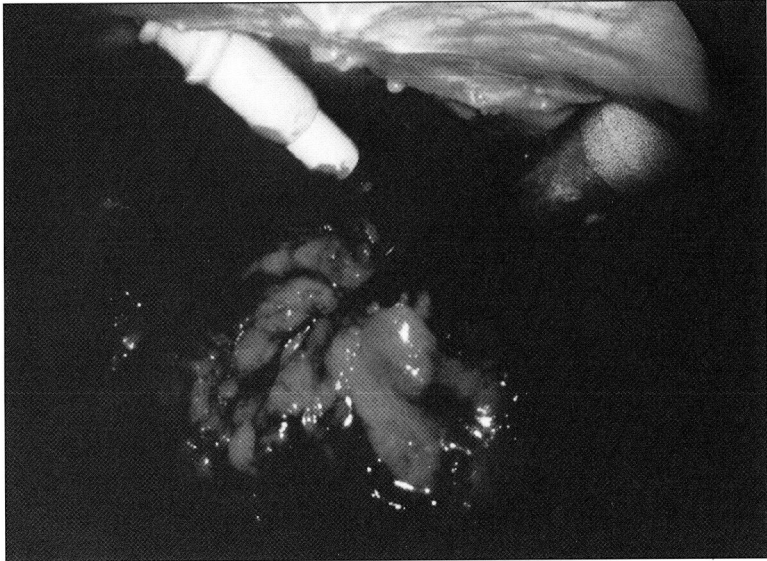

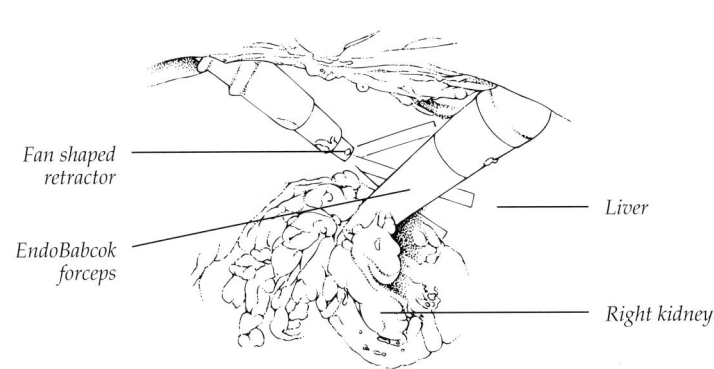

▶ **FIGURE 13-10.** (*See* Color Plate) Kidney dissection. Gerota's fascia is identified by its orange-yellow color, then incised to expose the renal surface. The plane between the fascia and the kidney surface is usually dissected easily with a combination of blunt and sharp dissection using endoshears connected to monopolar diathermy. In chronic pyelonephritis,

dissection of this plane may be difficult. In such cases, dissection of the kidney within its fascia at the extra-Gerotal plane may be carried out to avoid development of severe perirenal adhesions. To facilitate dissection of the upper pole, a fan-shaped retractor is passed through the fourth port to elevate the liver on the right side or the spleen on the left side.

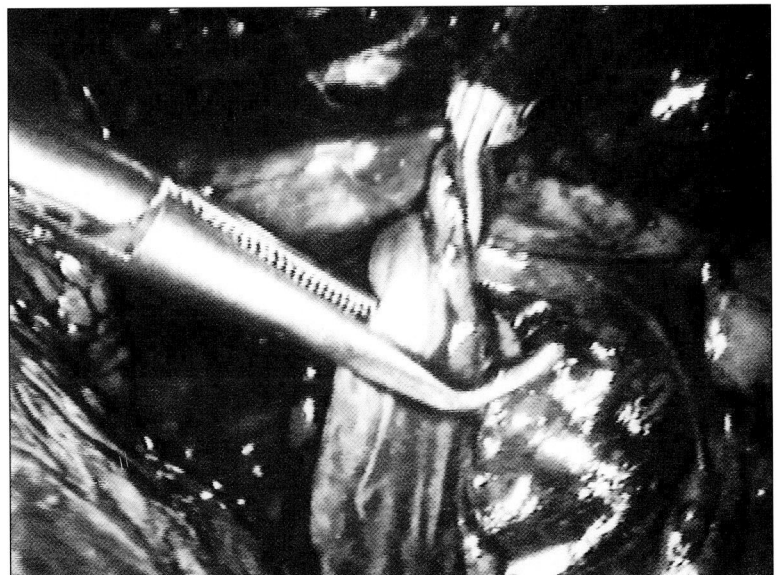

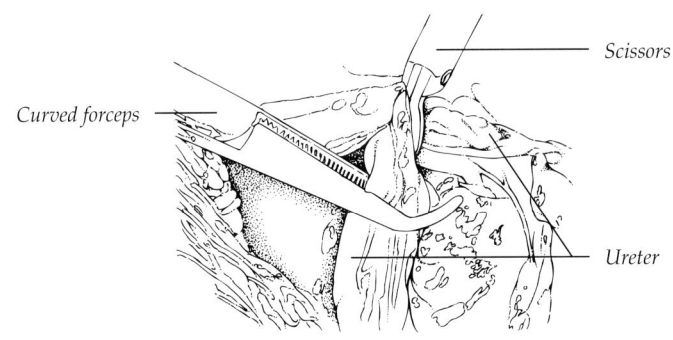

▶ **FIGURE 13-11.** (*See* Color Plate) Ureter identification and dissection. An EndoBabcock (United States Surgical Corp., Norwalk, CT) clamp is introduced through the fourth port to apply cephalad traction on the lower pole of the kidney. The upper ureter is thus easily identified below the kidney and anterior to the psoas muscle. By using electrosurgical

scissors, the periureteral fascia is dissected and the ureter is freed until it reaches the renal pelvis. It is then divided between 9-mm endoscopic clips if its caliber is normal. Otherwise, it could be ligated with endoscopic ligatures or clamped and incised with the endoscopic stapler.

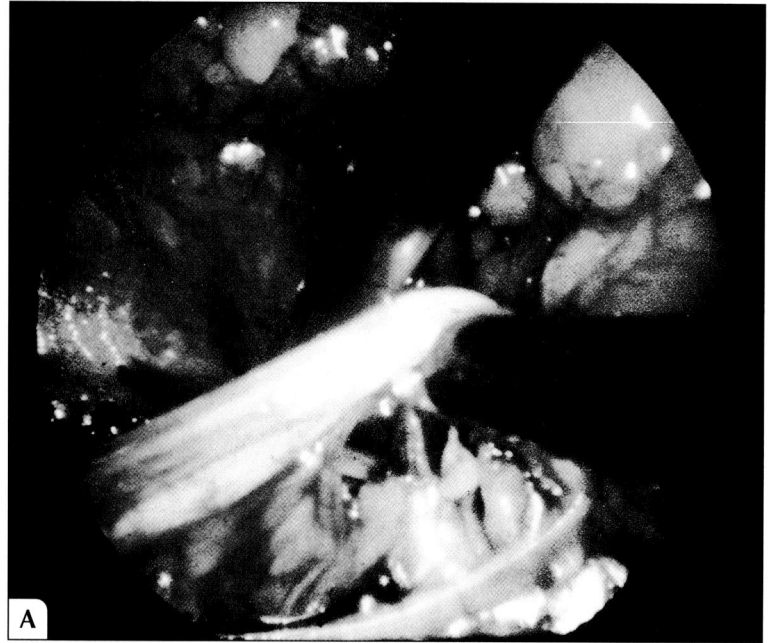

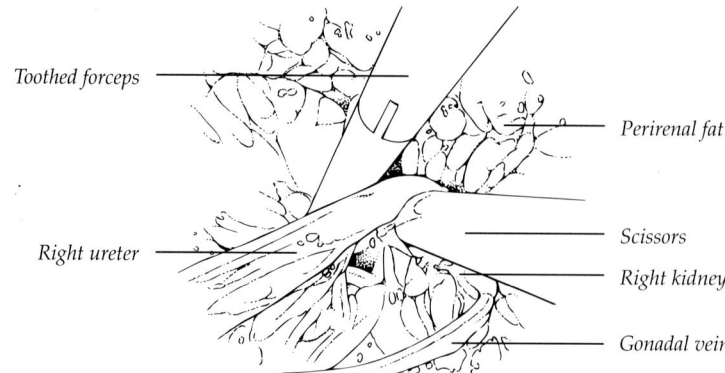

Labels on image 2: Toothed forceps, Perirenal fat, Scissors, Right kidney, Gonadal vein, Right ureter

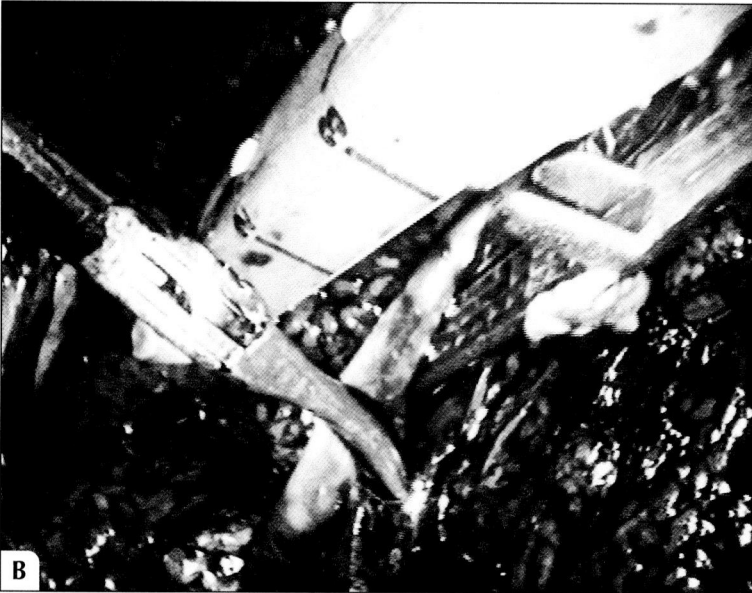

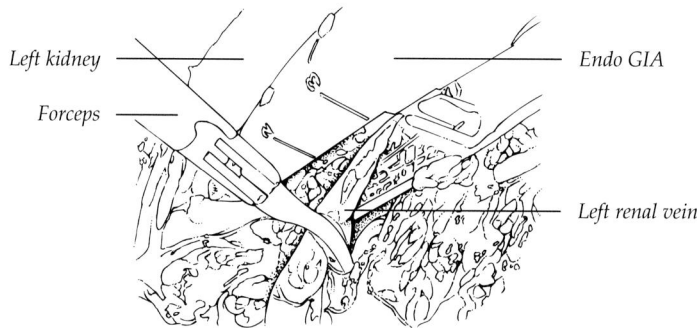

Labels on image 4: Left kidney, Endo GIA, Forceps, Left renal vein

A

B

▶ **FIGURE 13-12.** (*See* Color Plate) Control of the renal pedicle. **A,** A toothed forceps (5 mm) is introduced through the fourth port to grasp the proximal end of the divided ureter. With caudal and lateral traction on the proximal end of the divided ureter, the anterior surface and medial border of the renal pelvis are dissected to expose the renal vessels. Lateral traction along the medial aspect of the anterior surface of the kidney using endoscopic forceps passing though the fourth port helps to stretch the renal

hilum for further freeing, especially of the upper, lower, and posterior sides. A right-angled clamp can be very helpful. The renal vein appears first, followed by the renal artery posterosuperiorly. In most cases, the vein is too wide, so an endoscopic stapler is most useful. **B,** The stapler passes through the third port and is used for simultaneous stapling and division of this vein.

(*Continued on next page*)

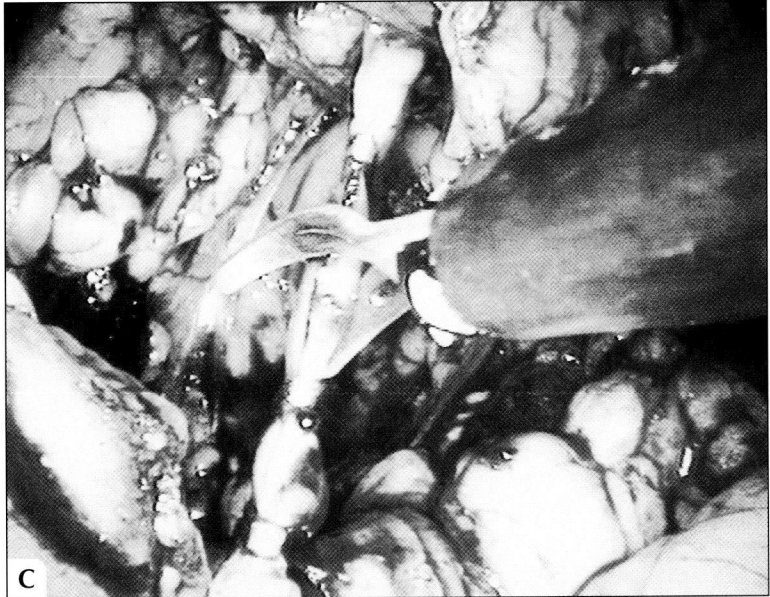

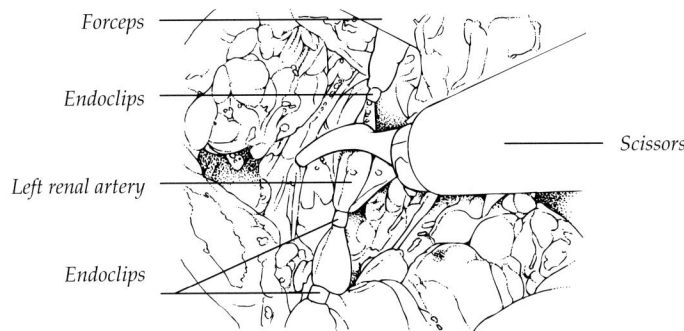

▶ **FIGURE 13-12.** (*Continued*) **C,** The renal artery is then secured between 9-mm endoscopic clips, and the artery is cut, leaving two to three clips toward the stump side. Sometimes, the vessels are surrounded by a dense fibrous reaction, and an attempt to separate the artery from the vein seems difficult and hazardous. In this situation, division of the renal pedicle en masse using the endoscopic stapler is safe, and the possibility of development of an arteriovenous fistula is remote due to the presence of

intervening dense tissue between the vessels. In some cases, the gonadal vein is identified either crossing the right ureter anteriorly or lying medially alongside the upper left ureter. Both can be dissected, clamped with a 9-mm endoscopic clip, and incised when necessary, but this must be done 2 cm away from the renal vein to avoid any problems with later application of the endoscopic stapler to the renal pedicle.

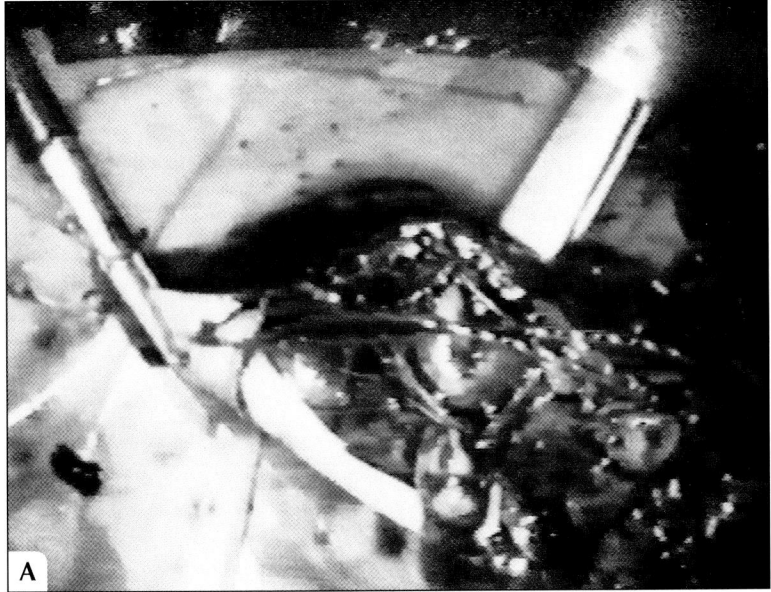

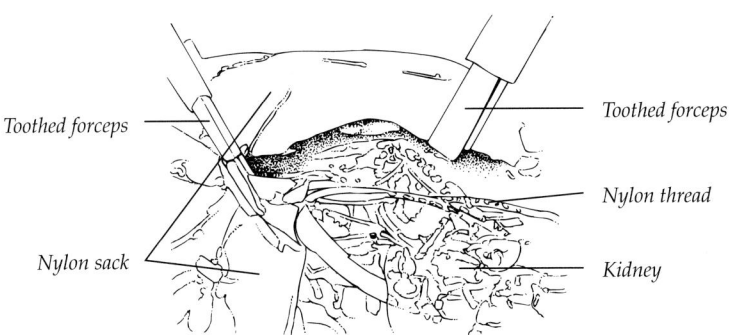

▶ **FIGURE 13-13.** (*See* Color Plate) Kidney entrapment and extraction. After complete dissection of the kidney, a 5 × 8 inch special sac is used for its entrapment (Lapsac, Cook Urological, Spencer, IN). The sac is folded around 5-mm forceps in a clockwise direction. The sac is introduced into the peritoneal cavity through the 12-mm port, thrown under the diaphragm, and unfolded in a counterclockwise direction. **A,** Two 5-mm toothed forceps are introduced through the third and fourth ports and are

used to catch the mouth of the bag at two marked points to keep it opened. A strong claw forceps or EndoBabcock clamp is passed through the 12-mm port to grasp the kidney and bring it into the sac. The nylon thread at the mouth of the sac is held by a grasper and is pulled to close the mouth by a pursestring action. The mouth of the sac is pulled out to the external surface of the abdominal wall through the site of the 12-mm port.

(Continued on next page)

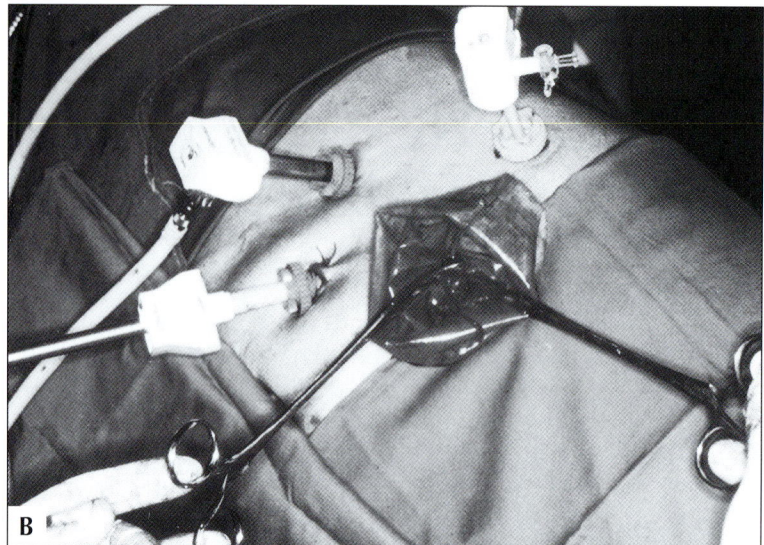

B

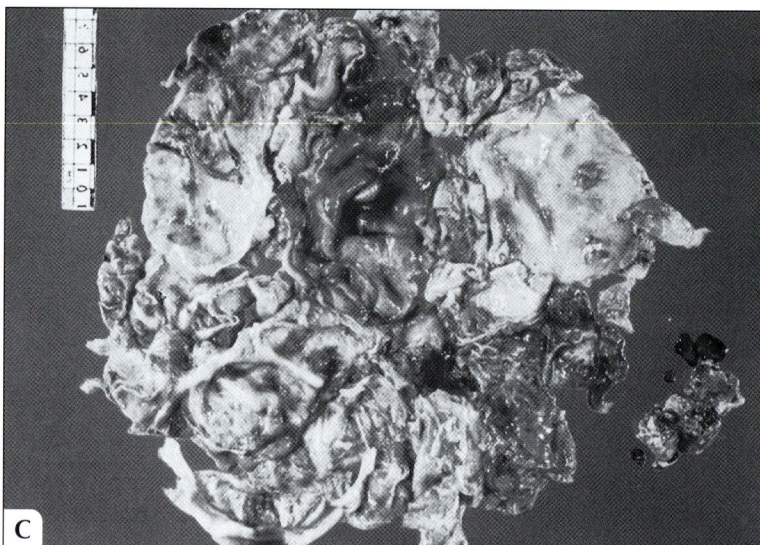

C

▶ **FIGURE 13-13.** (*Continued*) **B,** Blunt-ended scissors and strong surgical clamps are used to fragment the kidney inside the sac. **C,** It is extracted in sizable pieces suitable for histopathologic examination. In large hydronephrotic kidneys with thin parenchyma, the kidney could be totally extracted without fragmentation by using gentle gradual traction on renal tissue.

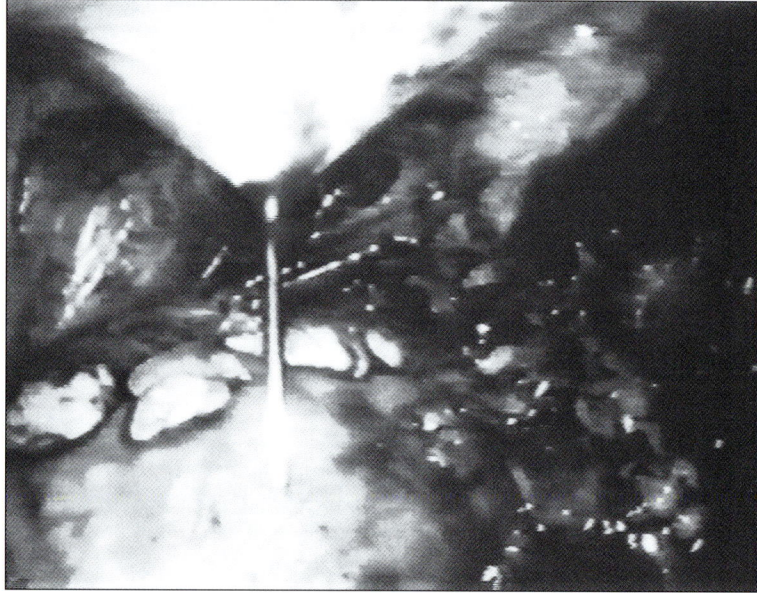

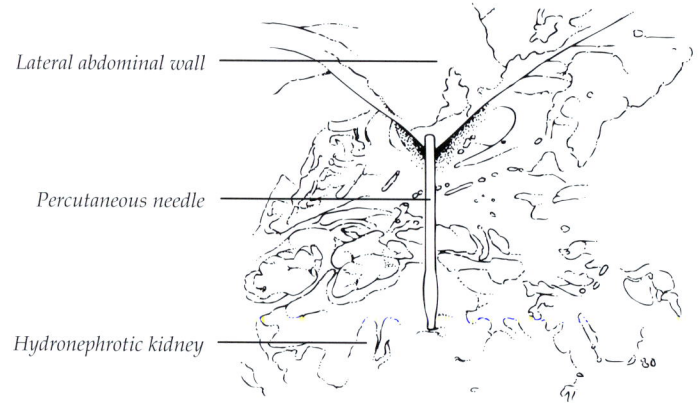

Lateral abdominal wall

Percutaneous needle

Hydronephrotic kidney

▶ **FIGURE 13-14.** (*See* Color Plate) Technical variations. Certain pathologic situations dictate some technical alterations. Sometimes, if the kidneys are small, the anatomic landmarks are obscure. To ensure safety, it is better to identify the ureter at the level of iliac vessels. Proximal dissection of the ureter will facilitate further dissection of the kidney and its vasculature.

For a large hydronephrotic kidney, dissection is facilitated by its tense surface and compressed surrounding atrophied fascia. Its fluid content is then aspirated. A laparoscopically guided percutaneous needle is inserted into the kidney, and the urine is evacuated completely. The working space then becomes wider. Moreover, this aspiration facilitates grasping and traction on the collapsed renal tissue and results in dramatic progress in the dissection and better pedicle control. In such a case, the ureter is dissected and cut in a later step.

Final Steps of the Procedure

Hemostasis
Tube drain
Removal of ports
Muscle closure
Skin closure

▶ **FIGURE 13-15.** Final steps. The final steps of the procedure include ensuring hemostasis, installing tube drainage, removing the ports, and closing the muscles and skin.

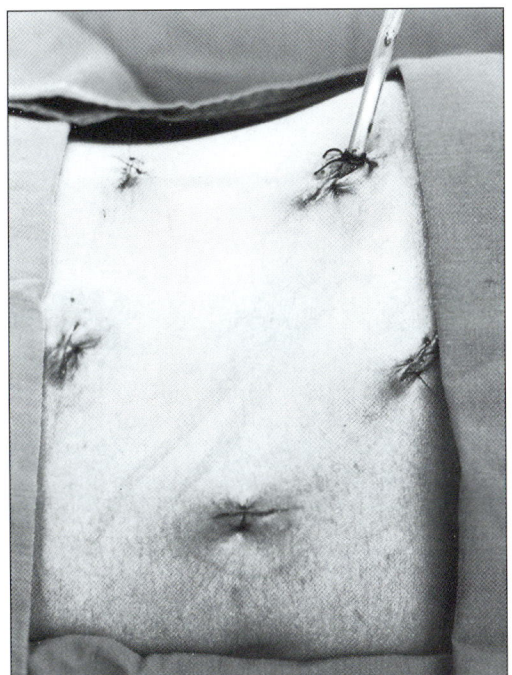

▶ **FIGURE 13-16.** Adequate hemostasis should be ensured after lowering the intra-abdominal pressure to 5 mm Hg to detect any minor venous bleeding. A 16-F tube drain is fixed at the site of the fourth port. All ports are removed under direct vision to detect any bleeding from port sites. The muscles should be meticulously approximated to avoid hernias at port sites, especially at the 10- and 12-mm ports. The skin incisions could be closed using nylon sutures or sterile strips.

TECHNIQUE OF RETROPERITONEAL
LAPAROSCOPIC NEPHRECTOMY

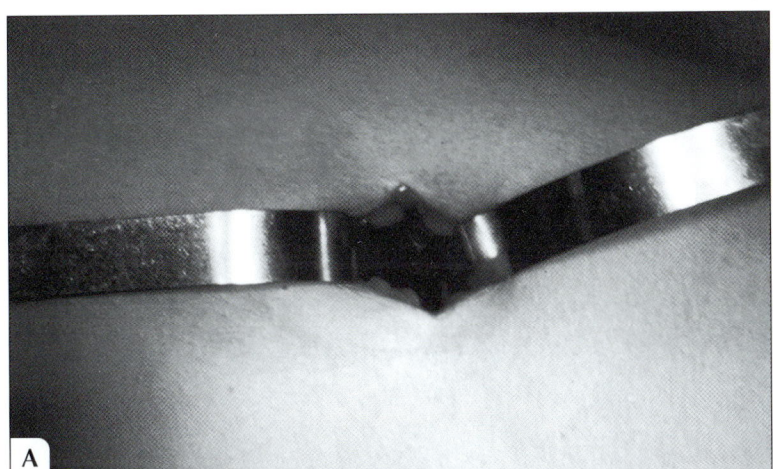

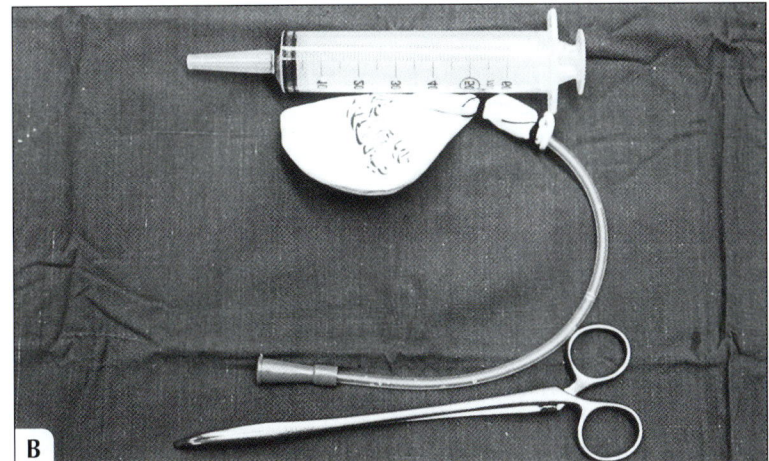

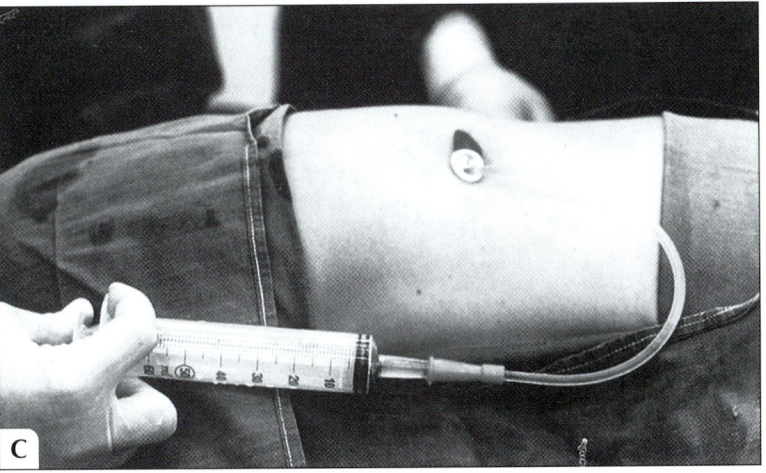

▶ **FIGURE 13-17.** Creation of the retroperitoneal space. The patient is put in the standard lumbar position. The surgeon stands at the dorsal side of the patient. A 2-cm subcostal incision is carried out one fingerbreadth below the tip of the last rib. **A,** This incision is deepened by either muscle cutting or muscle splitting until the white glistening lumbar fascia is identified. The fascia is sharply incised to reach the retroperitoneum. By blunt dissection using the index finger, a small retroperitoneal space is created to facilitate placement of the dissection balloon. **B,** In our institution, we use a simple toy balloon of 1.5 L capacity that is connected to an 18-F Nealon catheter using double ligatures of number 0 silk sutures. **C,** The balloon is introduced into the retroperitoneum, then inflated using 1.5 L of sterile saline. It is kept inflated for 5 to 10 minutes to allow for more dissection and hemostasis of the retroperitoneum. The balloon is then deflated and removed.

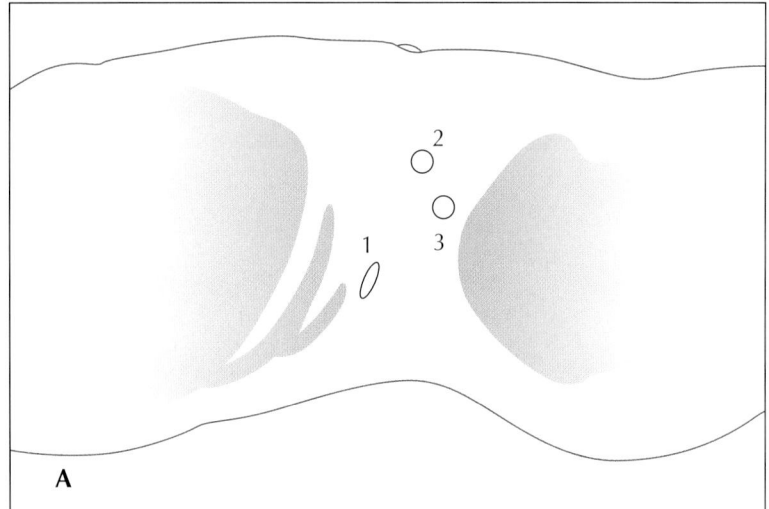

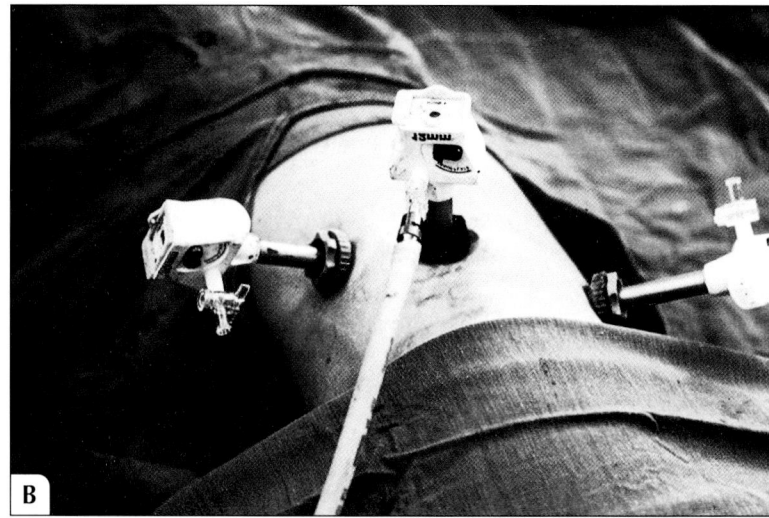

▶ **FIGURE 13-18.** Fixation of surgical ports. A Hasson blunt trocar (10 mm) is fixed at the site of the subcostal incision. To prevent gas leakage, the muscles around the port must be closed using simple sutures, and two mattress sutures (number 1 silk) must be used to close the skin incision and fix the port in place. CO_2 insufflation is started through this port to keep the pressure in the retroperitoneal space between 10 and 15 mm Hg.

The laparoscope is introduced through this port to facilitate fixation of another two ports under direct vision. The second port (12 mm) is fixed 10 cm anterior to the first port at the same subcostal line. **A,** The third port (10 mm) is fixed one fingerbreadth above the anterior superior iliac spine. **B,** The third port is used for the laparoscope, and the first and second ports are used for dissection and manipulations.

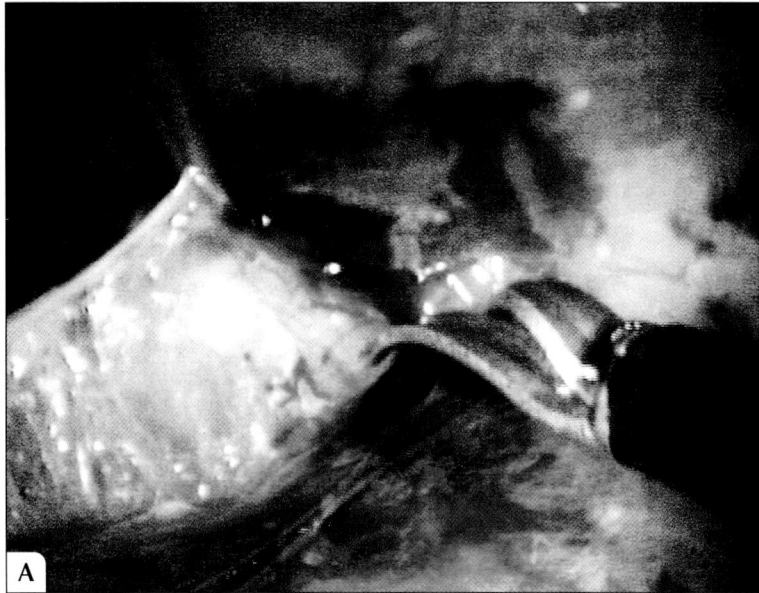

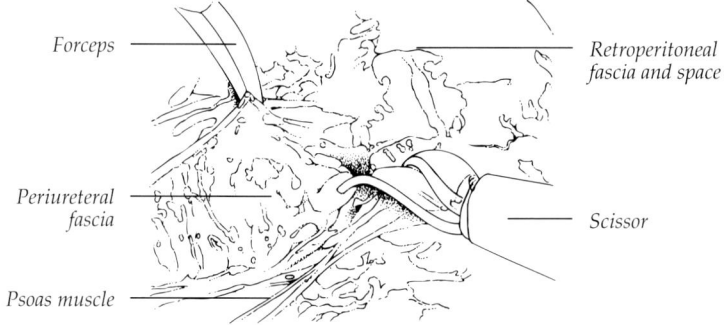

▶ **FIGURE 13-19.** (*See* Color Plate) Kidney dissection and extraction. When the perirenal fat is thin, the kidney is immediately visualized in the retroperitoneum. The kidney is dissected, and the procedure is completed as in the transperitoneal technique. In the majority of cases, Gerota's fascia

is thick, and the kidney is not easily identified. **A,** The only landmark in the field is the surface of the psoas muscle. The fibrous layer of Gerota's fascia is incised near the medial border of the muscle.

(*Continued on next page*)

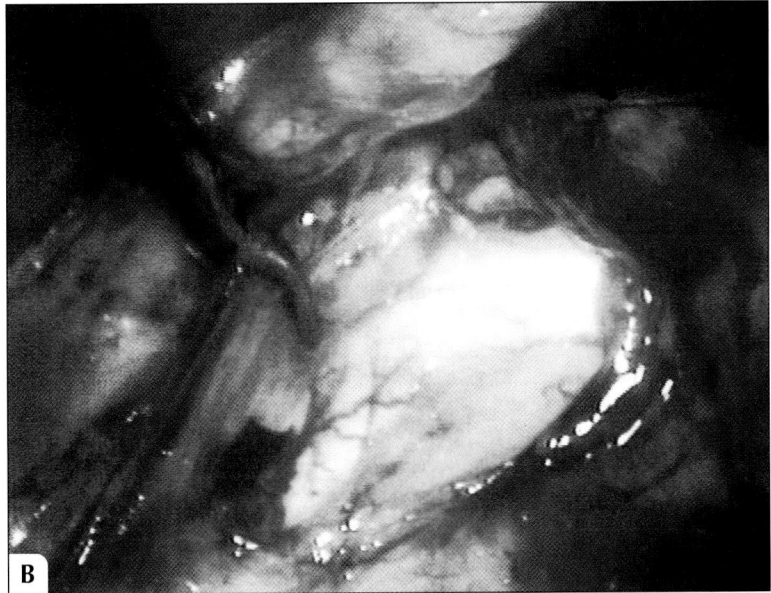

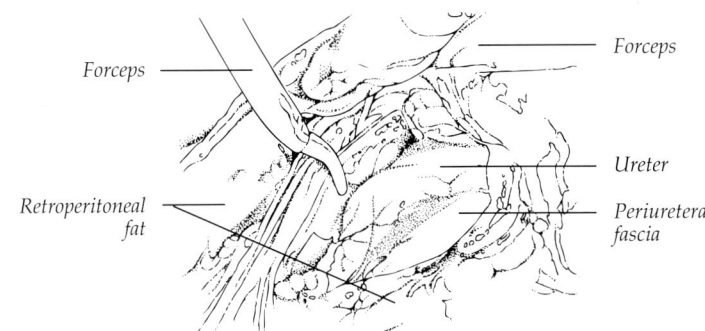

Forceps

Forceps

Retroperitoneal
fat

Ureter

Periureteral
fascia

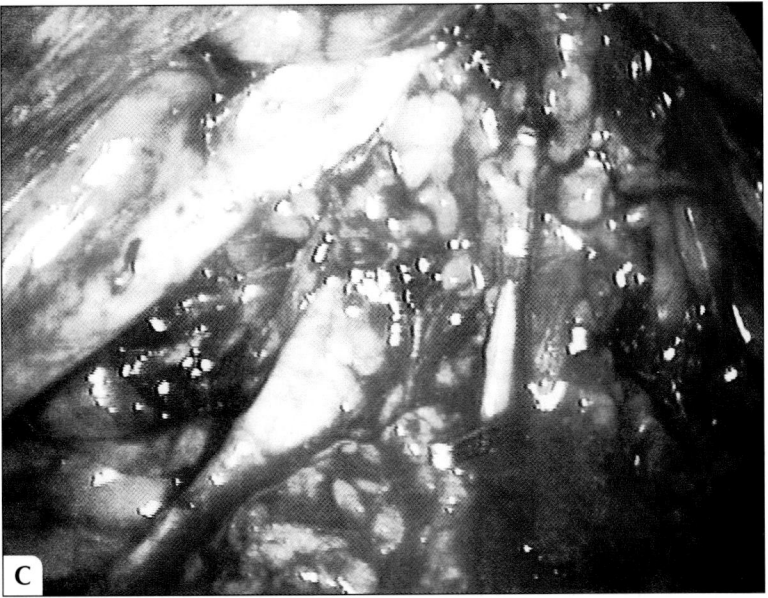

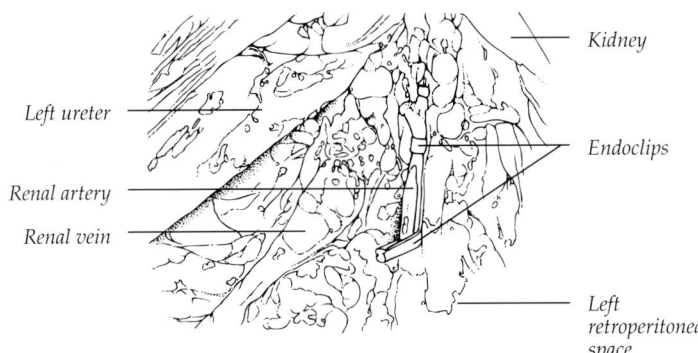

Kidney

Left ureter

Endoclips

Renal artery

Renal vein

Left
retroperitoneal
space

▶ **FIGURE 13-19.** (*Continued*) **B,** The incision is extended upward to expose the kidney and downward to expose the ureter. The ureter is divided between endoscopic clips. **C,** With lateral downtraction on the proximal ureter, the renal artery and vein are readily identified, and the ureter can be divided between endoscopic clips. The procedure is

completed as in transperitoneal nephrectomy. In the majority of cases, the kidney is usually extracted without fragmentation from the initial subcostal incision in view of its small size. With average-sized kidneys, entrapment and extraction are performed in a manner similar to the transperitoneal approach.

Postoperative Care

Antibiotics
Urethral catheter
Oral feeding
Tube drain
Hospital stay

▶ **FIGURE 13-20.** Postoperative care. The urethral catheter is removed the morning after surgery. The tube drain is removed within 48 hours. Oral feeding is restored after 24 hours. The patient receives oral antibiotics for 5 days. The mean hospital stay is 2.9 days, and patients are followed up to detect any delayed morbidity.

Complications of Laparoscopic Nephrectomy for Benign Disease

Type	Mansoura experience	US experience
Access related		
Abdominal wall hematoma or emphysema	1	1
Trocar injury to the kidney	0	1
Hernia at trocar site	4	1
Intraoperative		
Bleeding*		
Upper polar artery	1	0
Perirenal	2	0
Splenic laceration	0	1
Pneumothorax	0	1
Postoperative		
Gastrointestinal		
Ileus	0	3
Colonic perforation	1	0
Cardiopulmonary		
Heart failure	0	1
Atrial fibrillation	0	1
Pulmonary embolism	1	1
Pneumonitis	0	1
Genitourinary		
Urine retention	0	2
Epididymitis	0	1
Neurologic		
Peripheral nerve palsy	0	2
Confusion	0	1
Bleeding*		
Renal vein	1	0
Suprarenal area	2	0

All need laparotomy.

▶ **FIGURE 13-21.** Complications of laparoscopic nephrectomy for benign disease. In the United States, complications were encountered in 12% of cases in which laparoscopic nephrectomy had been performed for benign disease. In our series, complications were encountered in 7% of cases. This reflects the inclusion of the initial cases of five centers in the United States. Gill *et al.* [17] documented that 71% of the complications occurred in the initial 20 cases in these centers.

The learning curve effect is also evident; in our experience, half of the complications occurred in our initial 40 cases. The 7% incidence of complications is acceptable if compared with the inherent complications of open nephrectomy, about 10% of complications resulted in pleural injury, 12% in wound complications in flank incisions, 2.3% in splenic injury, and 1% in laparotomy for intestinal obstruction with a transperitoneal incision [15]. (*Data from* Eraky *et al.* [8] and Gill *et al.*[17].)

Mansoura Experience With Laparoscopic Nephrectomy*

Classification	Transperitoneal	Retroperitoneal
Cases, n	144	62
Age, y	13–17 (42)	9–58 (mean age 32)
Gender: male/female	84/60	40/22
Side: right/left	73/71	23/39
Kidney size	2.5 x 5 to 18 x 30	2.5 x 5 to 16 x 10
Disorder		
Hydronephrosis	89	8
Chronic pyelonephritis	47	24
End-stage renal disease	7	30
Renal hypoplasia	1	0
Success rate, n (%)	134 (93)	59 (95)
Conversion	To open surgery	To open surgery
Perirenal adhesions	5	2
Bleeding	4	0
Failure of entrapment	1	0
		(Transperitoneal approach)
Peritoneal tear	0	1
Operating time, min	75–420	45–270
Range (mean)	(176±48)	(108±27)
Hospital stay, d	2–12	2–5
Range (mean)	(2.9)	(2.4)

August 1992 to July 1997.

▶ **FIGURE 13-22.** Mansoura experience with laparoscopic nephrectomy. Between August of 1992 and July of 1997, 963 nephrectomies were performed at the Urology and Nephrology Center of Mansoura University. Of these nephrectomies, 392 cases were a donor nephrectomy, 138 cases were for malignant renal conditions, and 433 cases were for nonfunctioning kidneys having benign disease. Among the benign cases, 206 procedures were carried out using laparoscopic techniques: 144 through the transperitoneal route and 62 through the retroperitoneal approach.

Removal of neither right nor left kidney is associated with special technical difficulties. In the group undergoing retroperitoneal laparoscopic nephrectomy, more kidneys were removed from the left side because this group included 30 cases of chronic renal failure preparing for renal transplantation. The left kidneys in this group were removed through a retroperitoneal laparoscopic approach, although the right kidneys were removed through an open approach at the time of transplantation.

Due to the limited working space in the retroperitoneal approach, the removed kidneys were small to average in size. For big hydronephrotic kidneys (*eg,* in obese patients), or for kidneys harboring stones in which dissection may be difficult, the transperitoneal approach was preferred. The success rate of both approaches is high (93% to 95%). The relative increase in conversion to open surgery in the transperitoneal approach reflects the selection of more difficult cases for this approach.

The mean operative time for the transperitoneal approach (176 minutes) is longer than for retroperitoneal nephrectomy (108 minutes). This difference could be attributed to the fact that the retroperitoneal approach was not used until after the initial experience of more than 90 cases of transperitoneal nephrectomy. Moreover, big kidneys and difficult cases are usually selected for the transperitoneal route.

REFERENCES

1. Clayman RV, Kavoussi LR, Soper NJ, *et al.*: Laparoscopic nephrectomy: initial report of pelviscopic organ ablation in the pig. *J Endourol* 1990, 4:247–252.

2. Clayman RV, Kavoussi LR, Soper NJ, *et al.*: Laparoscopic nephrectomy: initial case report. *J Urol* 1991, 146:278–282.

3. Coptcoat MJ: Laparoscopy in urology: perspectives and practice. *Br J Urol* 1992, 69:561–567.

4. Coptcoat MJ, Joyce AD: Laparoscopic transperitoneal nephrectomy. In *Laparoscopy in Urology.* Edited by Coptcoat MJ, Joyce AD. London: Blackwell Scientific Publications; 1994:121–136.

5. Albala DM, Kavoussi LR, Clayman RV: Laparoscopic nephrectomy. *Semin Urol* 1992, 10:146–151.

6. Kerbl K, Clayman RV, McDougall EM, Kavoussi LR: Laparoscopic nephrectomy: the Washington University experience. *Br J Urol* 1994, 73:231–236.

7. Eraky I, El-Kappany H, Shamaa MA, Ghoneim MA: Laparoscopic nephrectomy: an established routine procedure. *J Endourol* 1994, 8:275–278.

8. Eraky I, El-Kappany H, Ghoneim MA: Laparoscopic nephrectomy: Mansoura experience with 106 cases. *Br J Urol* 1995, 75:271–275.

9. Elashry OM, Nakada SY, McDougall EM, Clayman RV: Laparoscopic for adult polycystic kidney disease: a promising alternative. *Am J Kidney Dis* 1996, 27:224–233.

10. Rassweiller J, Herkel TO, Frede T, *et al.*: Laparoscopic procedures in the upper retroperitoneum: the results of the first 150 cases. *J Endourol* 1995, 9:S103.

11. Ono Y, Katoh N, Kinukawa T, *et al.*: Laparoscopic nephrectomy, radical nephrectomy and adrenalectomy. Nagoya experience. *J Urol* 1994, 152:1962–1966.

12. Gaur DD: Laparoscopic operative retroperitoneoscopy: use of a new device. *J Urol* 1992, 148:1135–1139.

13. Riehle RA, Steckler R, Naslund EB, *et al.*: Selection criteria for the evaluation of living related renal donors. *J Urol* 1990, 144:845–848.

14. Weinstein SH, Navarre RJ, Loening SA, Corry RJ: Experience with live donor nephrectomy. *J Urol* 1980, 124:321–323.

15. Scott RF, Sezlman HM: Complications of nephrectomy: review of 450 patients and a description of a modification of the transperitoneal approach. *J Urol* 1966, 95:307–312.

16. Ruiz R, Novick AC, Braun WE, *et al.*: Transperitoneal live donor nephrectomy. *J Urol* 1980, 123:819–821.

17. Gill I, Kavoussi L, Clayman RV, *et al.*: Complications of laparoscopic nephrectomy in 185 patients: a multiinstitutional review. *J Urol* 1995, 154:479–483.

18. Gill IS, Carbone JM, Clayman RV, *et al.*: Laparoscopic live-donor nephrectomy. *J Urol* 1993, 149:149A.

19. Schulam PE, Kavoussi LR, Cheriff AD, *et al.*: Laparoscopic live donor nephrectomy: the initial 3 cases. *J Urol* 1996, 155:1857–1859.

20. Cava A, Roman J, Ganzalez-Quintela A, *et al.*: Subcutaneous metastasis following laparoscopy in gastric adenocarcinoma. *Eur J Oncol* 1990, 16:63–67.

21. Novick AC: Renal-sparing surgery for renal cell carcinoma. *Urol Clin North Am* 1993, 20:277–282.

Video-Controlled Renal Surgery

Walter Stackl
Clemens Hammer

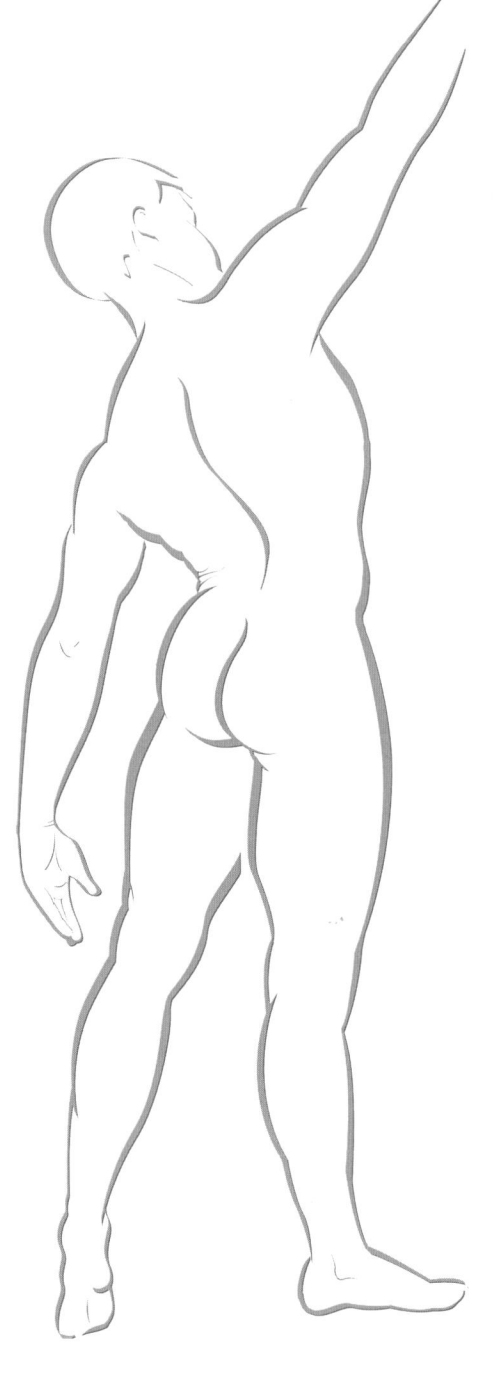

Although laparoscopic surgery of the kidney is time consuming and difficult to perform, it offers the advantages of small cosmetic incisions and rapid postoperative healing. Standard laparoscopic urologic surgery requires intraperitoneal access through maintenance of the laparoscopic cavity by constant CO_2 insufflation. It is associated with potential complications including gas embolism, cardiac arrhythmia, CO_2 absorption, acidosis, subcutaneous emphysema, bowel perforation, vascular injury, and perforation of solid organs [1]. Furthermore, conventional laparoscopy is not generally accepted because of training time and cost, use of unfamiliar instruments, instrument expense, and the periodic loss of pneumoperitoneum in more complex procedures, which also entails loss of exposure and time.

Open surgery is increasingly disliked by patients because of slow recovery and for cosmetic reasons. In 1993 we developed a gasless lumboscopy technique that allows minimally invasive surgery of the kidney combining the advantages of laparoscopy and open surgery [2]. Several gasless laparoscopy systems have been described. We use the Origin system, which is described in detail in this chapter. With a gasless technique, the complications of pneumoperitoneum and pneumoretroperitoneum can be avoided. Through a muscle-splitting incision the surgery can be performed by using conventional instruments. The laparoscopic control allows a small cosmetic skin incision and excellent magnification. Postoperative healing and pain are equal in conventional and gasless approaches, and both procedures are superior to open surgery in this regard. Therefore, video-controlled renal surgery through a mini-incision is cheaper, faster, and is easier to perform, teach, and learn than conventional laparoscopy.

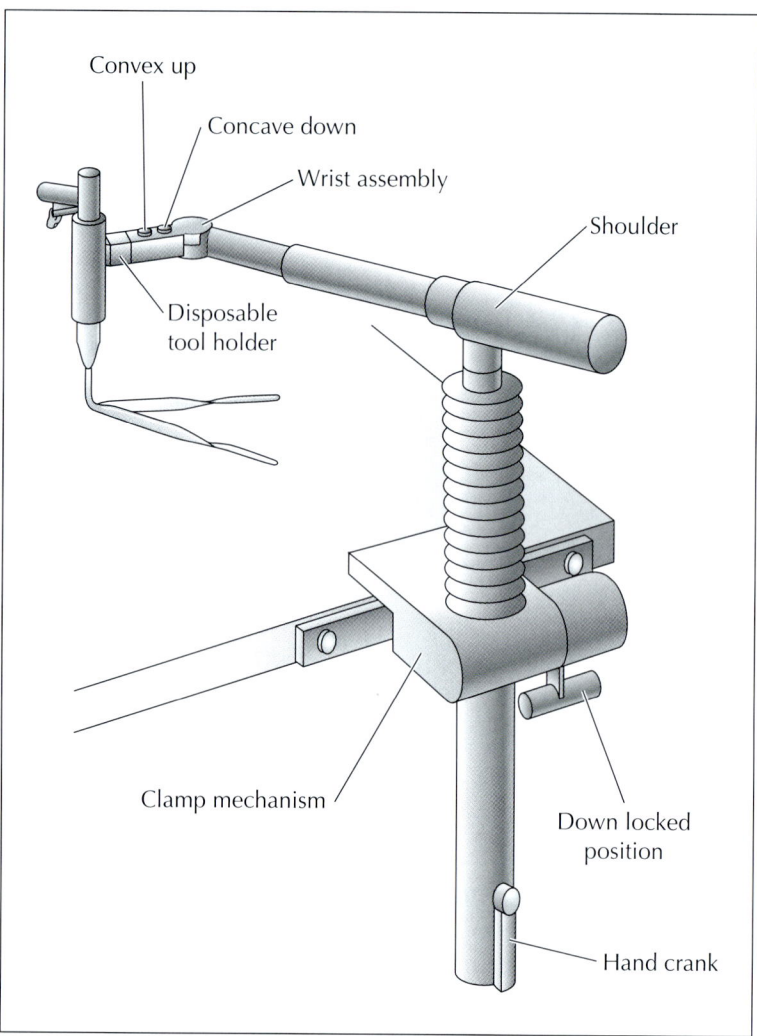

Convex up
Concave down
Wrist assembly
Shoulder
Disposable tool holder
Clamp mechanism
Down locked position
Hand crank

▶ **FIGURE 14-1.** A planar lift retractor (Laparolift, Origin Medsystems, Menlo Park, CA) that is used for video-controlled surgery of the kidney. The diagram shows the mechanical arm and fan-shaped retractor for abdominal wall distention. The retractor is connected to an electro-mechanical lifting arm that is attached to the side rail of the operating table. Controls on the mechanical arm provide for elevation of the abdominal wall or release of tension depending on the desires and needs of the operating surgeon. To prevent abdominal wall injury, a safety system allows only 13.6 kg (30 lb) of traction. The amount of lift roughly approximates the lifting force of pneumoperitoneum at 15 mm Hg.

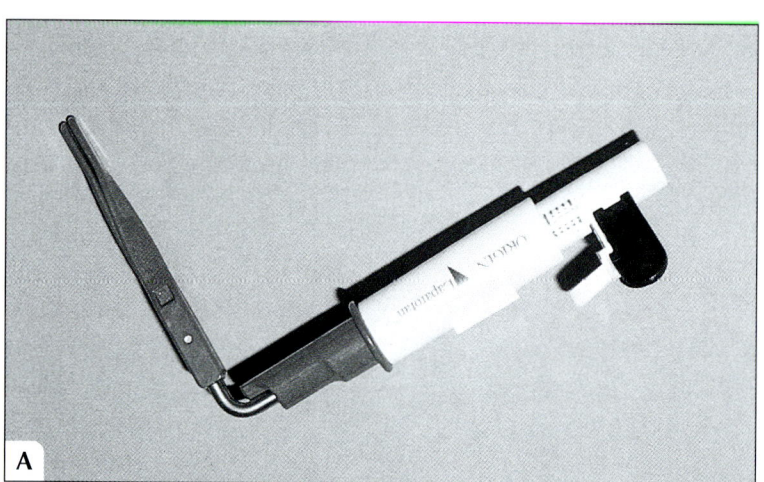
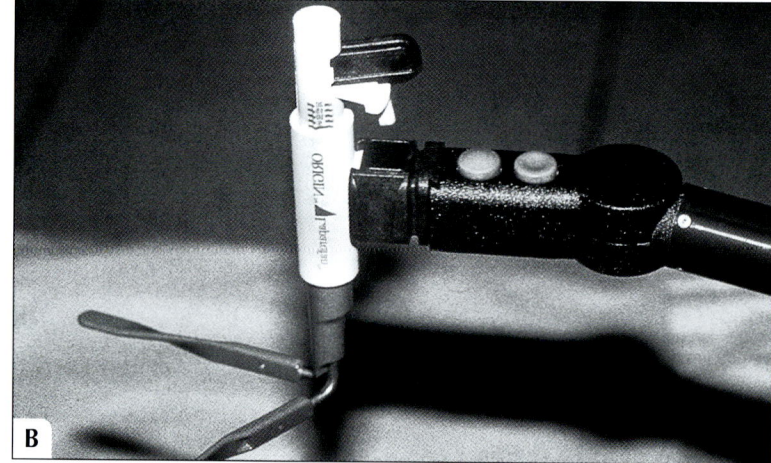

▶ **FIGURE 14-2.** Laparoscopic fan retractor. **A**, The closed fan retractor is inserted through the mini-incision. **B**, The 10-cm blades of the fan retractor are spread apart after insertion into the retroperitoneal cavity. The optimal location for the retractor varies from procedure to procedure. It can be located beneath the muscle wall or beneath Gerota's fascia.

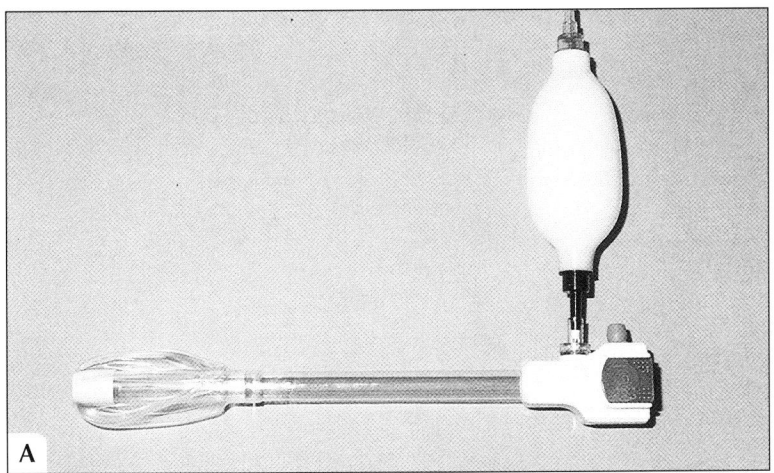

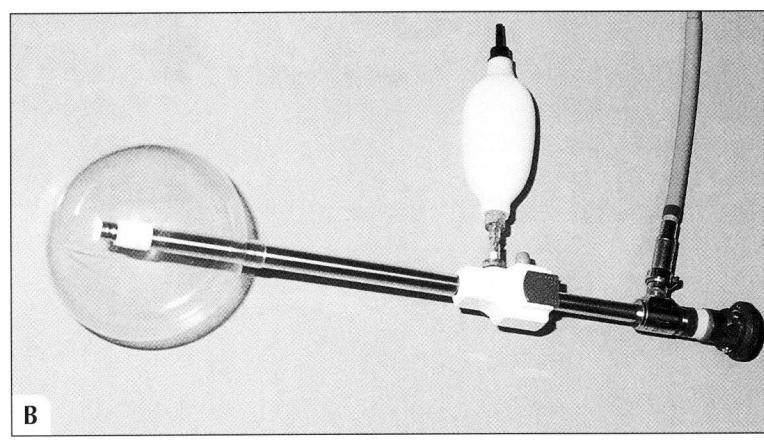

▶ **FIGURE 14-3.** Sphere-shaped distention balloon. **A,** The closed balloon is inserted through the mini-incision and inflated. **B,** The inflated spherical balloon provides a distention of 15 cm in diameter. Through its transparent silicone membrane it allows endoscopic control of the quality of the dilation.

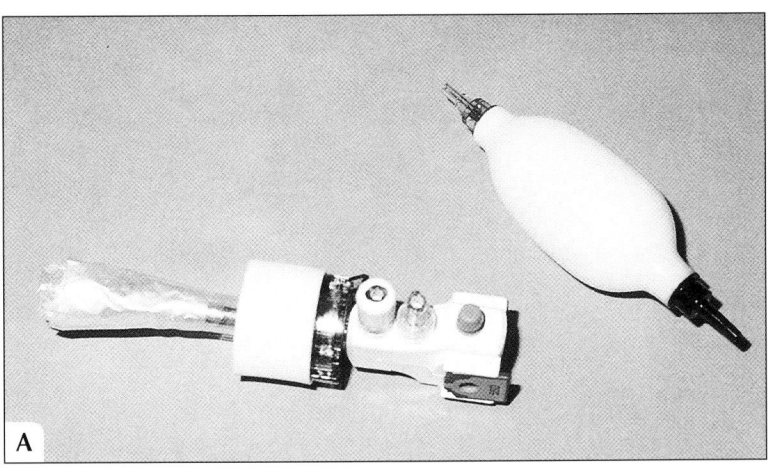

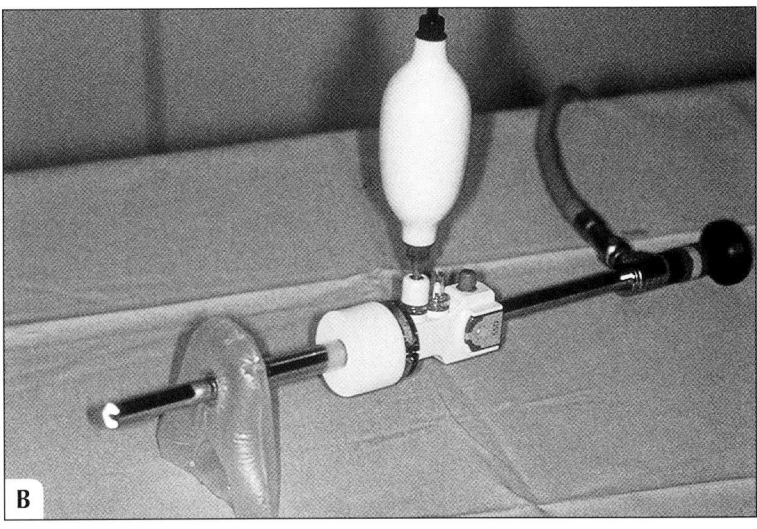

▶ **FIGURE 14-4.** Laparoscopic trocar. **A,** The laparoscopic trocar has a diameter of 1 cm. **B,** It is equipped with an integrated structural balloon, which serves as an inflatable retractor. This balloon provides helpful median retraction of the peritoneum.

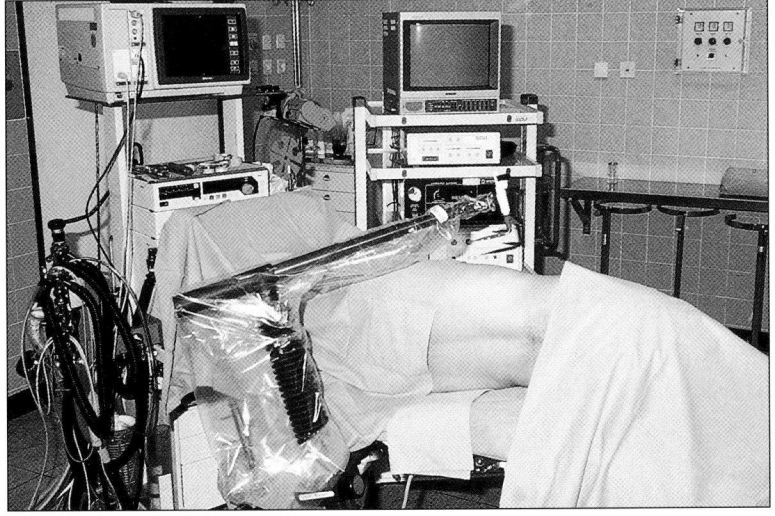

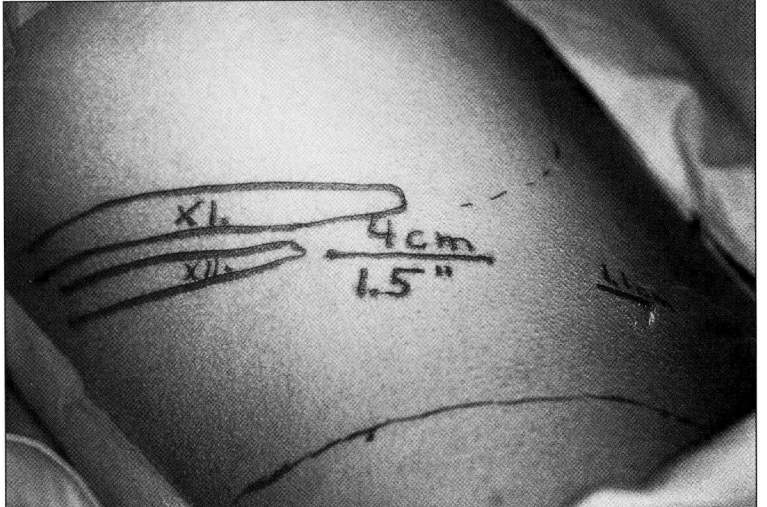

▶ **FIGURE 14-5.** The patient is placed in a standard flank position and is prepared and draped. The laparoscopic lift is mounted on the operating room table and covered with a sterile plastic sleeve.

▶ **FIGURE 14-6.** (*See* Color Plate) The skin is incised 3 to 5 cm starting at the tip of the 12th rib parallel to the 11th rib. A second incision 1.1 cm long is made medially to the first incision for the laparoscope port. Through this muscle-splitting incision the retroperitoneum is entered with the index finger, and extra space for the distention balloon is created with a sweeping motion.

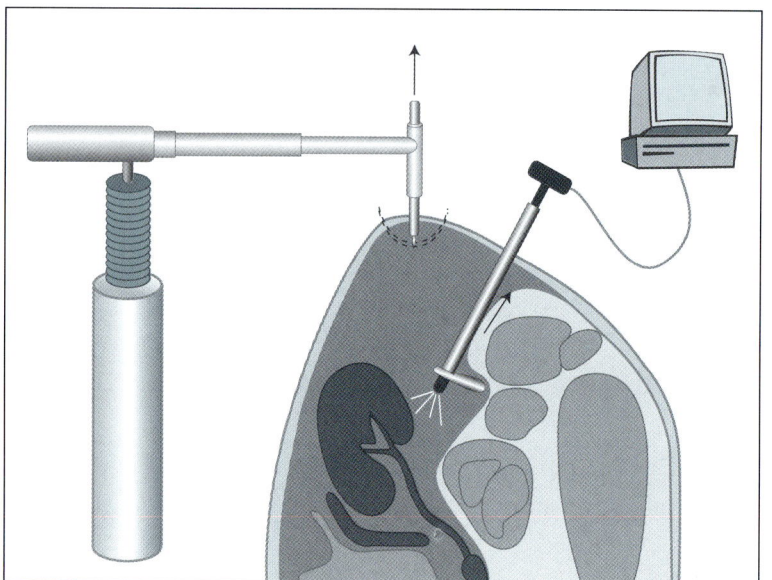

▶ **FIGURE 14-7.** Distention of the abdominal wall is created by the laparoscopic fan connected to the laparoscopic lift and by the structural balloon trocar for the laparoscope. The inflated balloon allows sufficient retraction of the peritoneum. This twofold retraction gives enough working space and compensates for the desirable effect of the pneumoretroperitoneum to compress the hollow viscera. In contrast to the dome-shaped exposure produced by gas insufflation, the mechanical abdominal wall lift system produces distention of the abdomen that resembles a truncated pyramid.

RENAL SURGERY USING VIDEO-CONTROLLED TECHNIQUES

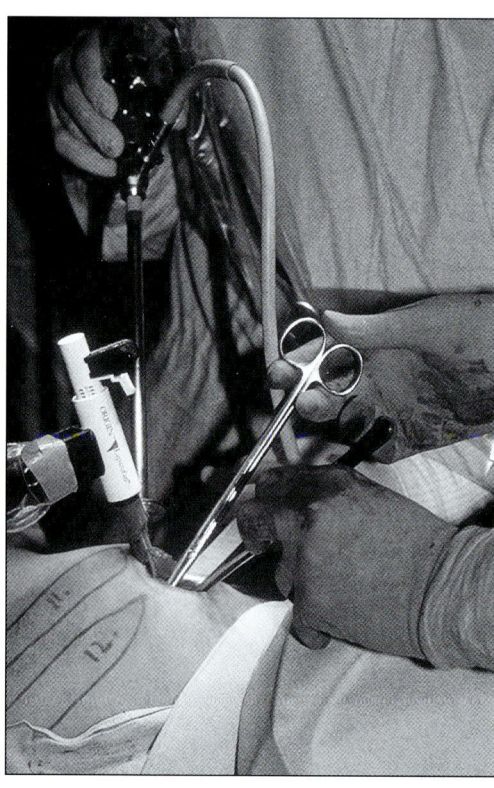

▶ **FIGURE 14-8.** (*See* Color Plate) Performance of video-controlled renal surgery. Because the gasless technique does not require an air-tight pneumoretroperitoneum, conventional instruments may be used routinely for surgery. This ability has advantages for both training and technique. High-volume suction and irrigation are easily accomplished. Also, under tactile guidance, a finger can be inserted through the mini-incision while visual control is obtained through the laparoscope. Conventional surgery facilitates reconstructive procedures such as pyeloplasties. Knots may be placed extracorporeally and then guided into place with the index finger.

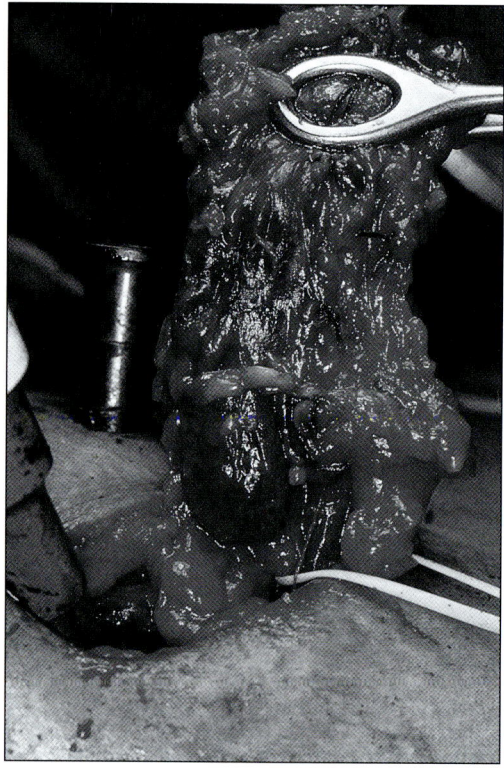

▶ **FIGURE 14-9.** (*See* Color Plate) Removal of complete kidney. A tremendous time-saving advantage of the mini-incision is the opportunity for the kidney to be saved in its entirety and sent to the pathologist. This advantage is especially important in tumor cases for staging and prevention of tumor cell–spilling.

Indications for Video-controlled Renal Surgery

Ideal	Relative
Nephrectomy	Tumors
Pyeloplasty	Nephropexy
Kidney biopsy	Pyelotomy
Renal cyst	Ureterotomy
Partial nephrectomy	

▶ **FIGURE 14-10.** Indications for video-controlled renal surgery. Nephrectomy of a small kidney is easy to perform with video-controlled renal surgery through mini-incision. Dismembered pyeloplasty, particularly in patients with crossing vessels, is another ideal indication [3]. Huge symptomatic cysts that cannot be approached by percutaneous techniques because of the proximity of bowel or other organs can be resected using this technique; partial nephrectomies can also be performed in nonfunctioning upper or lower systems in duplex kidneys. Kidney biopsy is indicated only if percutaneous biopsy techniques have failed. In keeping with oncologic principles, tumor surgery is reserved for highly selected cases. If extracorporeal shock wave treatment or endourologic procedures are not available or possible, video-controlled surgery is an option [4].

Patients Undergoing Video-controlled Renal Surgery*

Indication	Patients, n
Nephrectomy	35
Pyeloplasty	18
Nephroureterectomy	4
Renal cyst	5
Kidney biopsy	3
Partial nephrectomy	3

*A total of 68 patients, ranging from 3 to 78 years of age.

▶ **FIGURE 14-11.** Patients undergoing video-controlled renal surgery for various indications. The presented technique was performed successfully in 80% of patients. Operating time ranged between 0.45 and 3.4 hours with an average time of 1.8 hours. Compared with laproscopic surgery with gas, performed either transperitoneally or retroperitoneally, video-controlled renal surgery is definitely faster.

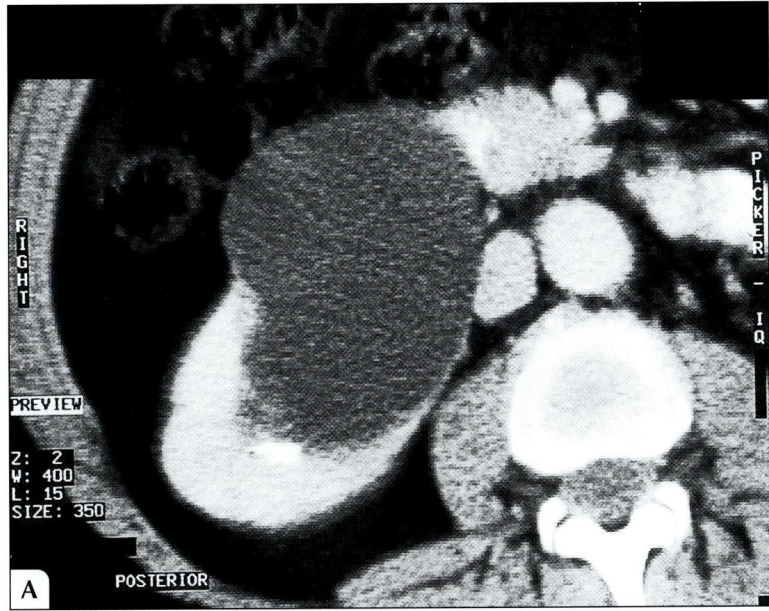

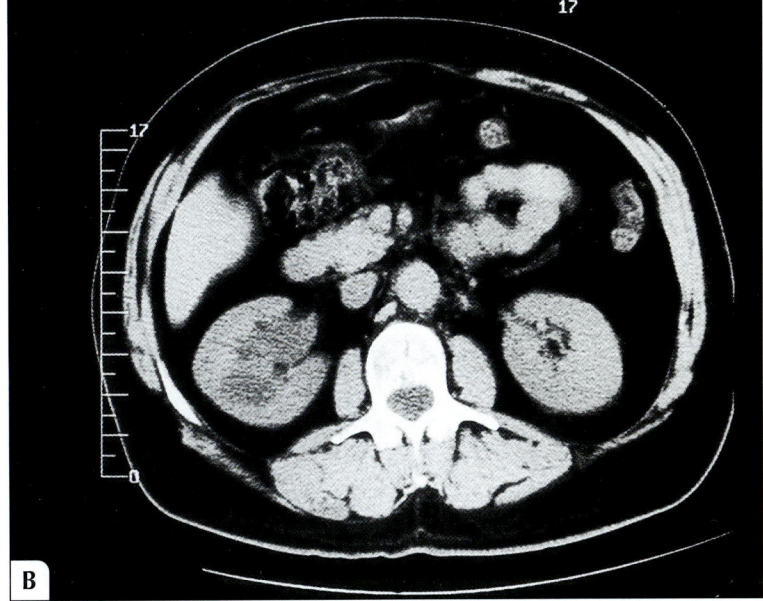

▶ **FIGURE 14-12.** Pre- and postoperative CT scans. **A,** A huge symptomatic renal cyst surrounded by bowel or kidney—a contraindication to percutaneous resection of the cyst wall. The resection of the cyst wall was performed under video control in 1 hour and 10 minutes. **B,** A follow-up CT scan 2 years later shows a perfect postoperative result with no perinephritic scarring.

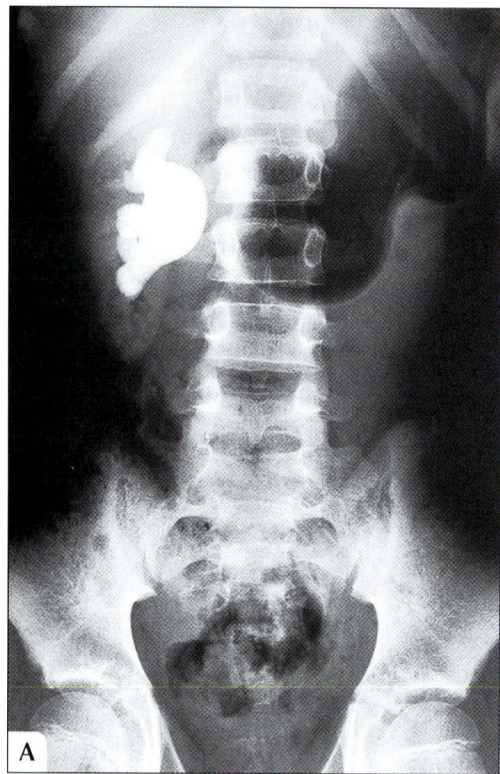 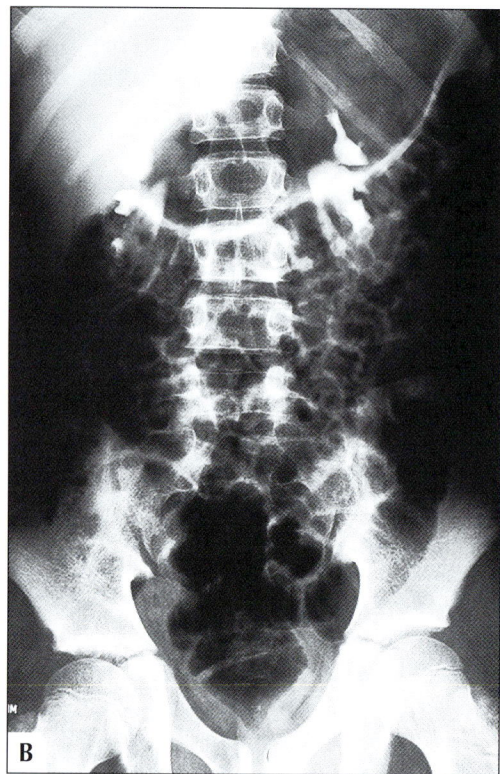

▶ **FIGURE 14-13.** Pre- and postoperative intravenous pyelogram in a 12-year-old boy. **A,** Late film (21 hours after dye injection) shows severe obstruction due to a crossing vessel. The anastomosis was performed using a 6.0 polydioxanone running suture. No stent or diversion was used. A retroperitoneal silicone drain was used for 24 hours. **B,** The follow-up film 6 months later shows a perfect result.

Conversion to Open Surgery

Reason for converting	Patients, n
Bleeding	7
Perirenal scar	9
Tumor in cyst	1
Huge hydronephrosis	3

A total of 20 of 112 patients had to be converted to open surgery.

▶ **FIGURE 14-14.** Failures. In 20 of 112 patients the procedure was converted to open surgery and was finished using a conventional surgical technique without further problems. It is easy to integrate the two incisions into a standard flank incision. Bleeding occurred in six patients, which may reflect a learning curve for the surgeons because it happened within the first 25 procedures we performed. Perirenal scar is not predictable, but because this technique can be converted easily to a conventional procedure, it is best to start with a mini-incision and video control. In one patient we found a small tumor in a renal cyst and converted to open surgery for oncologic reasons. In two patients with a huge hydronephrosis, we were not able to create sufficient space to perform surgery safely.

ADVANTAGES

Advantages of Video-controlled Renal Surgery Versus Open Surgery

Muscle-splitting incision
Excellent magnification
Rapid healing
Fast recovery
Short hospitalization
Minimal scars

▶ **FIGURE 14-15.** Advantages of video-controlled renal surgery versus conventional renal surgery. The size of the muscle-splitting incision is comparable with the incision for an appendectomy. There is no risk for herniation, and postoperative recovery is very fast. The video control provides excellent magnification, comparable with that in microsurgery.

Advantages of Video-controlled Renal Surgery Versus Conventional Laparoscopy

No puncture complications
No gas complications
Retroperitoneal approach
Conventional instruments
Conventional suturing
Easy conversion to open surgery
Harvesting of the intact kidney
Less time consuming
More cost effective
Shorter learning curve for surgeons

▶ **FIGURE 14-16.** Advantages of video-controlled renal surgery versus conventional laparoscopy. The presented technique is an ideal compromise between open surgery and laparoscopy with gas.

REFERENCES

1. Wolf GS, Stoller ML: The physiology of laparoscopy: basic principles, complications and other considerations. *J Urol* 1994, 152:294–302.

2. Hammer C, Baierlein M, Stackl W: Laparoskopisch kontrollierte minimal invasive Nierenchirurgie. *Akt Urol* 1996, 27:1.13, I–IV.

3. Stackl W, Baierlein M, Hammer C, Hasun R: Gasless lumboscopy–assisted pyeloplasty. *J Endourol* 1996, 10:S165.

4. Stackl W, Baierlein M, Hammer C, Hasun R: Gasless lumboscopy–assisted renal surgery. *J Urol* 1997, 157 (suppl):403.

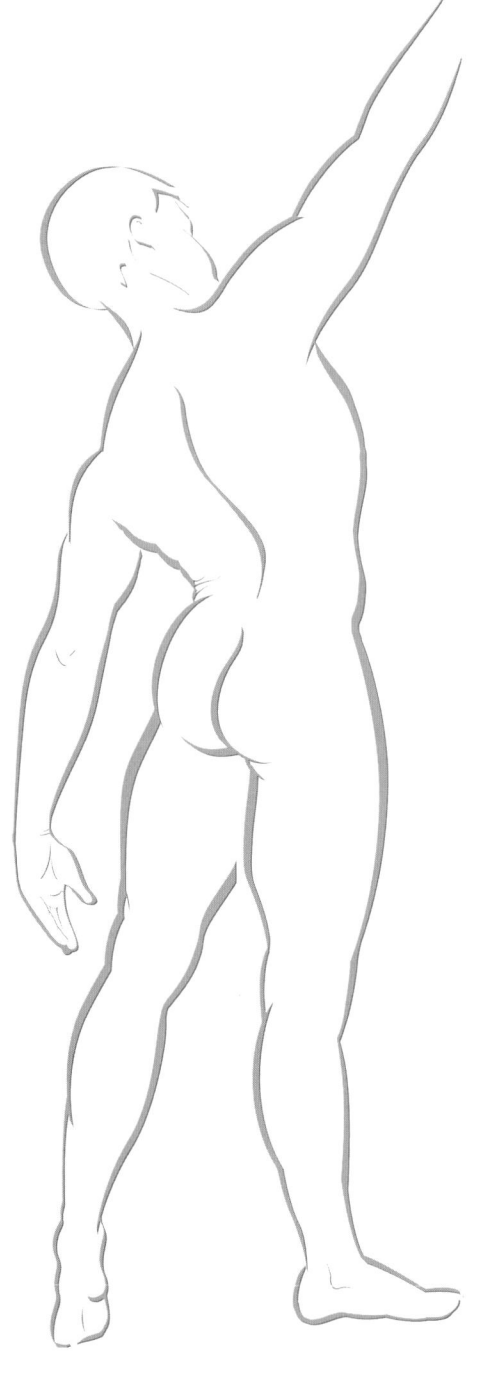

Endopyelotomy

Paul J. Van Cangh
Sylvain Nesa

15

NONCANCEROUS DISEASE SECTION

For several decades, open surgery has been recommended as the optimal therapy for ureteropelvic junction (UPJ) obstruction. Multiple techniques have been developed, and dismembered pyeloplasty is today considered the gold standard. Percutaneous techniques were developed in the early 1980s for the treatment of nephrolithiasis; the inherent advantage of these minimally invasive techniques was rapidly perceived and applied to the management of UPJ obstruction. As of 1983, isolated reports of endoscopic treatment began to appear under various names, such as percutaneous pyelolysis, percutaneous intubated ureterotomy, and endopyelotomy. Percutaneous approaches were later complemented by retrograde techniques performed initially under direct vision (ureterorenoscopy) and thereafter under indirect fluoroscopic control (dilation, disruption, and electroincision by inflatable balloons).

The basic principle underlying all these procedures is a full-thickness incision of the narrow segment down to the surrounding fat, including the adjacent proximal ureter and renal pelvis (literally performing an endoscopic ureteropyelotomy or endoureteropyelotomy), followed by prolonged stenting and drainage to allow regeneration of an adequate-caliber junction around the stent. The technique was first proposed in 1909 by the French urologist Joachim Albarran ("urétérotomie externe") and later popularized by Davis (intubated ureterotomy). Although confirmed by experimental and clinical data, their pioneer work remained underused in UPJ obstruction because of the excellent results of open pyeloplasty; both procedures necessitated an open operation. With the development of percutaneous surgery, which avoided the morbidity of an open operation, the interest in intubated ureterotomy was revived. To date, with long-term follow-up, satisfactory results are regularly obtained, although the final success rate remains somewhat inferior to that of open pyeloplasty [1–6]. Risk factors have been isolated, however, including the presence of vessels crossing the UPJ, redundancy of the renal pelvis, and disorders of renal function [7]. Better long-term results can now be expected with careful patient selection, matching the results of open pyeloplasty.

•• ANTEGRADE ENDOPYELOTOMY ••

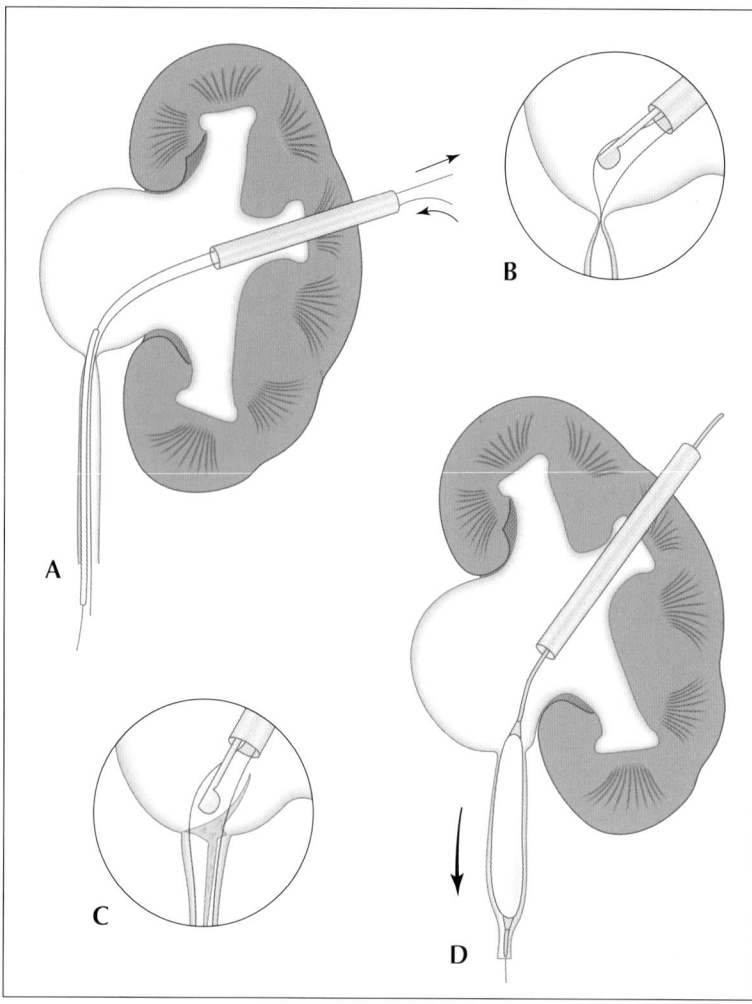

▶ **FIGURE 15-1.** Classic percutaneous technique. A retrograde open-end ureteral catheter is inserted and advanced through the ureteropelvic junction (UPJ). When this maneuver fails, the endoscopic route should be abandoned because further attempts to localize an impassable UPJ usually are unsuccessful, and unguided incision is dangerous and may result in total separation of the ureter. The patient then is positioned on the table in a position that is similar to that used for a classic percutaneous procedure, and a posterior calyx is punctured and catheterized. A middle or superior calyx should be selected to secure an adequate working angle. The tract is dilated, and the nephroscope is introduced. Secondary calculi are extracted at this stage. Extensive lithotripsy should be avoided in patients with a previous history of urinary tract infection or infectious stones because there is a significant risk of sepsis associated with urinary extravasation induced by the procedure. **A** and **B**, The UPJ is easily identified by the protruding retrograde ureteral catheter, and a second guidewire is introduced from above and lowered down into the ureter. **C**, The incision is made posterolaterally through the entire thickness of the pelvic wall, the UPJ, and the narrow portion of the proximal ureter as far down as necessary to visualize a normal-caliber lumen; vascular anatomic studies have shown that the lateral border of the UPJ is the safest place for incision [8]. **D**, When the exact length of the abnormal ureter is in doubt, a dilation balloon is inserted over a second guidewire and is inflated with contrast medium under fluoroscopic control; care should be taken to correct any residual narrowed areas.

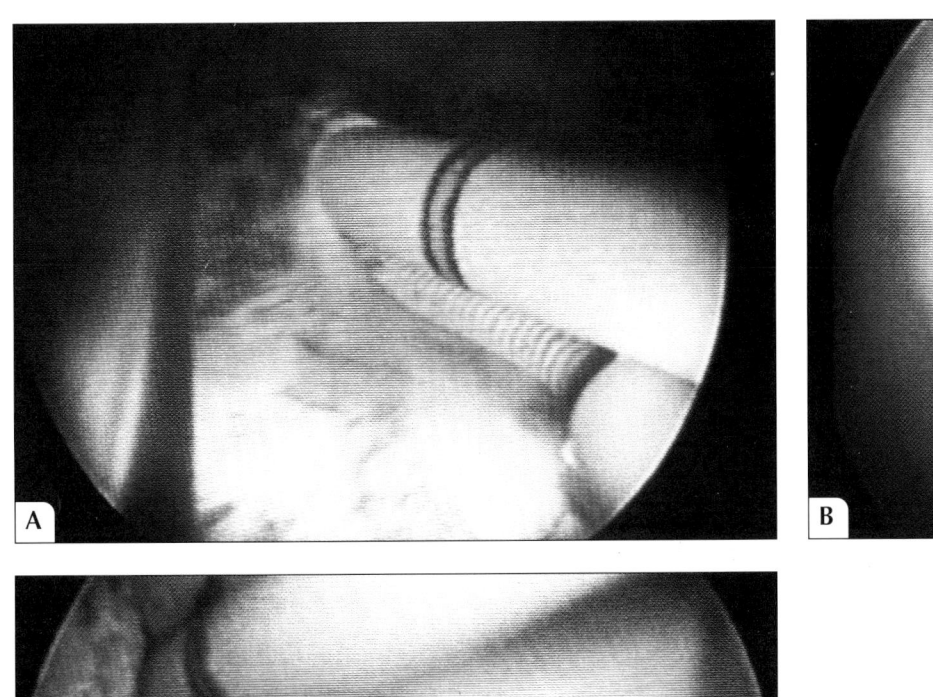

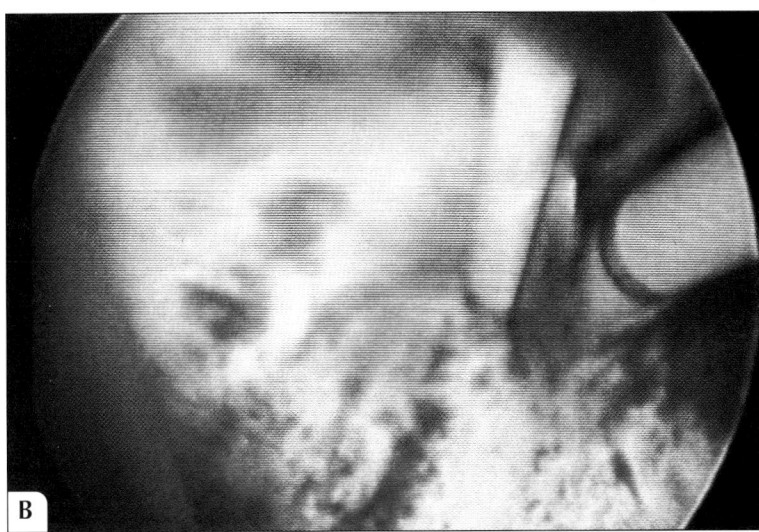

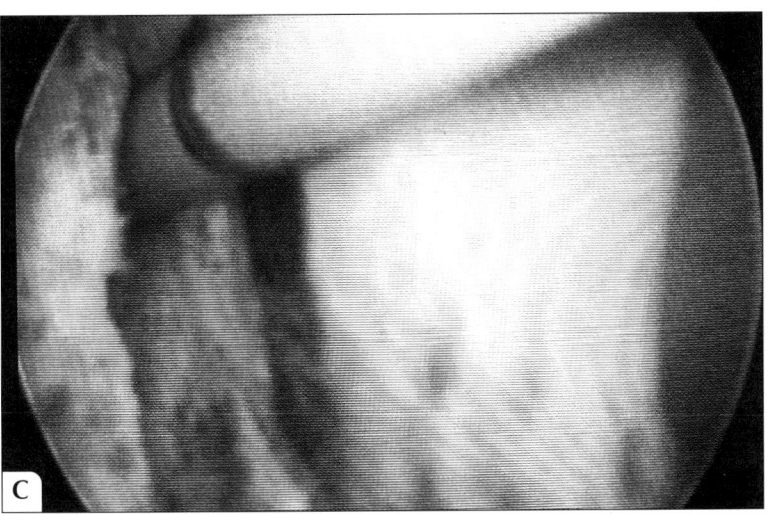

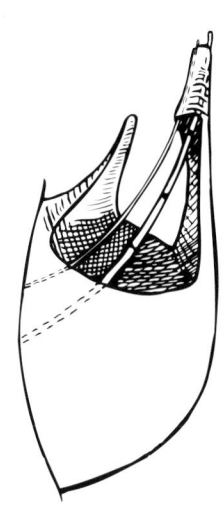

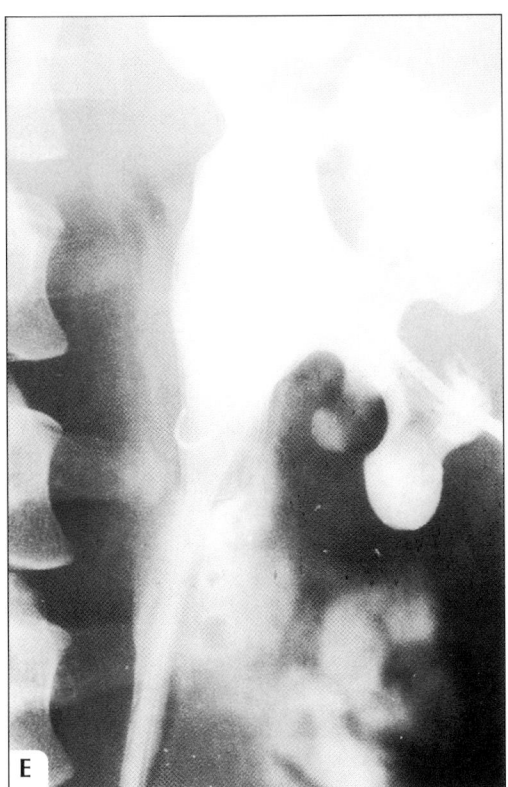

▶ **FIGURE 15-2.** (*See* Color Plate) Endoscopic views of the classic percutaneous technique. **A,** Endoscopic view showing the narrowed ureteropelvic junction (UPJ) from inside of the renal pelvis; the retrograde ureteral catheter and the second guidewire introduced from above are clearly seen. **B,** Endoscopic view of the cold knife in action. The use of a second guidewire is advantageous for straightening and stiffening the ureter to be incised. The cold knife literally is railroaded on the track. A full-thickness incision down to the surrounding fat must be performed. **C,** Endoscopic view from inside the renal pelvis looking into the ureter. The UPJ has been thoroughly opened and normal caliber proximal ureter has been reached. **D,** Line drawing of *panel C.* At this stage the results obtained with the endopyelotomy incision resemble those achieved with a Foley nondismembered pyeloplasty. Surrounding areolar tissue should be clearly visible. **E,** Extravasation of contrast medium under fluoroscopic control proves that the incision has been carried out at sufficient depth. The specific characteristics of the knife have little importance; equally successful results have also been obtained with electric and laser incision. Aggressive coagulation is, however, unwarranted.

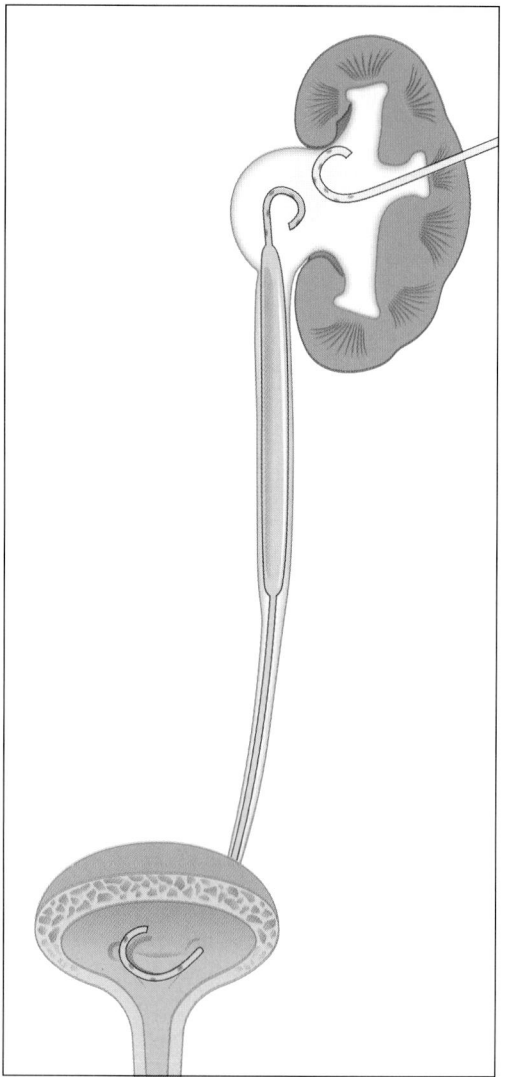

▶ **FIGURE 15-3.** A convenient stenting and drainage system consists of a 14/7 JJ stent traversing the incised uteropelvic junction. Other techniques can be used successfully, provided that drainage is adequate to prevent secondary fibrosis from persistent extravasation. A small nephrostomy tube remains in place for a few days until effective internal drainage is secured. The internal stent is removed in the outpatient clinic after 6 weeks.

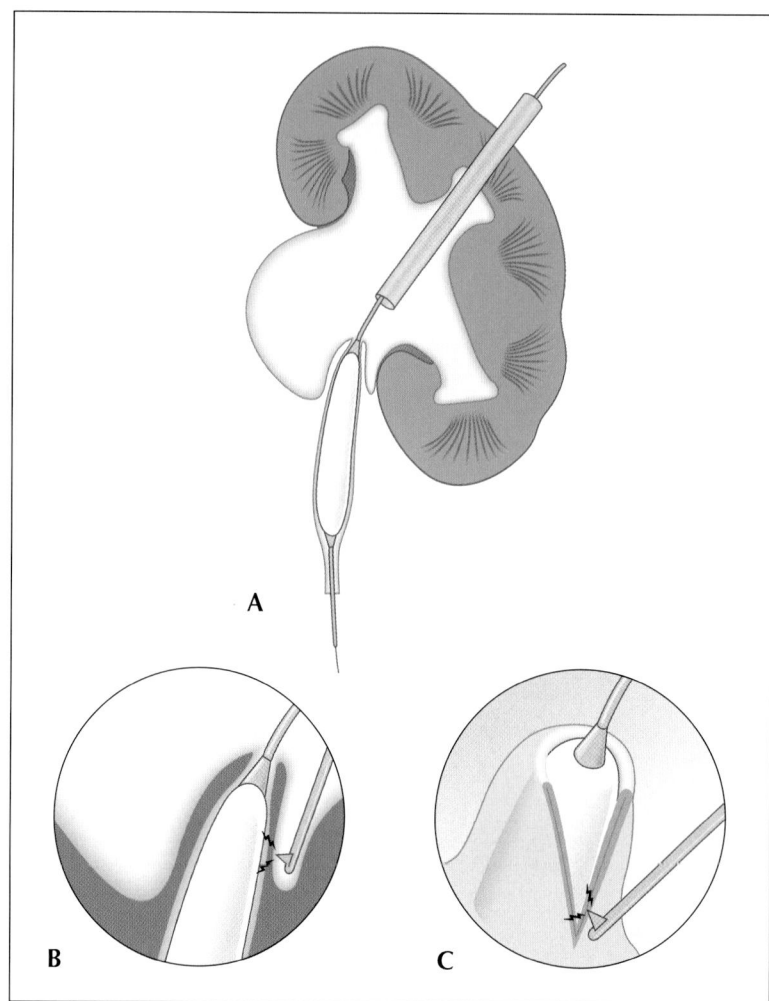

▶ **FIGURE 15-4.** **A** through **C,** Invagination technique. Incision of the ureteropelvic junction (UPJ) may be facilitated by a modification of the original technique [4]. Instead of a simple open-end ureteral catheter, a dilation balloon is used for the initial retrograde UPJ catheterization. After percutaneous access has been obtained, the balloon is inflated below the UPJ and attracted inside the renal pelvis by traction on the exteriorized guidewire, thereby invaginating the UPJ and the proximal ureter (*panel A*). The double layer of the invaginated pelvis and ureter is incised from inside the renal pelvis using electrocautery and a small-point electrode (*panels B and C*). When the balloon is deflated and removed from below, spontaneous reduction of the invagination occurs. If residual or additional narrowing is suspected, the balloon can be reinflated on its way out to calibrate the ureter. Drainage and stenting are identical to the classic percutaneous technique. The invagination technique facilitates the incision of the UPJ because the tissue is stabilized on the dilated balloon. It may also reduce the risk of damaging crossing vessels, although such complications have occurred.

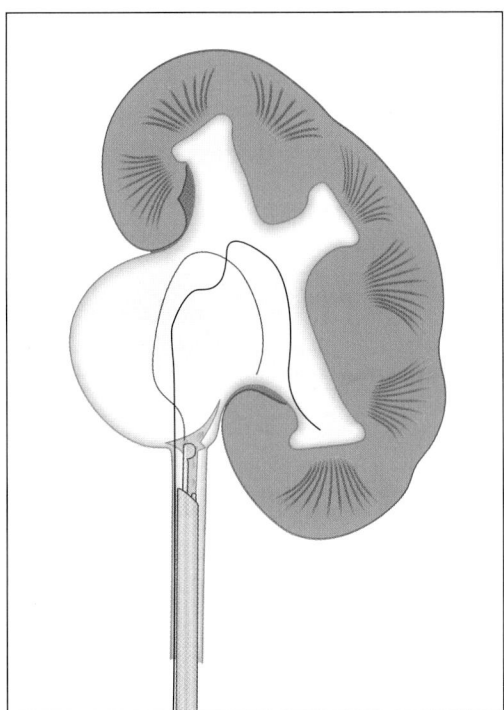

▶ **FIGURE 15-5.** Ureterorenoscopic approach. To reduce the invasiveness of the procedure, purely retrograde approaches have been devised. A small-caliber ureterorenoscope is advanced up to the level of the ureteropelvic junction (UPJ), and a posterolateral incision is performed under direct vision. The procedure is facilitated by the preliminary insertion of a JJ stent, which should remain in place 1 to 2 weeks to soften the ureter. This insertion, however, adds to the complexity of the procedure, which remains technically difficult, especially in male patients [9].

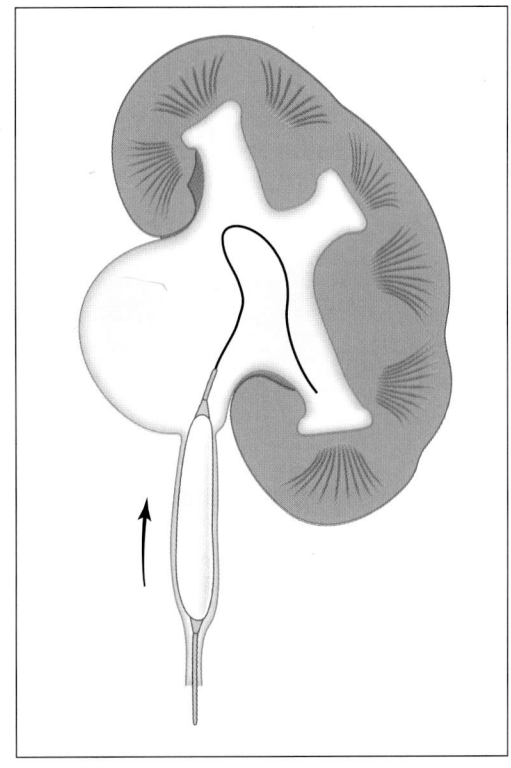

▶ **FIGURE 15-6.** Balloon dilation and rupture ("endoburst"). A retrograde ureteropyelogram delineates the upper collecting system. An angioplasty balloon is inserted over a guidewire and positioned across the ureteropelvic junction (UPJ) under fluoroscopic control. The balloon is inflated until waisting completely disappears and extravasation of contrast is observed. A simple dilation is insufficient; rupture of the narrowed area must be documented. Several inflation-deflation cycles are recommended to ensure that no residual narrowing remains. An endopyelotomy stent is inserted over the initial guidewire. Although initial skepticism prevailed, recent laboratory data have shown results equaling those of endopyelotomy [10].

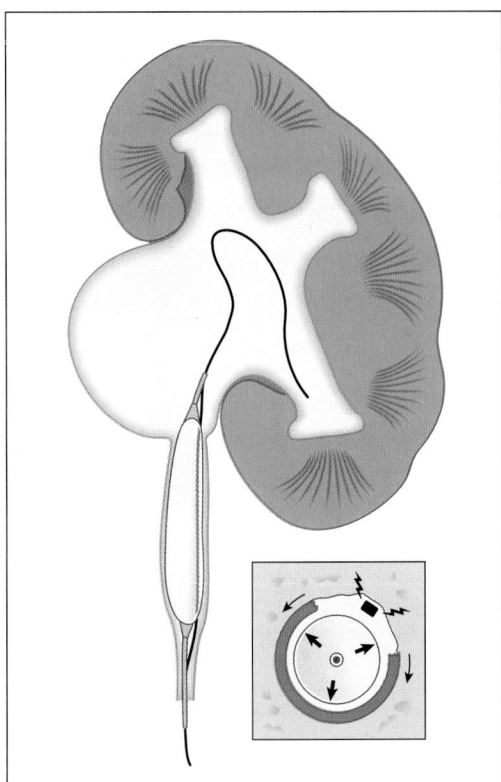

▶ **FIGURE 15-7.** Balloon electrocautery incision using the Acucise (Applied Medical Technologies; Laguna Hills, CA) endopyelotomy. The Acucise device consists of a low-pressure balloon fitted with an active electrosurgical wire over the 2-cm expandable portion of the balloon. The operative technique is rather similar to the endoburst. In this operation, however, the ureteropelvic junction (UPJ) is not forcefully disrupted but is cleanly cut by the electrosurgical wire that is activated during inflation of the balloon. It is necessary to see extravasation of contrast medium to ensure that the incision has been completed. When in doubt, flexible ureteroscopy and electrosurgical incision under direct vision are recommended. The technique is safe and reliable, especially when the surrounding vascular anatomy of the UPJ has been studied by preoperative spiral CT or endoluminal ultrasonography.

Retrograde approaches have the advantage of avoiding percutaneous nephrostomy and are thereby potentially less invasive than their percutaneous counterparts. Postoperative morbidity, duration of hospitalization, and delay in returning to full activity understandably favor strictly retrograde approaches. Their drawbacks include a sometimes less than ideal drainage system, relying only on the endopyelotomy stent, and the lack of direct visual control, which is essential for an exact incision and for efficient inspection in search of pulsation, indicating potential crossing vessels. In addition, associated disorders (*ie*, kidney stones) cannot be adequately treated via this route and are better approached percutaneously.

Results of Retrograde Endo(uretero)pyelotomy Techniques in Adults According to Type of Ureteropelvic Junction Obstruction

Technique	Procedure, n	Types I and II*	Device	Cutting mechanism	Success, %	Length of follow-up, mo
Balloon dilation and rupture (endoburst)						
O'Flynn [11]	31[†]	29 + 2	Balloon	Disruption	68	10 (3–30)
Mc Clinton [12]	42	33 + 9	Balloon	Disruption	80	18 (3–48)
Snow [6]	26	—	Balloon 36 F	Disruption	64	21 (3–44)
Cutting balloon (Acucise)						
Nadler [13]	28	23 + 5	Balloon	Cutting	81 (78 and 100)	33 (24–43)
Faerber [14]	32	27 + 5	Balloon	Cutting	87	14 (3–28)
Gelet [15]	(44) 38	29 + 19	Balloon	Cutting	76 (68 and 84)	12 (3–39)
Preminger [5]	66	52 + 14	Balloon	Cutting	77 (72 and 100)	8 (1–18)
Retrograde ureterorenoscopy						
Inglis [16]	2	0 +2	Rigid	Diathermy hook	100	4 and 12
Meretyk [17]	19	16 + 3	Rigid and flexible	Electrocautery	79	17 (4–36)
Chowdhury [18]	12	—	Rigid	Cold knife	83	4–18
Thomas [9]	49	40 + 9	Rigid	Cold knife and electrocautery	>90	15 (7–36)

*Type I—primary obstruction; type II—secondary obstruction.
[†]Twenty via antegrade approach.

▶ FIGURE 15-8. The results of endopyelotomy (see also Fig. 15-9). In the most recent series, antegrade and retrograde techniques obtain success rates in the same range; slightly better results have, however, been reported in secondary ureteropelvic junction (UPJ) obstruction, when using an antegrade technique. Results of several retrograde endopyelotomies fall somewhat short of those associated with contemporary open pyeloplasty (67% to 88% with endopyelotomy vs 95% with open pyeloplasty). Because most endopyelotomy series using different techniques achieve approximately the same results, selection criteria apparently play a major role. Risk factors have been identified. The presence of vessels directly crossing the UPJ stands out as a major prognostic factor of outcome; and the degree of hydronephrosis, the type of obstruction, and renal function also play a role, although of lesser importance [7,19].

Study	Procedures, n	Type of ureteropelvic junction obstruction	Type I, %	Success, %			Follow-up (mo)
		I (primary) + II (secondary)		Total	Type I	Type II	
Gupta [1]	401	235 + 166	59	85	82	89	51 (6–144)
Kunkel [2]	143	63 + 80	44	76	81	73	12 (6–43)
Van Cangh [20]	123	100 + 23	81	71	68	83	62 (6–153)
Cuzin [4]	81	44 + 37	54	84	86	81	37 (mean)
Kletscher [21]	50	39 + 11	78	88	90	82	12 (4–74)
Combe [22]	49	37 + 12	48	78	75	84	16 (3–36)
Meretyk [23]	23	12 + 11	52	78	75	91	22 (2–39)
Perez [24]	17	7 + 10	41	88	86	90	14 (4–40)
Total	887	537 + 350	61	81	79	84	—

▶ **FIGURE 15-9.** Results of antegrade endopyelotomy in adults according to type of ureteropelvic junction obstruction.

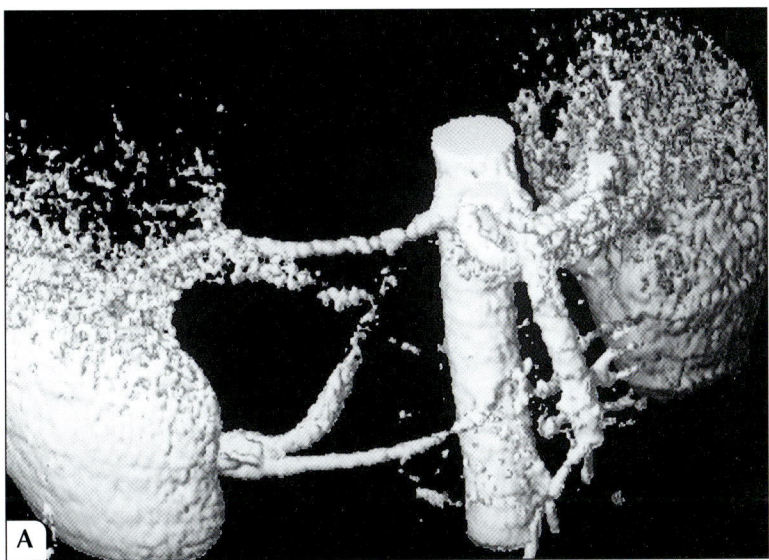

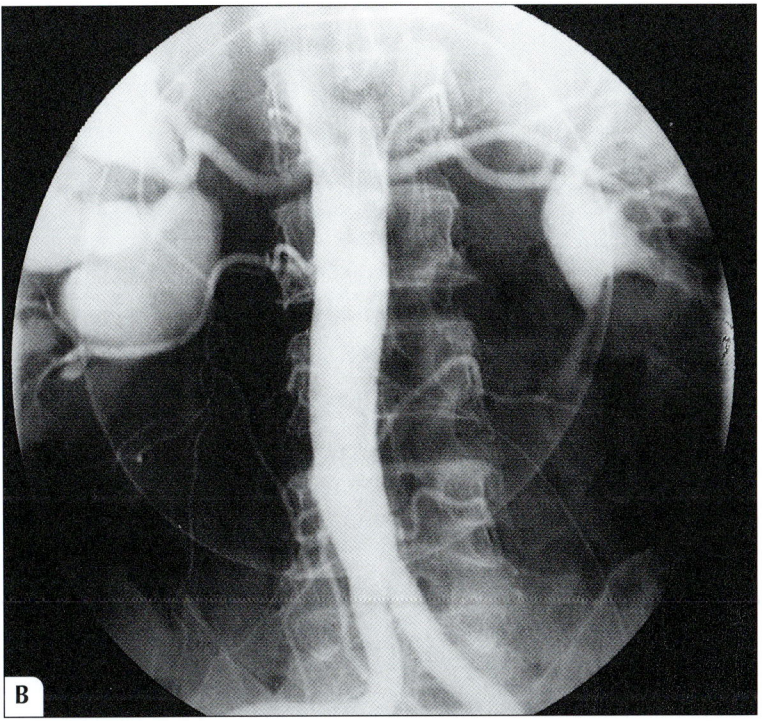

▶ **FIGURE 15-10.** The presence of a crossing vessel should be ascertained preoperatively because it significantly influences the outcome. Modern diagnostic techniques such as spiral CT (**A**) and endoluminal ultrasonography have replaced more invasive procedures such as angiography (**B**). When a crossing vessel has been documented, a classic endopyelotomy is likely to provide inadequate results, especially in the presence of a large renal pelvis, or may even promote recurrence [3,19]. When a small artery or a venous channel is encountered, consideration can be given to transection of the crossing vessel. If a major vessel is present, an alternative treatment, such as open or laparoscopic pyeloplasty, is preferable [25,19].

With careful attention to operative details, endopyelotomy produces outstanding results with minimal morbidity. Present retrograde techniques, which avoid the morbidity of percutaneous access and achieve comparable success, are promising.

Prognostic factors such as crossing vessels and high-grade hydronephrosis have been identified. We believe that with better definition of the indications, the outcome will improve further and will match open pyeloplasty results in well-selected patients. In the absence of vessels crossing the ureteropelvic junction and a massively dilated renal pelvis, a 95% success rate can be expected.

REFERENCES

1. Gupta M, Tuncay OL, Smith A: Open surgical exploration after failed endopyelotomy: a 12-year experience. *J Urol* 1997, 157:1613–1619.

2. Kunkel M, Korth K: Endopyelotomy: long-term follow-up of 143 patients. *J Endourol* 1990, 4:109–115.

3. Van Cangh PJ, Wilmart JF, Opsomer RJ, *et al.*: Long-term results and late recurrence after endoureteropyelotomy: a critical analysis of prognostic factors. *J Urol* 1994, 151:934–937.

4. Cuzin B, Abbar M, Dawahra M, *et al.*: 100 endopyélotomies percutanées: techniques, indication, résultats. *Prog Urol* 1992, 2:559–569.

5. Preminger GM, Clayman RV, Nakada SY, *et al.*: A multicenter clinical trial investigating the use of a fluoroscopically controlled cutting balloon catheter for the management of ureteral and ureteropelvic junction obstruction. *J Urol* 1997, 157:1625–1629.

6. Snow TM, Wells IP, Hammond JC: Balloon rupture and stenting for pelviureteric junction obstruction: abolition of waisting is a prognostic marker. *Clin Radiol* 1994, 49:708–710.

7. Van Cangh PJ, Nesa S: Endopyelotomy: prognostic factors and patient selection. *Urol Clin North Am* 1998, 25:281–288.

8. Sampaio FJB, Favorito LA: Ureteropelvic junction stenosis: vascular anatomical background for endopyelotomy. *J Urol* 1993, 150:1787–1791.

9. Thomas R, Monga M, Klein EW: Ureteroscopic retrograde endopyelotomy for management of ureteropelvic junction obstruction. *J Endourol* 1996, 10:141–145.

10. Pearle MS, Moon YT, Endicott RC, *et al.*: Comparison of retrograde endopyelotomy and Endoballoon rupture of the ureteropelvic junction in a porcine model. *J Urol* 1994, 152:2232–2239.

11. O'Flynn K, McKelvic G, Steyn J: Endoballoon rupture and stenting for pelviureteric junction obstruction technique and early results. *Br J Urol* 1989, 64:572–574.

12. McClinton S, Steyn JH, Hussey JK: Retrograde balloon dilatation for pelvi-ureteric junction obstruction. *Br J Urol* 1993, 71:152–155.

13. Nadler RB, Rao GS, Pearle MS, *et al.*: Acucise endopyelotomy: assessment of long term durability. *J Urol* 1996, 156:1094–1097.

14. Faerber GJ, Richardson TD, Farah N, *et al.*: Retrograde treatment of ureteropelvic junction obstruction using the ureteral cutting balloon catheter. *J Urol* 1997, 157:454–458.

15. Gelet A, Combe M, Ramackers JM: Endopyelotomy with the Acucise cutting balloon: early clinical experience. *Eur Urol* 1997, 31:389–393.

16. Inglis JA, Tolley DA: Ureteroscopic pyelolysis for pelvi-ureteric junction obstruction. *Br J Urol* 1986, 58:250–252.

17. Meretyk I, Meretyk S, Clayman RV: Endopyelotomy: comparison of ureteroscopic retrograde and antegrade percutaneous techniques. *J Urol* 1992, 148:775–783.

18. Chowdhury SD, Kerogbon J: Rigid ureteroscopic endopyelotomy without external drainage. *J Endourol* 1992, 6:357–360.

19. Kumon H, Tsugawa M, Hashimoto H, *et al.*: Impact of 3-dimensional helical computerized tomography on selection of operative methods for ureteropelvic junction obstruction. *J Urol* 1997, 158:1696–1700.

20. Van Cangh PJ, Nesa S, Galeon M, *et al.*: Vessels around the ureteropelvic junction: significance and imaging by conventional radiology. *J Endourol* 1996, 10:111–119.

21. Kletscher BA, Segura JW, Leroy AJ, *et al.*: Percutaneous antegrade endoscopic pyelotomy: review of 50 consecutive cases. *J Urol* 1995, 153:701–704.

22. Combe M, Gelet A, Abdelrahim AF, *et al.*: Ureteropelvic invagination procedure for endopyelotomy (Gelet technique): results of 51 consecutive cases. *J Endourol* 1996, 10:153–157.

23. Meretyk I, Meretyk S, Clayman RV: Endopyelotomy: comparison of ureteroscopic retrograde and antegrade percutaneous techniques. *J Urol* 1992, 148:775–783.

24. Perez LM, Friedman RM, Carson CC: Endoureteropyelotomy in adults. *Urology* 1992, 39:71–76.

25. Van Cangh PJ, Nesa S: Endoureteropyelotomy atlas. *Urol Clin North Am* 1996, 4:43–58.

Laparoscopic Pyeloplasty

Günter Janetschek

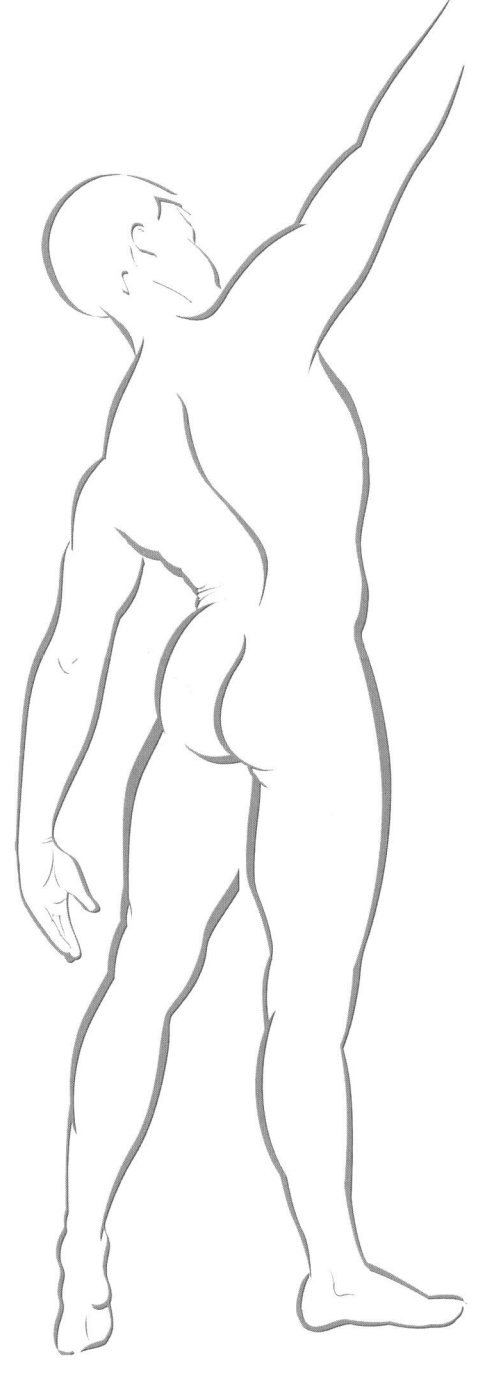

Hydronephrosis due to congenital ureteropelvic junction (UPJ) obstruction is one of the anomalies more commonly seen in children. Owing to the wide-spread use of ultrasound imaging in fetuses, nearly all cases can now be recognized and diagnosed in the perinatal period [1]. In children, UPJ obstruction is typically caused by an intrinsic lesion in the ureteropelvic wall, although secondary obstruction due to crossing vessels is a relatively rare finding. Despite the availability of minimally invasive alternatives, pyeloplasty by open surgical means is still the standard procedure in small children.

In adults, the situation is quite different. In this group of patients, primary intrinsic stenosis occurs only in exceptional cases, although the incidence of crossing vessels has been reported to be approximately 67% [2,3]. Whether these vessels are the underlying cause of UPJ obstruction, however, or just an incidental finding of no clinical significance is still a matter of discussion. In a given case, either of these may be correct. Obstruction in adults with previously normal collecting systems who are diagnosed with crossing vessels at the UPJ is most likely caused by these vessels. The same etiologic factor can be assumed in intermittent hydronephrosis, which is frequently associated with crossing vessels [4]. The obstructive nature of crossing vessels is also confirmed by surgical studies reporting good results with simple displacement or transection of the crossing vessels, leaving the ureteropelvic junction itself intact [5,6]. On the other hand, it is a well-known fact that in a great number of patients, removal of the crossing vessels does not suffice to repair the stenosis, because an intrinsic stenosis is present as well [7]. Again, this can be interpreted in several ways. The intrinsic stenosis could be due to the continuous pressure exerted by crossing vessels. It is also conceivable, however, that mild primary intrinsic stenosis requires the additional component of the pelvis descending over the lower-pole vessels, thereby aggravating the obstruction. In other cases, the crossing vessels may not contribute to the obstruction at all. So long as open surgery was the only method available for the repair of UPJ obstruction, the role of crossing vessels in the etiology of obstruction was of minor importance, because it did not have any impact on therapy. Now that the different techniques of endopyelotomy and laparoscopic pyeloplasty provide attractive, efficacious, and less harmful alternatives, crossing vessels are a major concern in preoperative assessment [8]. One has to be aware, though, that the presence of crossing vessels increases the risks of endopyelotomy. Serious complications resulting from bleeding vessels have been reported by several authors [9–12]. Furthermore, there seems to be a close association between the presence of crossing vessels, recurrent obstruction, and poor long-term outcome for endopyelotomy; a long-term success rate of only 42% was reported in patients presenting with crossing vessels [13]. For this indication, laparoscopy can be highly recommended because it allows for management of crossing vessels as in open surgery [14]. Simple intrinsic stenoses might also be treated with laparoscopy, but equal results can probably be obtained with endopyelotomy, which is even less invasive, at least if performed in a retrograde fashion. For this reason, thorough preoperative assessment of the underlying cause of the obstruction is essential to select the most appropriate technique for a given patient. Even if the presence of crossing vessels is not considered relevant to the surgical strategy, careful preoperative evaluation may still contribute to a better understanding of the results.

Intra-arterial angiography is highly accurate in detecting small arterial branches, but it is an invasive technique that does not visualize crossing veins. Alternatively, endoluminal ultrasonography, which is also invasive [6], and spiral CT scanning, a noninvasive technique, can be used and have been reported to yield good results. Color Doppler ultrasound to assess UPJ obstruction preoperatively is cost effective, efficient, easily available, and uses nonionizing radiation. The sensitivity and specificity of contrast-enhanced ultrasound scanning were reported to be 95% and 100%, respectively [15].

Retroperitoneoscopy allows for ready and direct access to the UPJ [16]. It provides only limited working space, however, and therefore complicated reconstructive procedures become even more difficult [14]. The conventional transperitoneal approach involves reflection of the ipsilateral colon, which is quite time consuming [17]. In addition, this approach has the disadvantage that vessels crossing dorsal to the ureteropelvic junction may interfere with the repair, since they have to be transposed ventrally by dismembered pyeloplasty. When ventrally crossing vessels are encountered, some authors transpose the renal pelvis anteriorly, which (albeit facilitating the repair) may compromise the long-term results, because the crossing vessels are brought into an unphysiologic position. To overcome these problems, we have modified the transperitoneal approach in several ways [14]. The peritoneum is incised lateral to the colon and along the spleen or liver up to the diaphragm. The colon is not dissected at all. The same space is opened as in retroperitoneoscopy, and subsequently the kidney is rotated anteromedially approximately 180°, thus providing direct access to the renal pelvis. Conversely, when performing laparoscopic pyeloplasty in a patient with a horseshoe kidney, there is no need to reflect the kidney because the renal pelvis is in a ventral position already [14]. More recently, we have further simplified this approach. On the right side, an incision is made in the peritoneum cranial and parallel to the colonic flexure and the transverse colon, which allows for easy and quick exposure of the ureteropelvic junction. On the left side, the junction is approached via an incision in the mesentery of the colonic flexure, thus avoiding mobilization of the colon. With this new, simplified approach, exposure of the ureteropelvic junction is faster than in retroperitoneoscopy. In addition, it has the advantage of being well suited to nondismembered pyeloplasty (described later). To transpose a dorsally crossing vessel by means of dismembered pyeloplasty (Anderson-Hynes–plasty), we still prefer to dissect and rotate the kidney medially, which provides ample working space for the reconstruction.

Dismembered pyeloplasty is the preferred technique, which can be applied in most settings [18]. Laparoscopy can be performed with the same technique as for open surgery [3,14]. Laparoscopic dismembered pyeloplasty is technically difficult and demanding, however, which is why up to now the procedure has been limited to a few specialized centers. Therefore, we have been on the lookout for alternatives that would help make pyeloplasty less difficult without compromising its efficacy. In most urology textbooks, various types of nondismembered pyeloplasty are described, each of which has specific advantages and applications [19,20]. In terms of surgical technique, the different methods of nondismembered pyeloplasty are probably better suited to laparoscopy, provided the indications are clearly defined. The procedure described by Davis (a longitudinal incision through the stenotic junction, which is then stented) is the simplest technique [21]. Antegrade and retrograde endopyelotomies, two widely used techniques that are also based on Davis' principles, were shown to yield good results [22]. In 1894, Fenger used a similar longitudinal incision, which was then closed with several interrupted sutures placed in a transverse manner [23]. This technique, which allows for watertight closure of the ureter, yielded good results and was quite popular in Europe several decades ago. The so-called Fenger-plasty is technically easy and therefore well suited to laparoscopy.

Several studies document that the morbidity associated with laparoscopic pyeloplasty is significantly lower than that for open pyeloplasty, which results in a short hospital stay and rapid convalescence [3,14]. Although other minimally invasive procedures such as retrograde endopyelotomy carry an even lower morbidity rate than laparoscopy, the success rates of incisional endoscopic techniques are 10% to 20% lower than those of reconstructive methods [24]. Hence, laparoscopic pyeloplasty is clearly superior to both open surgery and endopyelotomy in terms of overall morbidity and successful outcome, its only drawback being the long and steep learning curve.

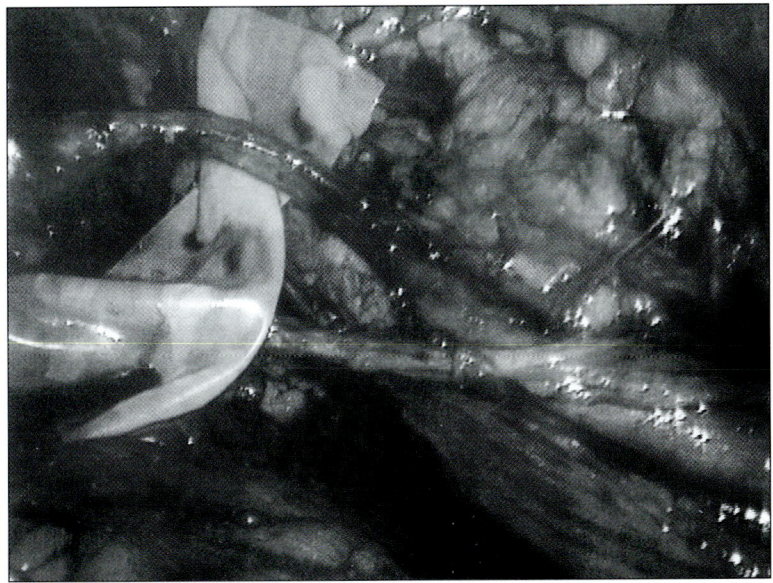

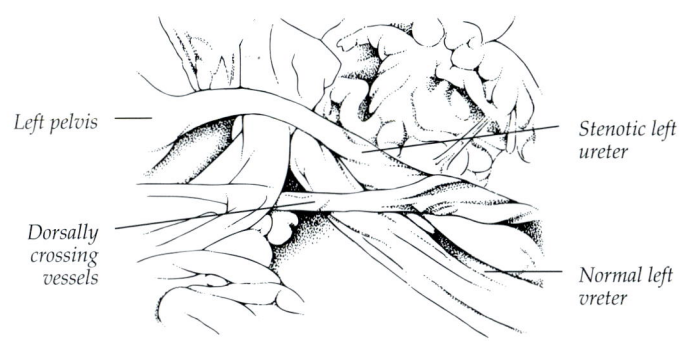

▶ **FIGURE 16-1.** (*see* Color Plate) Ventral transperitoneal approach, kidney rotated medially 180° (left side), showing long intrinsic stenosis and dorsally crossing vessels. Intrinsic stenoses are more common in children than in adults. A short stenosis may be repaired with nondismem-

bered pyeloplasty, but a long stenosis as seen here is best repaired with dismembered pyeloplasty (Anderson-Hynes) [18–20]. In this case, there are also dorsally crossing vessels, which have to be transposed ventrally by means of dismembered pyeloplasty.

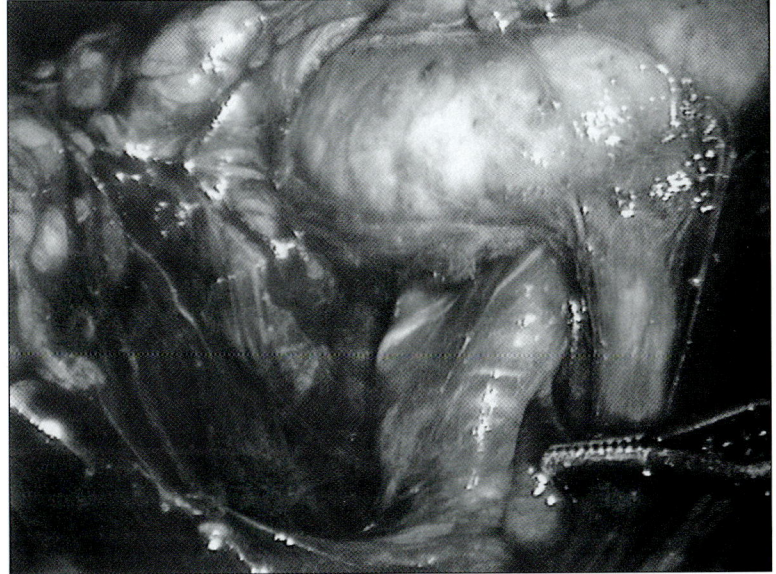

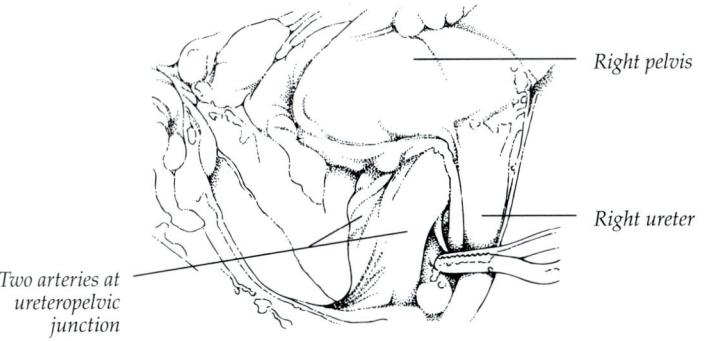

▶ **FIGURE 16-2.** (*see* Color Plate) Retroperitoneoscopic approach (right side), showing ventrally crossing arteries. As in the majority of cases, the crossing vessel at the ureteropelvic junction in this patient was found in a ventral position. It is difficult to assess preoperatively whether the obstruction is exclusively caused by these vessels or whether there is an additional

intrinsic stenosis. Transection of crossing vessels, although technically easy, should not be performed. In all instances, we displace ventrally crossing vessels cephalad, interpose a pedicle flap obtained from Gerota's fascia, and perform a Fenger-plasty. Only after incision of the ureteropelvic junction does it become obvious whether an intrinsic stenosis is present as well.

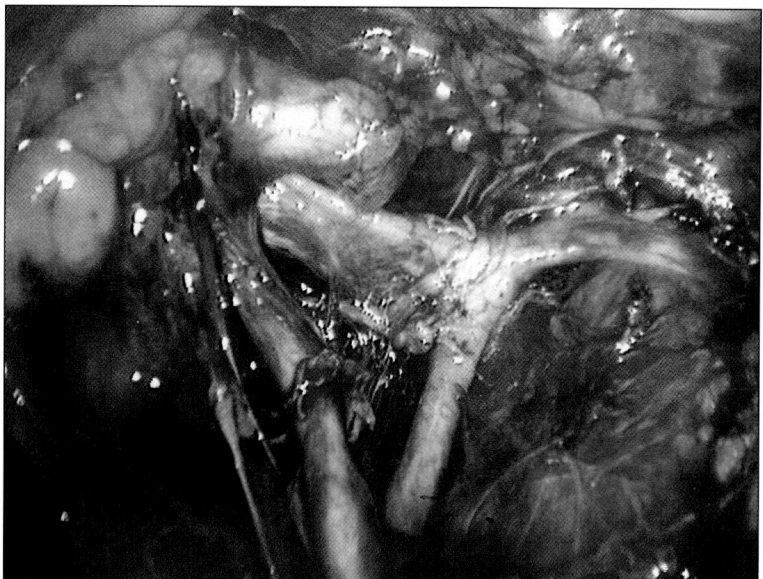

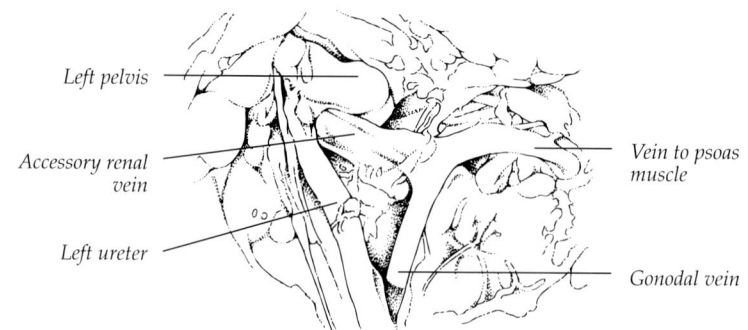

▶ **FIGURE 16-3.** (*see* Color Plate) Ventral transperitoneal approach, kidney rotated medially 180° (left side), showing ventrally crossing vein. This ventrally crossing vein was the cause of the obstruction. Although

crossing veins are difficult to identify preoperatively, they can in most cases be detected with color Doppler ultrasound, which in this setting is even more reliable than angiography [15].

DIAGNOSIS

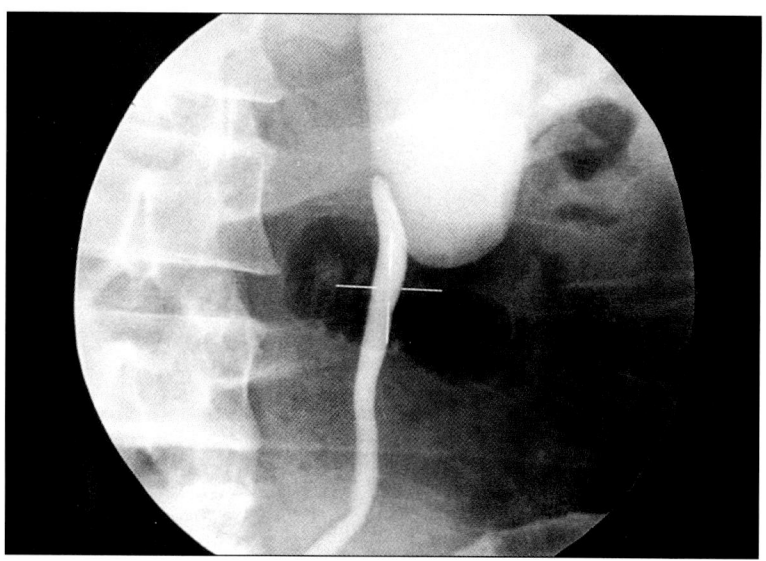

▶ **FIGURE 16-4.** Retrograde pyelography (left side). As in this patient, high-inserting ureters can cause obstruction. In this setting, most urology textbooks recommend a nondismembered type of pyeloplasty [19,20].

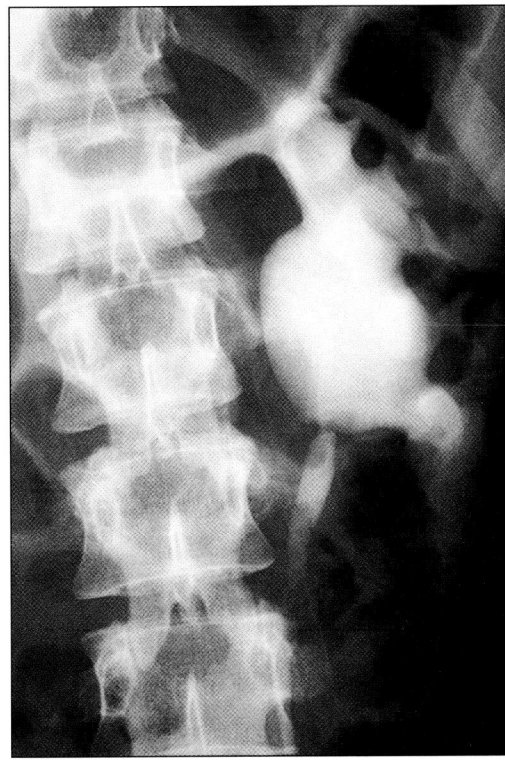

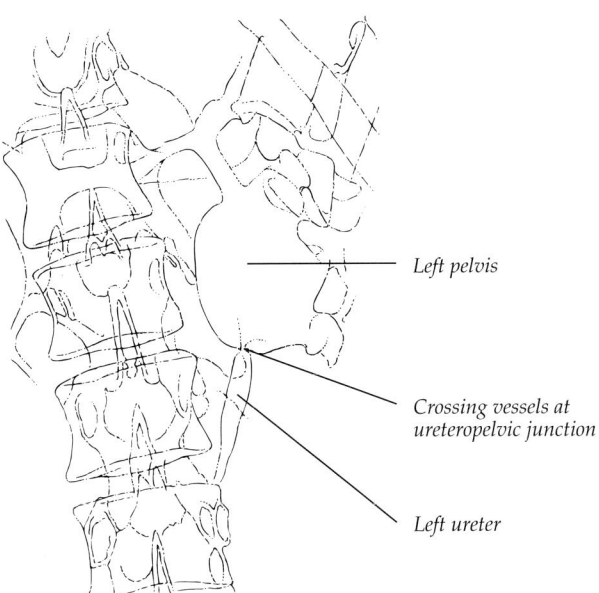

Left pelvis

Crossing vessels at
ureteropelvic junction

Left ureter

▶ **FIGURE 16-5.** Retrograde pyelography (left side). In this case, the obstruction at the ureteropelvic junction was caused by a crossing artery. Because this

obstruction is not much different from that shown in Fig. 16–4, additional imaging modalities are needed to identify or exclude crossing vessels.

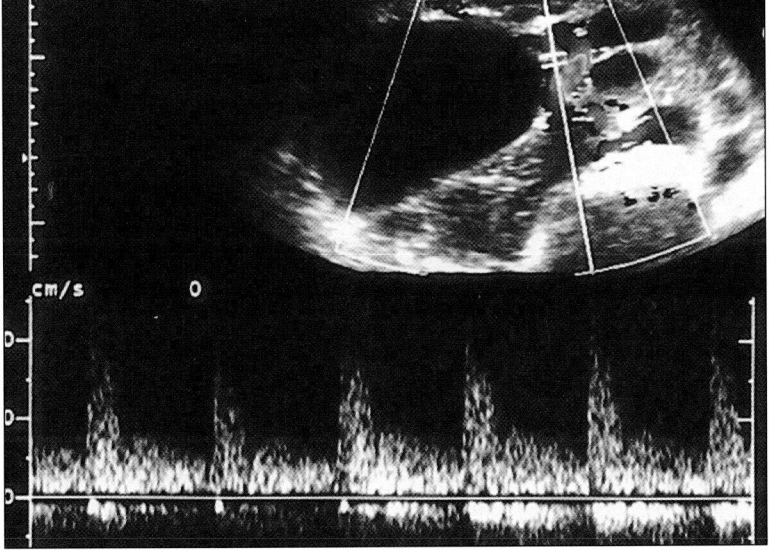

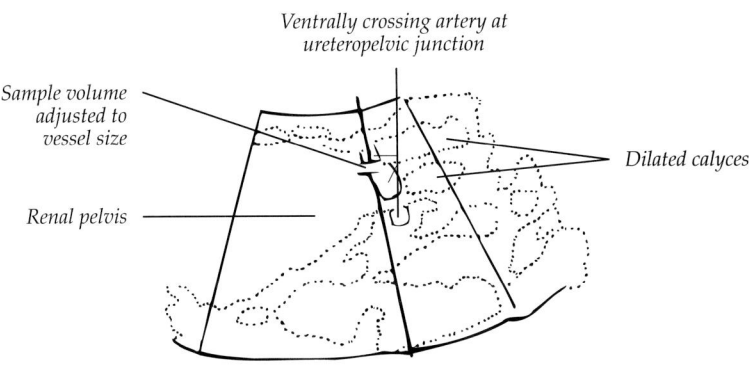

Ventrally crossing artery at
ureteropelvic junction

Sample volume
adjusted to
vessel size

Dilated calyces

Renal pelvis

▶ **FIGURE 16-6.** (*see* Color Plate) Color Doppler ultrasound. In our hands, abdominal ultrasonography has been proven to be the best technique for visualizing crossing vessels at the ureteropelvic junction; on contrast-enhanced scanning using a special ultrasound contrast medium, the sensitivity and specificity were 95% and 100%, respectively [15]. Ultrasound

allows for differentiation between vessels crossing ventrally or dorsally (color Doppler) and between arteries and veins (pulsed Doppler). Accurate preoperative diagnosis enables the surgeon to select the most appropriate approach (direct transperitoneal or rotation of the kidney) and the most suitable technique (nondismembered or dismembered pyeloplasty) [25].

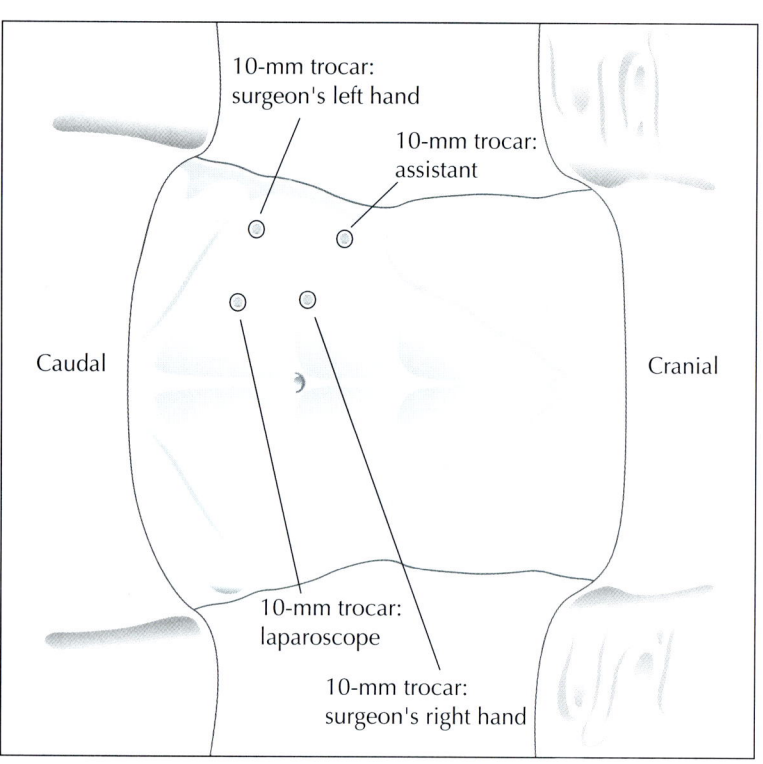

10-mm trocar:
surgeon's left hand

10-mm trocar:
assistant

Caudal

Cranial

10-mm trocar:
laparoscope

10-mm trocar:
surgeon's right hand

▶ **FIGURE 16-7.** Trocar positions for the direct and the modified transperitoneal approach (right side). The trocar for the laparoscope is placed pararectally several centimeters below the umbilicus. The precise position of this trocar depends on the location of the ureteropelvic junction, which is marked while placing a stent preoperatively. The two ports for the surgeon are in the right lower abdomen (left hand) and pararectally above the umbilicus (right hand). A fourth trocar (held by the assistant) is placed laterally just below the costal margin. Only 10-mm trocars are used.

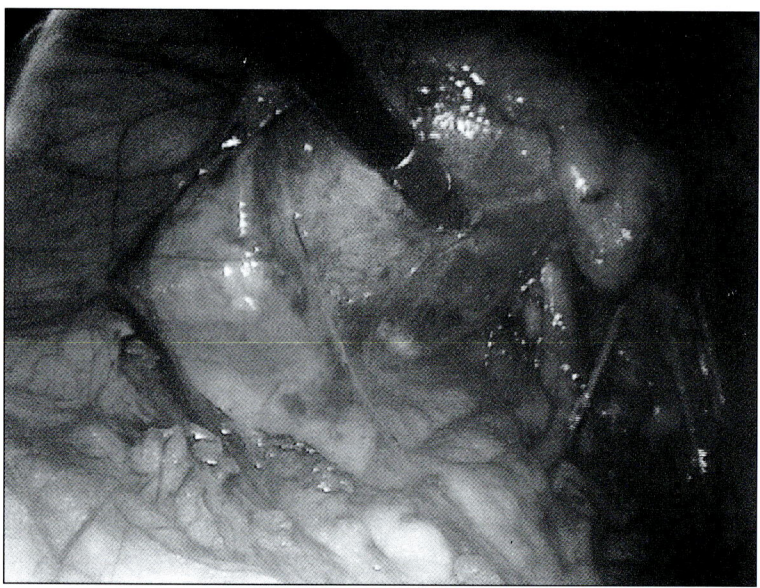

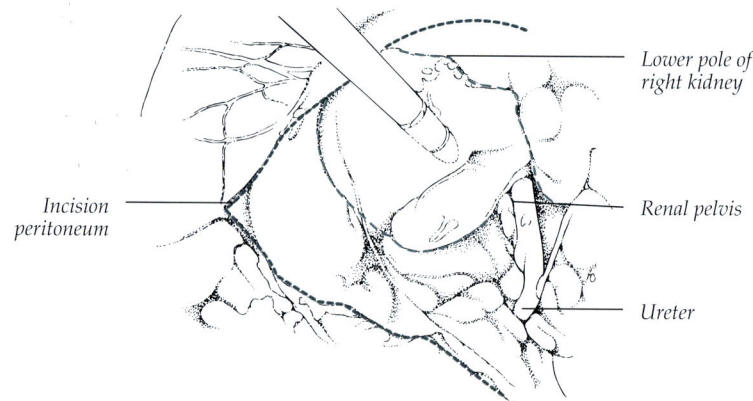

Lower pole of
right kidney

Incision
peritoneum

Renal pelvis

Ureter

▶ **FIGURE 16-8.** (*see* Color Plate) Direct transperitoneal approach (right side). The patient is placed in a 45° lateral position so that by rotating the table, the patient can be brought into the supine position as well as a 90° lateral position. The peritoneum is incised cephalad and parallel to the right colonic flexure and transverse colon. Following this,

only a little dissection is necessary to identify the ureter lateral to the vena cava. The ureter is followed in a cephalad direction as far as the ureteropelvic junction. For better exposure, the peritoneum overlying the ureter may be incised as well. The colon is not dissected at all. This approach is best combined with a Fenger-plasty.

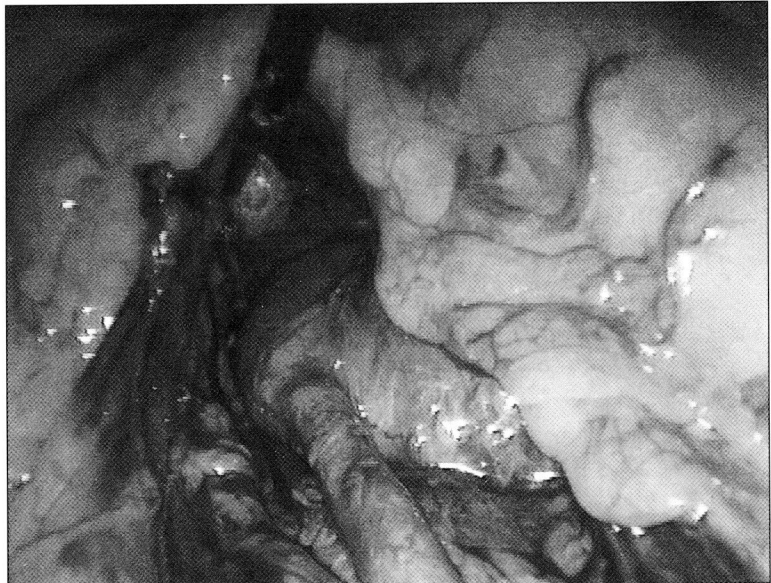

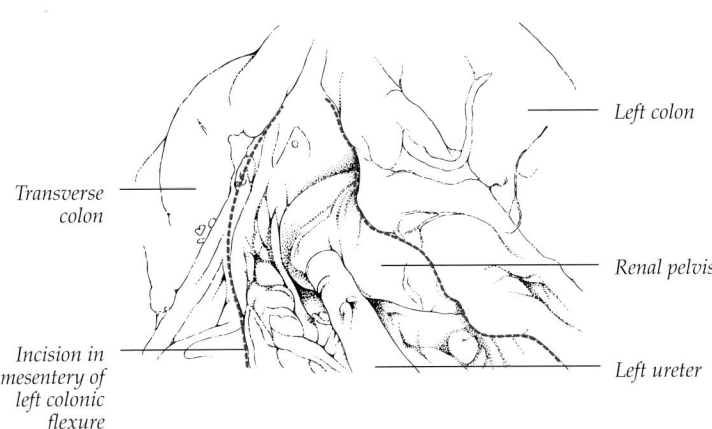

Transverse colon

Left colon

Renal pelvis

Incision in mesentery of left colonic flexure

Left ureter

▶ **FIGURE 16-9.** (*see* Color Plate) Direct transperitoneal approach (left side). In thin patients, the proximal ureter can be seen shining through the peritoneum at the base of the mesentery of the left colonic flexure. Frequently, the hydronephrotic pelvis can also be seen causing the colonic

mesentery to bulge. The mesentery is incised along the ureter up to the renal pelvis in a cephalad direction, where larger vessels are usually not encountered. This approach allows for easy and fast exposure of the ureteropelvic junction.

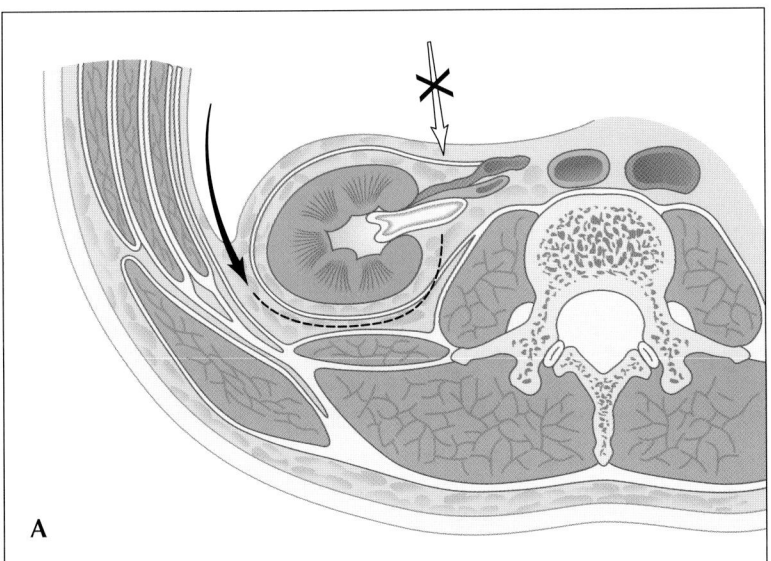

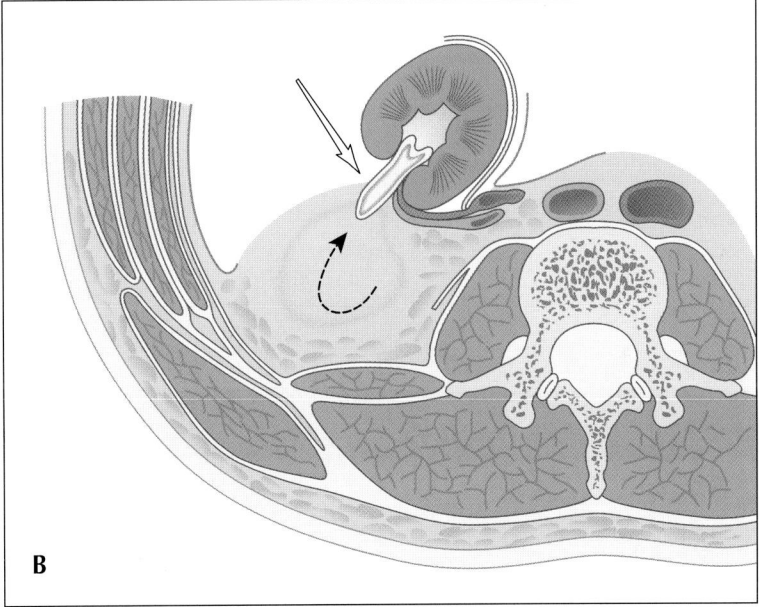

A

B

▶ **FIGURE 16-10.** Modified transperitoneal approach (right side). The patient's position on the operating table is the same as for the direct transperitoneal approach. **A,** The peritoneum is first incised lateral to the colon; then the incision is extended from just above the pelvic brim beyond the colonic flexure along the liver (the spleen on the left side) up to the diaphragm. Next the layer between Gerota's fascia and the lateral

and dorsal abdominal walls is opened. **B,** Following this dissection, the kidney is rotated anteromedially approximately 180°, thus permitting direct access to the renal pelvis. In dismembered pyeloplasty, we prefer the modified approach because it provides ample working space for the difficult task of suturing. (*From* Janetschek *et al.* [14].)

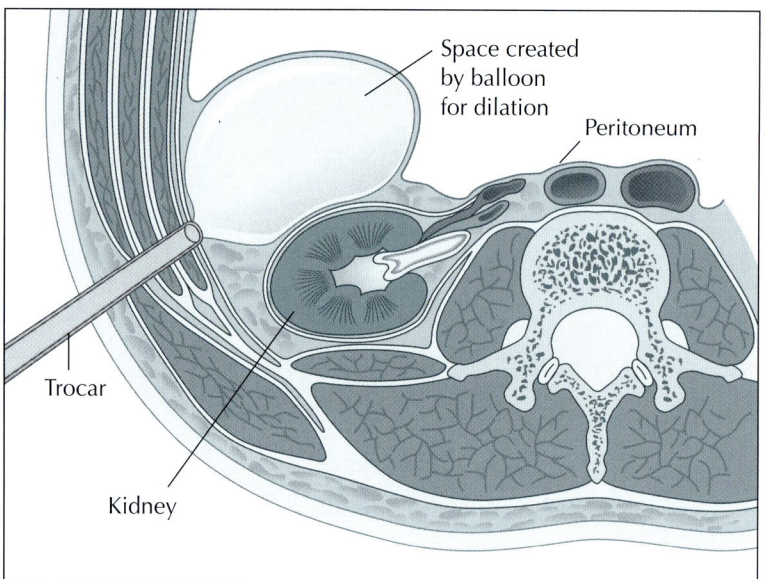

FIGURE 16-11. Retroperitoneoscopic approach (right side). This technique was previously described in detail [16]. A balloon is introduced into the retroperitoneum through a small muscle-splitting incision below the tip of the 12th rib and inflated to open up the retroperitoneal space. With the patient in a lateral position, only little dissection is required to gain access to the ureteropelvic junction, but there is also very little space to perform complicated reconstructive procedures. On the right side, we restrict this approach to patients who have had prior transperitoneal surgery, but our preferred approach on the left side now has become retroperitoneoscopy.

Labels on figure: Space created by balloon for dilation; Peritoneum; Trocar; Kidney

PYELOPLASTY

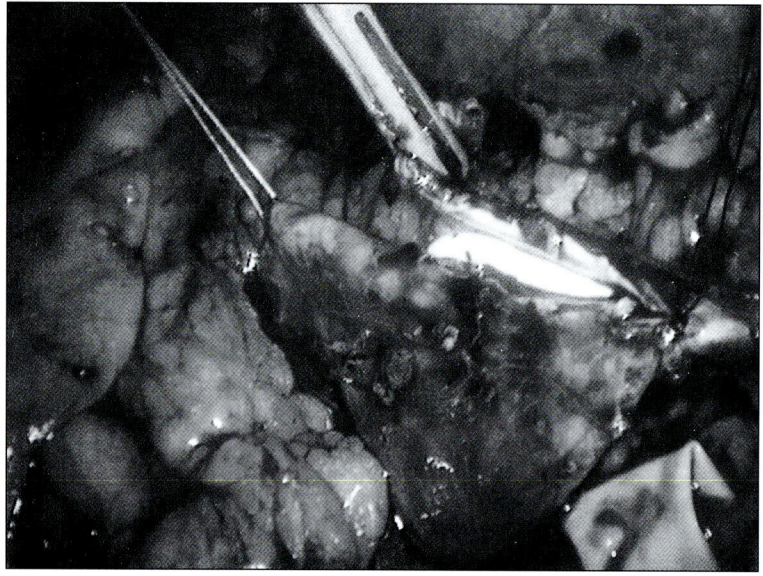

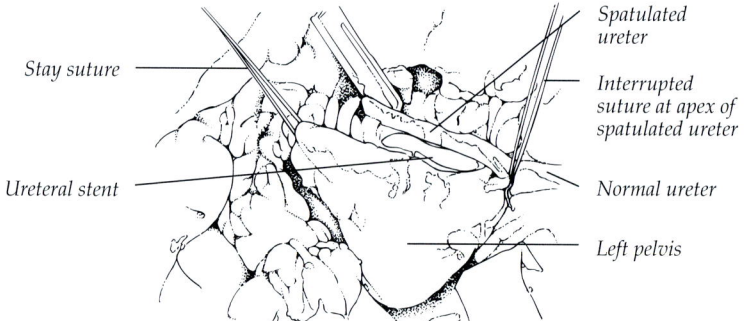

Labels on figure: Stay suture; Ureteral stent; Spatulated ureter; Interrupted suture at apex of spatulated ureter; Normal ureter; Left pelvis

FIGURE 16-12. (*see* Color Plate) Dismembered pyeloplasty. The ureter is stented preoperatively. The technique is essentially the same as in open surgery. A stay suture may be placed to facilitate exposure. Following transection of the ureteropelvic junction, the ureter is spatulated. If the pelvis is redundant, it is trimmed. The anastomosis is started with a 4-0 polydioxanone suture, which is placed both at the apex of the spatulated ureter and at the most dependent aspect of the renal pelvis. The suture is tied extracorporeally and is delivered with a knot pusher. Subsequently, a running 4-0 polyglactin suture is placed on either side; the beginning of the suture is tied intracorporeally, and its end is secured with an absorbable clip (Lapra-Ty; Ethicon Inc., Somerville, NJ). Finally, the cut edges of the renal pelvis superior to the ureteral anastomosis are reapproximated with another suture or with the help of an endoscopic suturing device.

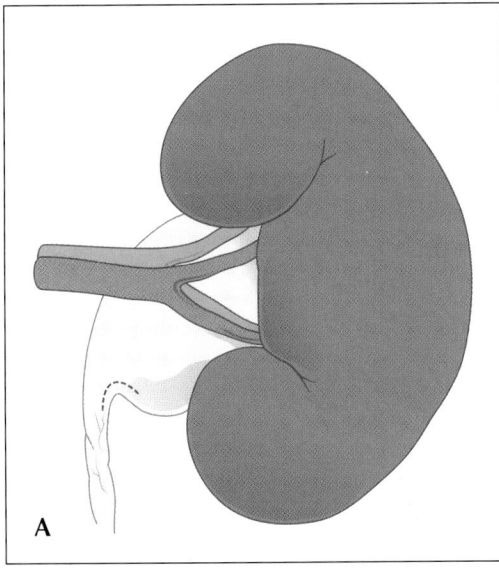

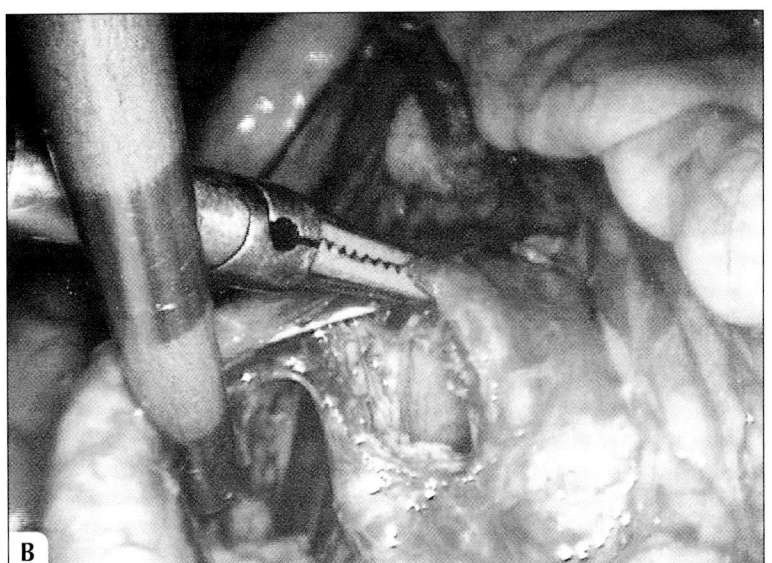

▶ **FIGURE 16-13.** Fenger-plasty (left side).
A, Analogous to endopyelotomy, a longitudinal incision is made through the stenotic uretero-pelvic junction. A ureteral stent is placed preoperatively. If a ventrally crossing vessel is encountered, it is freed and displaced cephalad.
B, (*see* Color Plate) Intraoperative site.

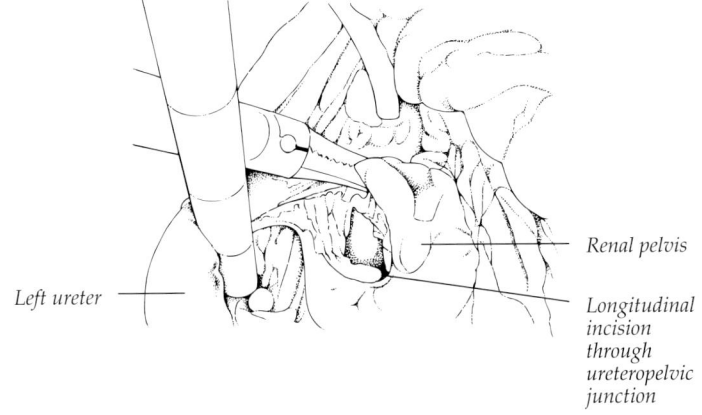

Renal pelvis

Left ureter

Longitudinal incision through ureteropelvic junction

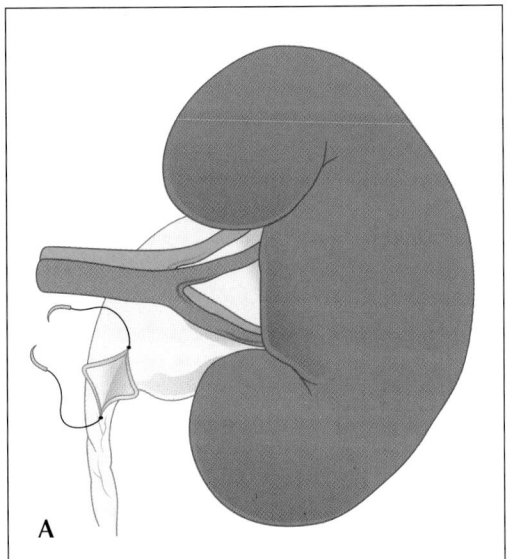

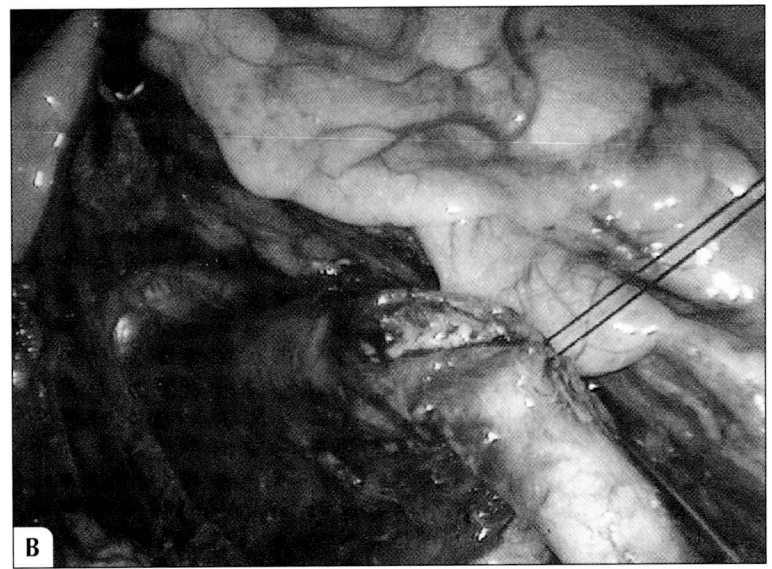

▶ **FIGURE 16-14.** Fenger-plasty (left side).
A, As a second step, the longitudinal incision is closed in a transverse fashion with one to three extracorporeally tied interrupted sutures (4-0 polydioxanone suture). **B,** (*see* Color Plate) Intraoperative site.

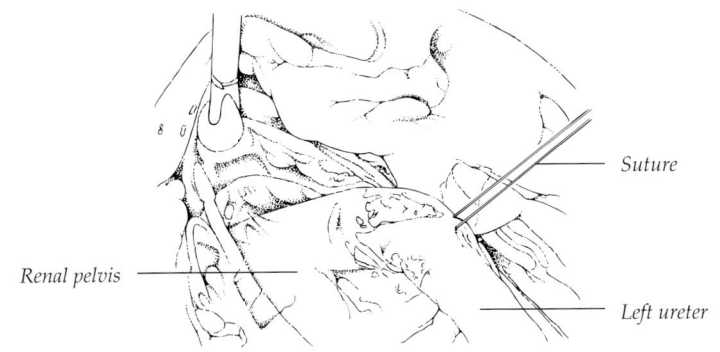

Suture

Renal pelvis

Left ureter

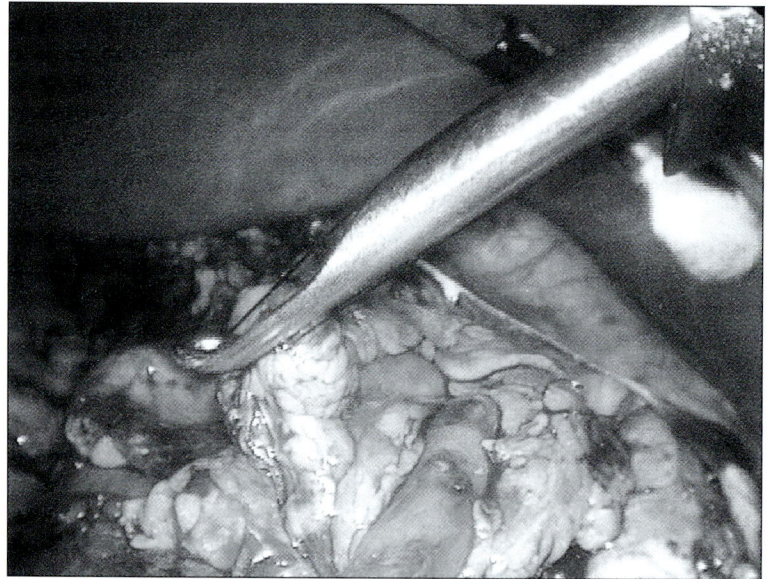

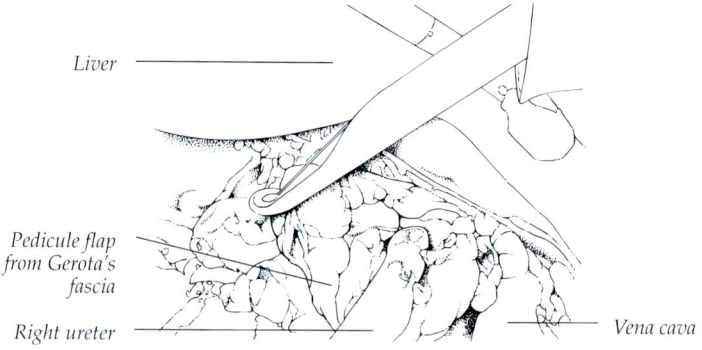

Liver

Pedicule flap
from Gerota's
fascia

Right ureter

Vena cava

▶ **FIGURE 16-15.** (*see* Color Plate) Fenger-plasty (right side). Finally, the plasty is covered with a pedicle flap of fatty tissue obtained from Gerota's fascia. This flap also helps to displace crossing vessels.

SUTURING TECHNIQUE

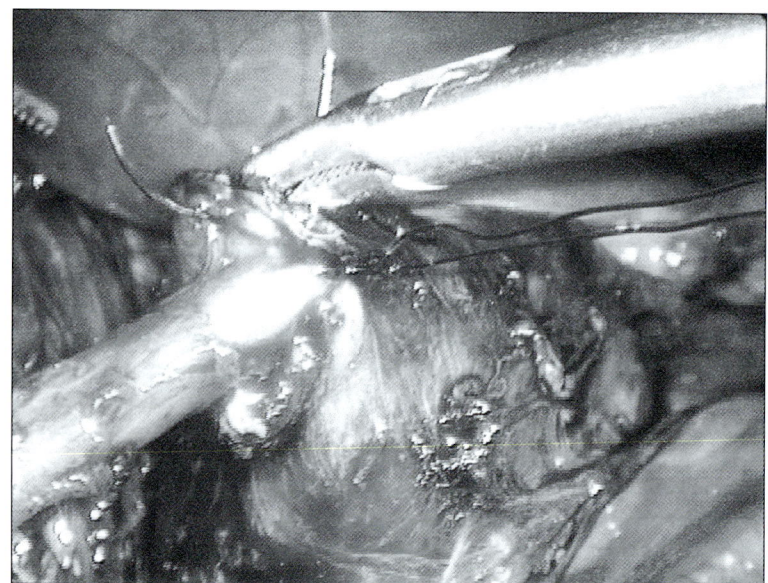

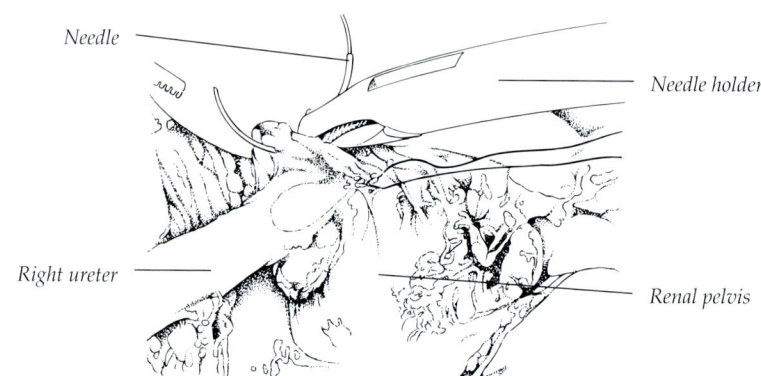

Needle

Needle holder

Right ureter

Renal pelvis

▶ **FIGURE 16-16.** (*see* Color Plate) Laparoscopic suturing. Straight needles and ski-needles have been developed specifically for laparoscopy, yet we prefer curved needles, which are also used in open surgery. One has to make sure, however, that the needle is not too large to be passed through the trocar without difficulty; we recommend the use of a suture introducer. The suture size is 4-0. We prefer polydioxanone suture (PDS) to polyglactin, because extracorporeally tied knots have better gliding properties when PDS is used together with a knot pusher. Running sutures are secured with an intracorporeal knot or an absorbable suture clip.

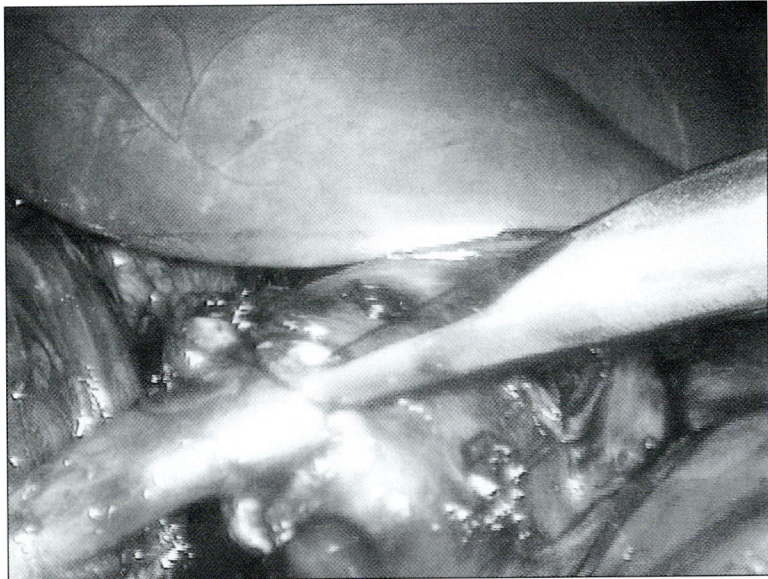

▶ FIGURE 16-17. (*see* Color Plate) Knot pusher. Knot-tying is the most difficult part of laparoscopic suturing. A knot pusher is very helpful in performing this task. The knots are tied extracorporeally, as in open

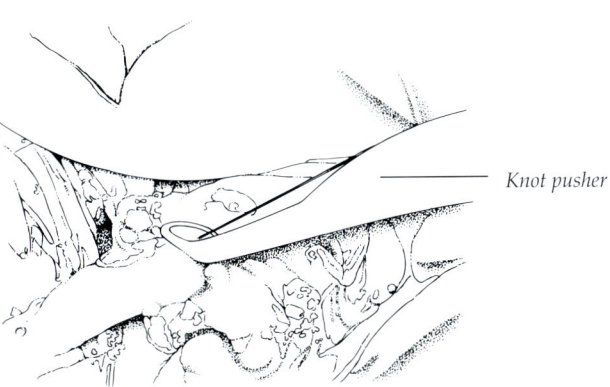

surgery; the knot pusher takes over the role of the surgeon's finger and helps to deliver the knot and lock it in place.

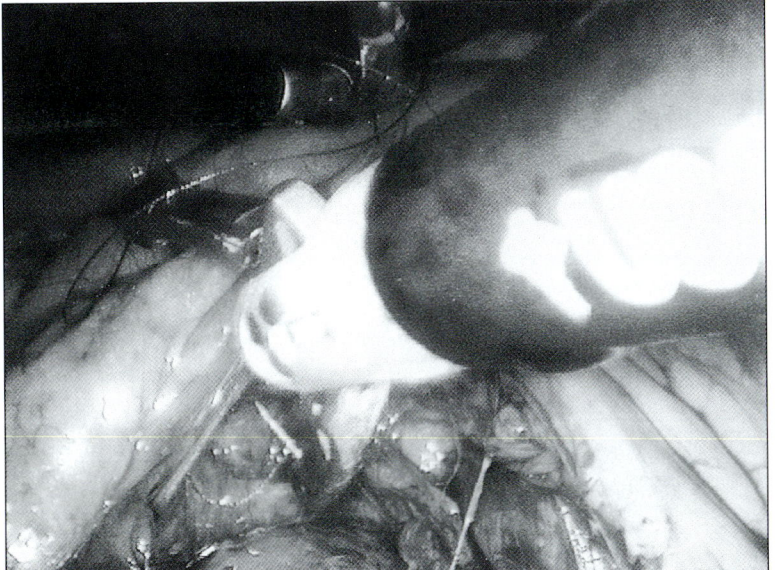

▶ FIGURE 16-18. (*see* Color Plate) Use of a laparoscopic suturing device. The Endostitch (United States Surgical Corp., Norwalk, CT) greatly facilitates laparoscopic suturing. We feel that suture placement is

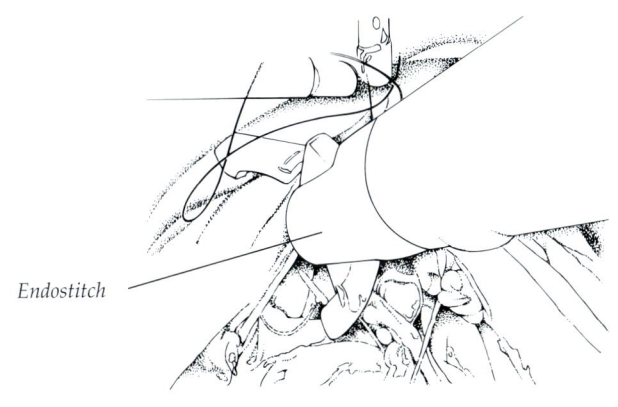

far less accurate than with a curved needle, however, because the needle is short and straight, and the suture is not threaded at the end of the needle but in the middle of the needle.

Postoperative Management

First oral intake	24 h
Ambulation	24 h
Drainage	2 d
Indwelling catheter	4 d
Postoperative hospitalization	4–5 d
Ureteral stent	4–6 wk

▶ FIGURE 16-19. Postoperative management. First, an antibiotic is given. The patient is started on a clear liquid diet 24 hours after surgery, which is advanced as tolerated. Ambulation is resumed on the first postoperative day. The drain is usually removed on the second postoperative day. The transurethral catheter is left in place 4 days to avoid reflux resulting from the ureteral stent. The postoperative hospital stay is 4 to 5 days. The ureteral stent is removed 4 to 6 weeks after surgery.

Survey of the Literature

Study	Patients, n	Approach, n/n		Pyeloplasty, n/n		Conversion rate, %	Success rate, %
		Transperitoneal	Retroperitoneal	Dismembered	Nondismembered		
Schuessler et al. [26]	5	5/5	0	5/5	0	0	80
Recker et al. [27]	5	5/5	0	4/4	0	20	100
Brooks et al. [24]	2	12/12	0	12/12	0	0	97
Moore et al. [3]	30	30/30	0	26/30	4/30	0	97
Puppo et al. [28]	11	0	11/11	6/6	0	45	100
Janetschek et al. [14]	11	10/11	1/11	8/11	3/11	0	100
Janetschek et al. [29]	19	18/19	1/19	0	19/19	45	100

▶ **FIGURE 16-20.** Success and conversion rates. A survey of the literature allows several interesting observations. Less than 100 procedures have been documented. Most of them were performed transperitoneally by means of dismembered pyeloplasty. The conversion rate is low, and the success rate is very good, comparable with that of the gold standard of open surgery.

REFERENCES

1. Brown T, Mandell J, Lebowitz RL: Neonatal hydronephrosis in the era of ultrasonography. *AJR Am J Roentgenol* 1987, 148:959–963.

2. Lowe FC, Marshall FF: Ureteropelvic junction obstruction in adults. *Urology* 1984, 23:331–335.

3. Moore RG, Averch TD, Schulam PG, *et al.*: Laparoscopic pyeloplasty: experience with the initial 30 cases. *J Urol* 1997, 157:459–462.

4. Hoffer FA, Lebowitz RL: Intermittent hydronephrosis: a unique feature of ureteropelvic junction obstruction caused by a crossing renal vessel. *Radiology* 1985, 156:655–658.

5. Balfour J, Metcalfe J, Campbell J, *et al.*: Results of treatment of hydronephrosis. *J Urol* 1964, 92:188–191.

6. Keeley FX, Bagley DH, Kulp-Hugues D, Gomella LG: Laparoscopic division of crossing vessels at the ureteropelvic junction. *J Endourol* 1996, 10:163–168.

7. Henline RB, Hawes CJ: Uretero-pelvic obstructions: symptoms and treatment: report of 62 operations. *JAMA* 1948, 137:777–786.

8. Smith AD: Should open pyeloplasty be abandoned? [editorial] *J Urol* 1997, 157:467–468.

9. Meretyk L, Meretyk S, Clayman RV: Endopyelotomy: comparison of ureteroscopic retrograde and antegrade percutaneous techniques. *J Urol* 1992, 148:775–783.

10. Cassis A, Brannen GE, Bush WH, *et al.*: Endopyelotomy: review of results and complications. *J Urol* 1991, 146:1492–1495.

11. Malden ES, Picus D, Clayman RV: Arteriovenous fistula complicating endopyelotomy. *J Urol* 1992, 148:1520–1523.

12. Streem SB, Geisinger MA: Prevention and management of hemorrhage associated with cautery wire balloon incision of ureteropelvic junction obstruction. *J Urol* 1995, 153:1904–1906.

13. Van Cangh PJ, Wilmart JF, Opsomer RJ, *et al.*: Long-term results and late recurrence after endoureteropyelotomy: a critical analysis of prognostic factors. *J Urol* 1994, 151:934–937.

14. Janetschek G, Peschel R, Altarac S, Bartsch G: Laparoscopic and retroperitoneoscopic repair of ureteropelvic junction obstruction. *Urology* 1996, 47:311–316.

15. Frauscher F, Janetschek G, Helweg G, *et al.*: Crossing vessels at the ureteropelvic junction: detection with contrast-enhanced color doppler US. *Radiology* 1999, 210: 727–731.

16. Potempa DM, Janetschek G, Rassweiler J: Retroperitoneoscopy. In *Laparoscopic Surgery in Urology.* Edited by Janetschek G, Rassweiler J, Griffith DP. New York: Thieme-Verlag; 1996:212–230.

17. Chen RN, Moore RG, Kavoussi LR: Laparoscopic pyeloplasty. *J Endourol* 1996, 10:159–161.

18. Anderson JC, Hynes W: Retrocaval ureter; case diagnosed preoperatively and treated successfully by a plastic operation. *Br J Urol* 1949, 21:209–214.

19. Hensle TW: The correction of ureteropelvic junction obstruction. In *Operative Urology.* Edited by Marshall FF. Philadelphia: WB Saunders Co; 1991:469–476.

20. DeWeerd JH: Ureteropelvioplasty. In *Urologic Surgery,* edn 3. Edited by Glenn JF. Philadelphia: JB Lippincott; 1983:227–252.

21. Davis DM: Intubated ureterostomy: a new operation for ureteral and ureteropelvic stricture. *Surg Gynecol Obstet* 1943, 76:513–523.

22. Motola JA, Badlani GH, Smith AD: Results of 212 consecutive endopyelotomies: an 8-year followup. *J Urol* 1993, 152:453–456.

23. Fenger C: Konservative Operation f¸r renale Retention infolge von Strikturen oder Klappenbildung am Ureter. *Langenbecks Arch Chir* 1900, 52:528–535.

24. Brooks JD, Kavoussi LR, Preminger GM, Schuessler WW: Comparison of open and endourologic approaches to the obstructed ureteropelvic junction. *Urology* 1995, 46:791–795.

25. Kumon H, Tsugawa M, Hashimoto H, *et al.*: Impact of 3-dimensional helical computerized tomography on selection of operative methods for ureteropelvic junction obstruction. *J Urol* 1997, 158:1696–1700.

26. Schuessler WW, Grune MT, Tecuanhuey LF, Preminger GM: Laparoscopic dismembered pyeloplasty. *J Urol* 1993, 150:1795–1799.

27. Recker F, Subotic B, Goepel M, Tscholl R: Laparoscopic dismembered pyeloplasty: preliminary report. *J Urol* 1995, 153:1601–1604.

28. Puppo P, Perachino M, Ricciotti G, *et al.*: Retroperitoneoscopic treatment of ureteropelvic junction obstruction. *Eur Urol* 1997, 31:204–208.

29. Peschel R, Janetschek G, Bartsch G: Laparoscopic non-dismembered pyeloplasty [abstract VII–6]. *J Endourol* 1997, 11(suppl 1):S82.

Management of Perirenal Fluid Collections

Paolo Puppo
Massimo Perachino

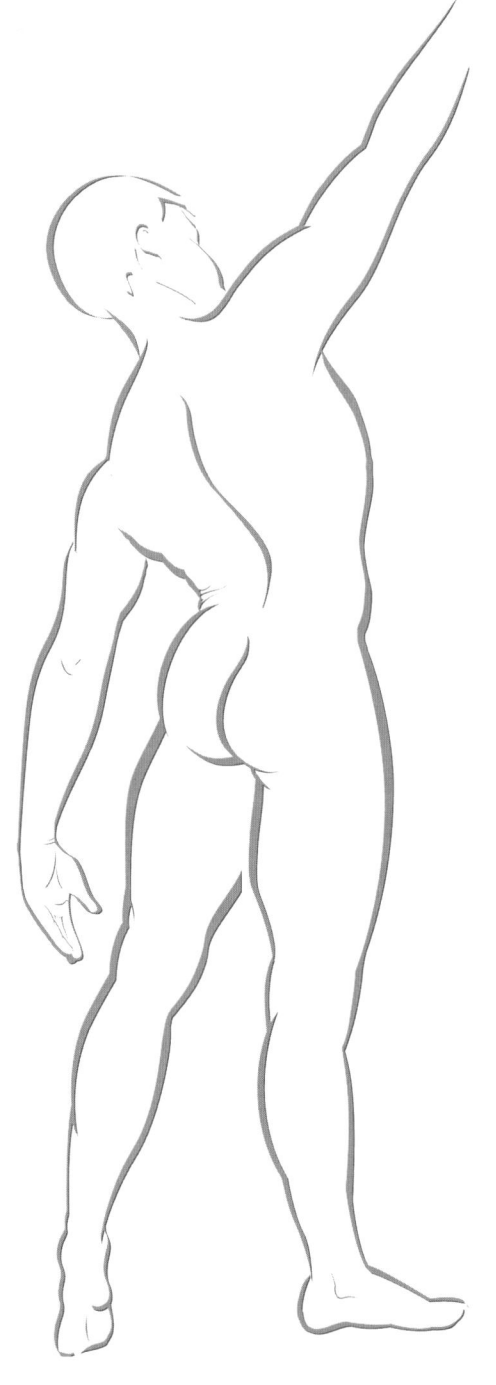

The perirenal space may be involved with diseases that arise within or outside it. Extraperitoneal fluid collections consist of blood, pus, urine, lymph, or pancreatic fluid [1–3]. Except for acute or subacute hemorrhage, these different collections of fluid are indistinguishable on computed tomography (CT) scans or with ultrasound. The presence of extraluminal gas usually indicates an abscess caused by gas-forming organisms or an enteric communication. Urinomas tend to be cystic, whereas hematomas may be solid, cystic, or a combination of both, depending on the stage of clot breakdown. Ultrasound offers an accurate, noninvasive, radiation-free means of following the presence and course of perinephric hematomas resulting from blunt trauma. Although sonography can show extraperitoneal fluid collections, it is much less effective than CT. Sonography is hampered by overlying bowel gas and, more important, cannot show fascial planes [4,5,6]. After intravenous injection of contrast medium, however, enhancement of adjacent organs may make it difficult to recognize the high attenuation of retroperitoneal blood [7]. Retroperitoneal hemorrhage can be detected and localized to any of the extraperitoneal compartments by using CT.

URINOMA

A perirenal urinoma results from renal or ureteral obstruction or from iatrogenic or accidental trauma associated with urine extravasation (*eg*, neoplasm, surgical ligation, or calculus disease). Extravasation of urine into the perirenal space is usually caused by a forniceal rupture [4–6,8,9]. The symptoms and signs of a urinoma may include vague abdominal or flank discomfort and sometimes a palpable mass. There may be a delay of several months between the causative event and presentation and diagnosis. CT scan is the optimal study to define the extent of the urinoma and its relationship to surrounding structures [4,5,7]. Percutaneous perirenal drainage associated with internal or external urine drainage is the management of choice; open surgery is rarely needed.

PERINEPHRIC ABSCESS

Perinephric abscesses are soft tissue or fluid masses that displace or deform the renal contour, sometimes with formation of gas bubbles [10–14]. The CT findings are those of chronic hydronephrosis. Stones may be present in the collecting system, which usually contains fluid of density greater than urine. Renal abscesses also may be present. Abdominal ultrasound serves as an excellent screening test and should be the first imaging study performed when a perinephric abscess is suspected [10]. CT scanning provides more detailed information about the size, content, and extent of the retroperitoneal process, making it the diagnostic procedure of choice [12,13].

Small perirenal abscesses may be treated with percutaneous drainage and antibiotic therapy [10,11]. The drainage catheter is removed when clinical improvement, decreased drainage, and significant shrinkage of the abscess cavity are noted. Surgical management is required for large and multiloculated abscesses; for those with thick, purulent material; for recurrent abscesses; and for patients with a nonfunctioning kidney in whom nephrectomy has to be performed. Moreover, surgical correction of any obstructive processes must be considered to alleviate underlying causes of abscess.

With a fluid collection, drainage is the first treatment of choice. Under ultrasound or CT guidance, a percutaneous drain is placed in the most dependent aspect of the fluid collection [15–17]. The aspirated fluid is sent for the following tests: creatinine determination, blood cell count, culture and sensitivity testing, and, when indicated, amylase evaluation. The creatinine content of a urinoma should be high, similar to that of the urine. If there is no longer a communication with the collecting system and no ongoing obstruction, drainage usually ceases after 48 to 72 hours. In prolonged drainage, placement of an indwelling ureteral stent and urethral catheter or a percutaneous nephrostomy generally provides diversion sufficient for spontaneous closure of the fistulous tract [14]. An open surgical approach is warranted for débridement and closure of the fistulous tract when there is devitalized tissue [14,18,19]. When the drainage has ceased, if there is still a large cavity with no demonstrable communication with the collecting system, then ethanol sclerotherapy or repeat electrocoagulation can be used to facilitate collapse of the cavity [14].

HEMATOMA

Hematoma formation in the perirenal space may be due to either traumatic or spontaneous causes, usually with the kidney as the source organ. The most common traumatic causes include motor vehicle accidents and iatrogenic mechanisms, such as percutaneous renal surgery, renal biopsy, or extracorporeal shock wave lithotripsy (ESWL) [20–29].

•• HEMATOMA DUE TO RENAL TRAUMA ••

The mechanism of injury to the kidney is classified as blunt or penetrating. Blunt trauma is more common, accounting for 80% to 90% of injuries. It results from automobile accidents, falls, contact sports, assaults, and personal violence. Gunshot and stab wounds cause up to 20% of renal injuries and represent the most common causes of penetrating injury [29].

Accurate radiographic staging, preferably with CT scanning, is essential to planning treatment because it differentiates lacerations and contusions and allows precise classification of the laceration according to the criteria of the American Association for Surgery of Trauma [26]. Nonoperative treatment of penetrating renal lacerations seems to be appropriate in hemodynamically stable patients without associated injuries. Grade 2 injuries can be treated nonoperatively, but grade 3 and 4 injuries are associated with a significant risk of delayed bleeding if treated expectantly. Exploration should be considered if laparotomy is required for other injuries [29].

The simple drainage of a hematoma should never indicate an early surgical approach because most hematomas will undergo spontaneous reabsorption. Delayed surgery should always be advised in hemodynamically stable patients without concomitant abdominal injuries.

SPONTANEOUS HEMORRHAGE

There are several spontaneous causes of perirenal hemorrhage. Malignant renal lesions, mostly adenocarcinomas, have been reported in association with spontaneous retroperitoneal hemorrhage. Although fewer than 1% of patients with renal carcinoma present with retroperitoneal bleeding [20–23], it is the most common cause of spontaneous retroperitoneal hemorrhage because of its overall relative incidence. Other renal diseases associated with spontaneous retroperitoneal hemorrhage include pyelonephritis with or without renal or perirenal abscess, other renal inflammatory disorders, and renal vascular disease [25–27,30–33].

The adrenal gland is also a source of spontaneous retroperitoneal hemorrhage. In most cases, clinically significant hemorrhage from an adrenal source occurs in the setting of severe stress (eg, pregnancy, trauma, sepsis, or burns). Massive bleeding has also been reported in association with adrenal tumors, including pheochromocytoma and adrenal carcinoma; other rare causes of spontaneous retroperitoneal hemorrhage include diseases of the pancreas and primary or metastatic retroperitoneal tumors [25].

Currently, based on clinical findings and the use of modern imaging modalities, a diagnosis of spontaneous retroperitoneal hemorrhage can be made and the underlying cause determined before surgical exploration in most cases [27]. Management of patients with spontaneous retroperitoneal hemorrhage depends on a high index of suspicion, an awareness of etiologic factors, an aggressive and systematic diagnostic approach, and the specific cause. Patients with spontaneous retroperitoneal hemorrhage in the setting of a systemic coagulopathy or systemic vasculitis should be managed conservatively because an obvious bleeding source is almost never found at the time of exploration [26]. If the CT scan reveals a renal tumor, the possibility of angiomyolipoma must be considered. When a diagnosis of angiomyolipoma is made, especially in the setting of tuberous sclerosis (with its high frequency of bilateral involvement), a renal-sparing approach, usually in the form of a partial nephrectomy, may prove optimal [21]. If a solid malignant tumor is identified, treatment is chosen accordingly.

NORMAL ANATOMY

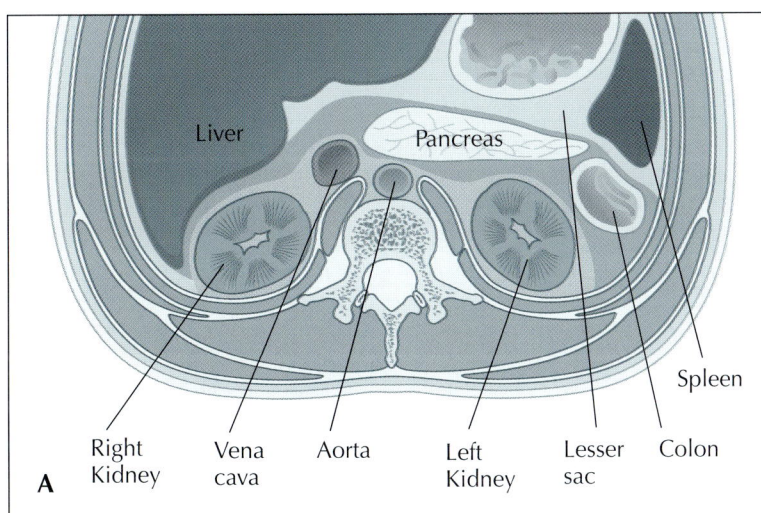

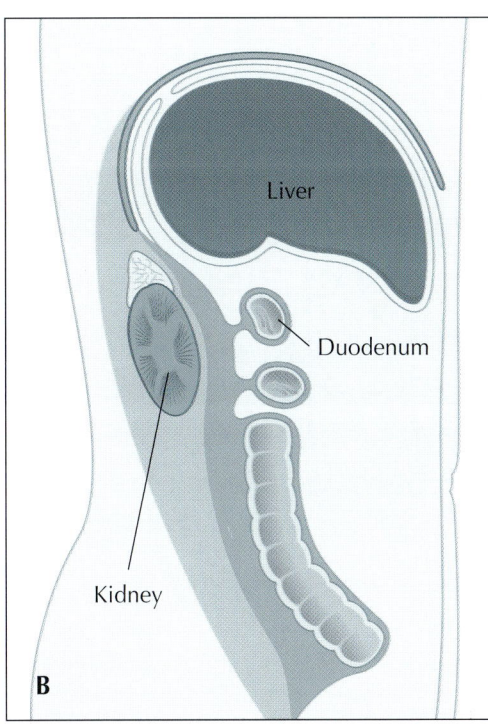

FIGURE 17-1. Normal anatomy of the perirenal space. Each of the perirenal spaces is an inverted cone of tissue that lies lateral to the lumbar spine and is limited by the anterior renal fascia, also known as Gerota's fascia or the fascia of Toldt, and the posterior renal fascia (Zuckerkandl's fascia). These are dense, elastic connective tissue sheaths that are generally less than 2 mm thick. The perirenal space contains the kidney, adrenal glands, renal vessels and collecting system, and a variable amount of fat.

The anterior perirenal space, lying between the posterior parietal peritoneum anteriorly and the anterior renal and lateroconal fascia posteriorly, contains most of the pancreas and the retroperitoneal portions of the duodenum, ascending colon, and descending colon. Little fat is present in this compartment. The posterior perirenal space, situated between the poste-

rior renal fascia and the lateroconal fascia anteriorly and the transversalis fascia posteriorly, contains a moderate amount of fat and is most notable for its absence of contained organs [1,2]. **A,** Axial view. **B,** Sagittal view.

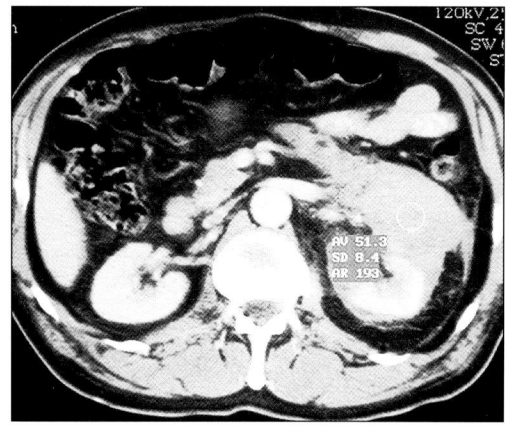

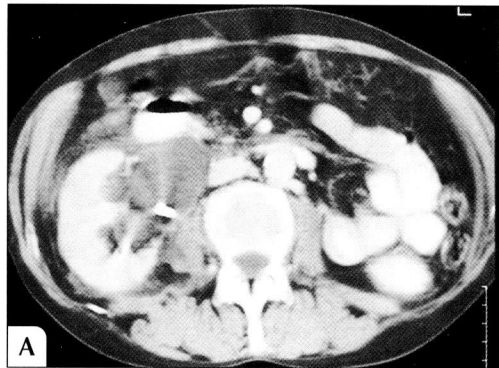

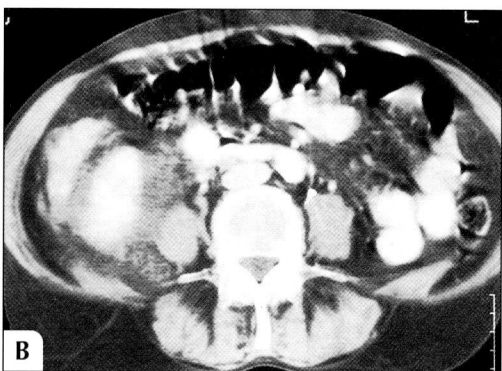

▶ **FIGURE 17-2.** CT scanning with extraperitoneal fluid collection. Extraperitoneal fluid collections may consist of blood, pus, urine, lymph, or pancreatic fluid. Except for acute or subacute hemorrhage, these collections are indistinguishable on CT scans. The presence of extraluminal gas usually indicates an abscess caused by gas-forming organisms or an enteric communication. Retroperitoneal hemorrhage can be detected and localized to any of the extraperitoneal compartments by using CT, as in this figure. Normal CT anatomy is visible on the right side and a large hematoma on the left. The densitometry of the fluid suggests its nature [3].

▶ **FIGURE 17-3.** **A** and **B,** Urinoma. As stated previously, perirenal urinoma results from renal or ureteral obstruction or from iatrogenic or accidental trauma associated with urine extravasation (*eg,* neoplasm, surgical ligation, calculus disease). Extravasation of urine into the perirenal space is usually caused by a forniceal rupture.

Three mechanisms associated with urinoma formation are a forniceal or a transcapsular tear of the renal parenchyma that extends to the calyx or pelvis, failure of the injury to heal or seal off before significant amounts of urine leak out, and concomitant ureteral obstruction. Inflammation and fibrosis at the site of leakage can lead to ureteral obstruction, progressive hydronephrosis, and ultimately loss of renal function. Sometimes, urinomas may extend into the mediastinum and pleural space [20].

Symptoms and signs of a urinoma may include vague abdominal or flank discomfort and sometimes a palpable mass. There may be a delay of several months between the causative event and presentation and diagnosis. In a left-sided collection, the most important entity in the differential diagnosis is a pancreatic pseudocyst [4].

CT scanning is the optimal study to define the extent of the urinoma and its relationship to surrounding structures. The wall of the urinoma may be thickened and smooth; the density of the urinoma is -10 to +30 Hounsfield units [4]. Homogeneous enhancement of the urinoma implies a functioning kidney and the presence of a communication between the urinoma and the collecting system.

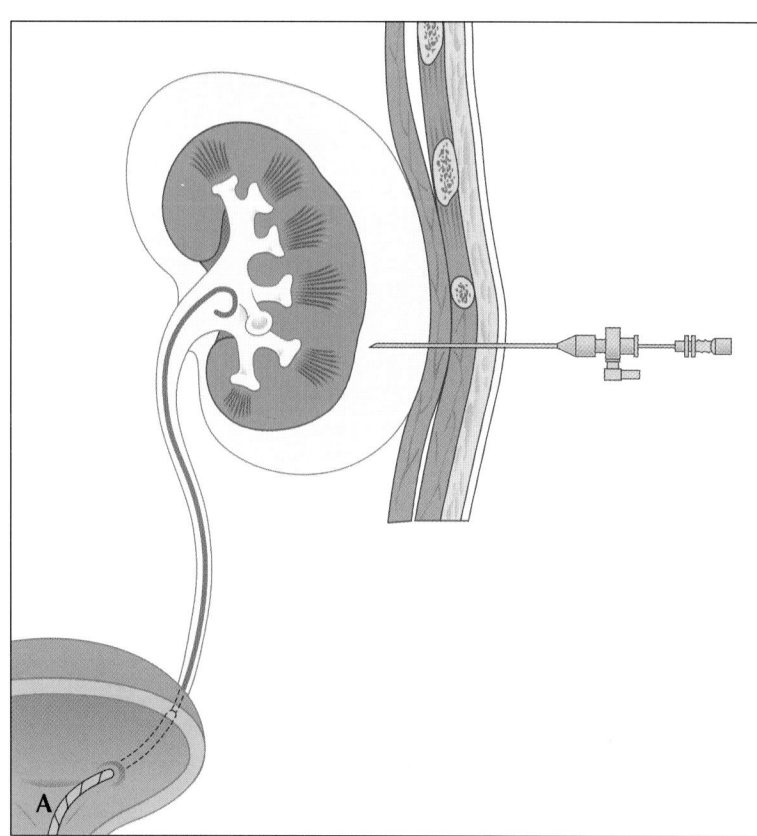

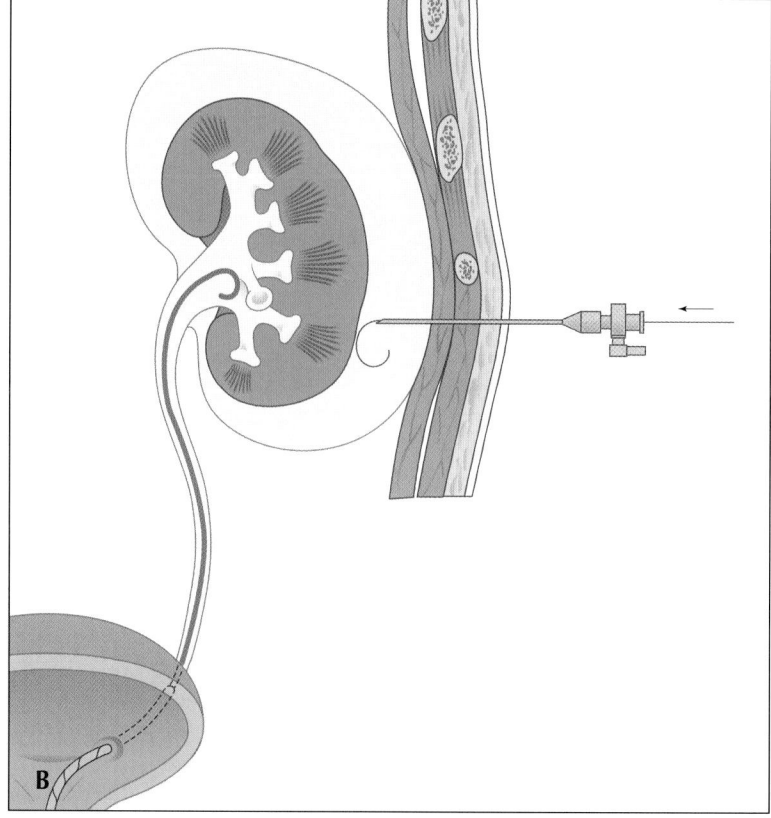

▶ **FIGURE 17-4.** Percutaneous drainage of a fluid collection in the retroperitoneum. Under ultrasound or CT guidance, a 10- to 14-F urinary drainage catheter (**A**) [10,11,15–19] and a 7-F ureteral pigtail catheter (**B**) or a percutaneous nephrostomy tube are placed.

(Continued on next page)

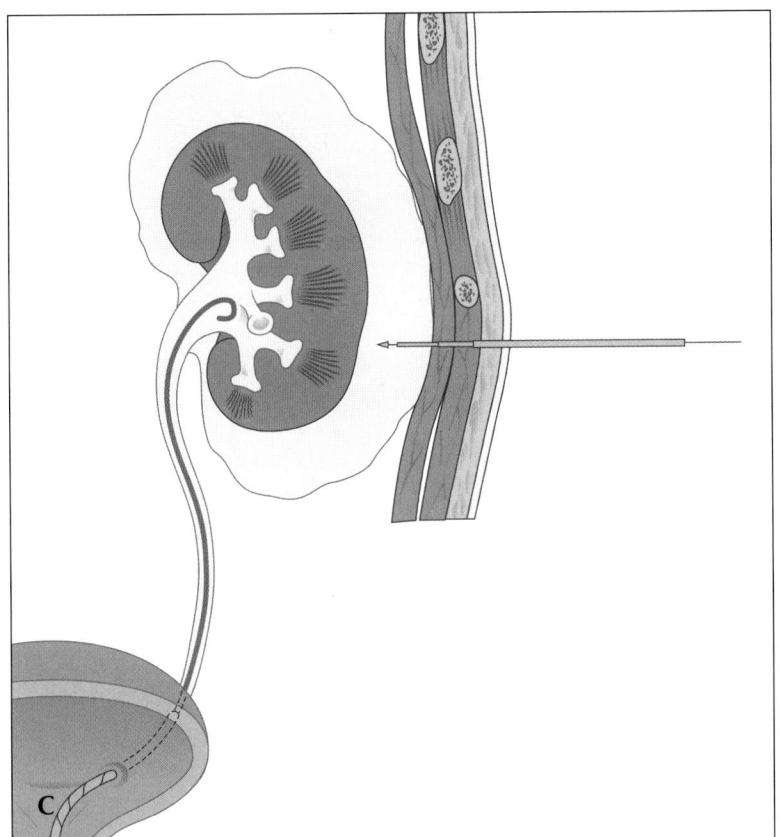

FIGURE 17-4. (*Continued*) A coaxial dilation system (**C**) allows the physician to insert a 14-F nephrostomy tube through a 16-F sheath. The perirenal tube is left in place until radiographic studies show the sponta-neous closure of the fistulous tract. A JJ stent is generally left in place for some weeks to prevent relapse of leakage (**D**).

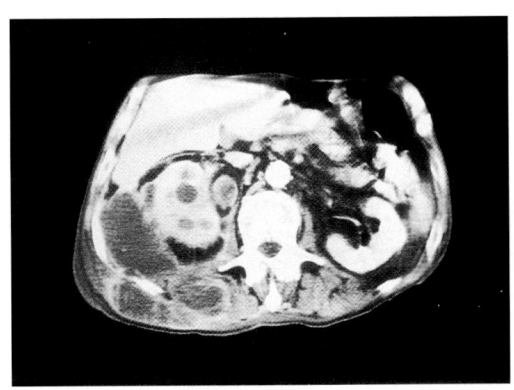

FIGURE 17-5. Diagnosis of perinephric abscess. CT scanning provides more detailed informa-tion about the size, content, and extent of the retroperitoneal process, making it the diagnostic procedure of choice in the evaluation of retroperitoneal abscess [12]. Typical findings include the demonstration of air–fluid levels within the mass and the frequent extension of the process along fascial planes, which may even reach the pelvis. The accuracy of CT scanning has been as high as 96% [13].

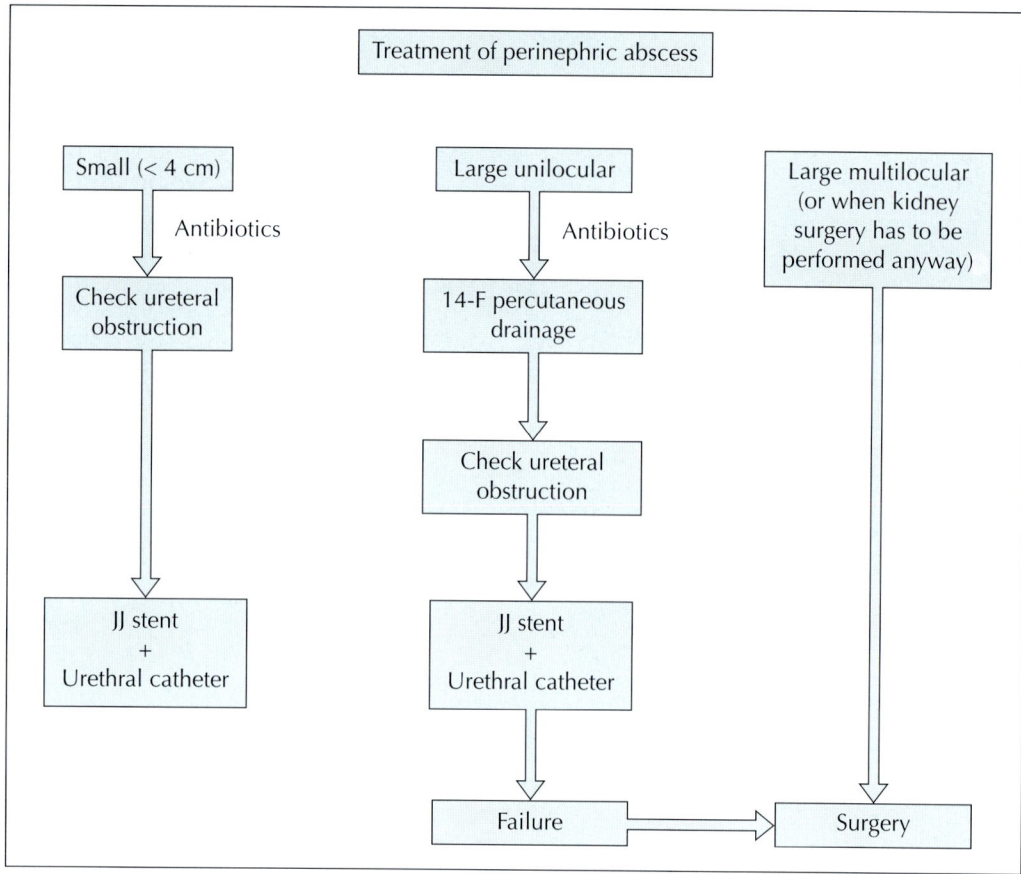

Treatment of perinephric abscess

FIGURE 17-6. Treatment of perinephric abscess. Small retroperitoneal abscesses may be treated with percutaneous drainage and antibiotic therapy [10,11,18]. The basic principles of percutaneous drainage of retroperitoneal abscesses are the evaluation of the extent of the abscess by CT scanning; identification of a safe, extraperitoneal, percutaneous window; diagnostic aspiration; and placement of an indwelling catheter for drainage of the abscess cavity. Multilocular abscesses may also be treated by using multiple drainage catheters [14]. The drainage catheter is removed when clinical improvement, decreased drainage, and significant shrinkage of the abscess cavity are noted.

Surgical management is required for large or multiloculated abscesses; for those with thick, purulent material; for recurrent abscesses; and for patients with a nonfunctioning kidney in whom nephrectomy has to be performed. Moreover, surgical correction of any obstructive processes must be considered to alleviate an underlying cause of abscess [19].

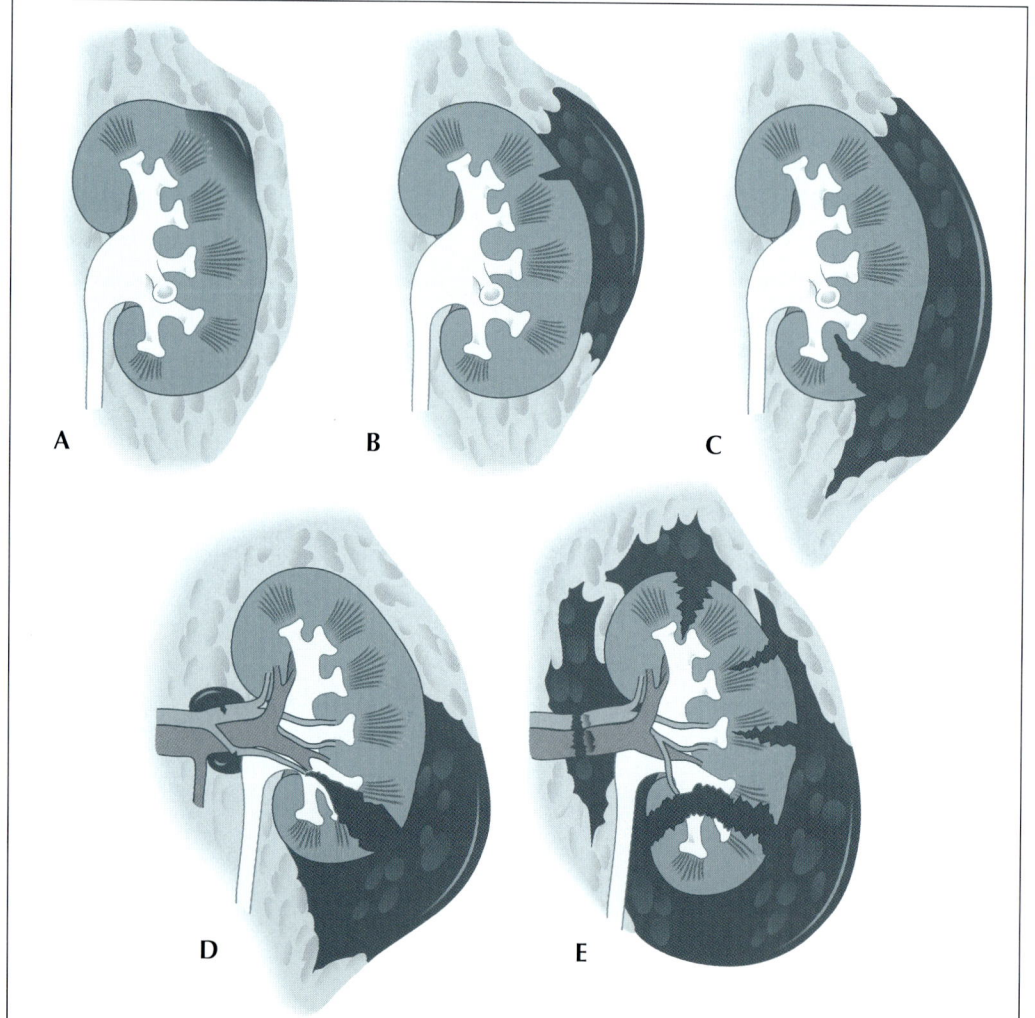

FIGURE 17-7. Classification of renal injuries. Renal injuries can be classified according to the American Association for Surgery of Trauma [28] into five large groups. **A,** Renal contusions, which are subcapsular hematomas associated with an intact renal capsule and collecting system. **B,** Minor lacerations, which are superficial cortical disruptions less than 1 cm in depth that do not involve the deep renal medulla or collecting system. **C,** Parenchymal lacerations greater than 1 cm in depth without collecting system rupture or urinary extravasation. **D,** Parenchymal laceration extending through the renal cortex, medulla, and collecting system or main renal artery or vein injury with contained hemorrhage. **E,** Completely shattered kidney or avulsion of main renal artery or vein that devascularizes the kidney.

Gross or microscopic hematuria is usually present [29]. These patients often have abdominal tenderness, bony fractures, and flank contusions. A palpable abdominal mass with associated shock may be indicative of a rapidly developing retroperitoneal hematoma from a major renal parenchymal or renal vascular injury.

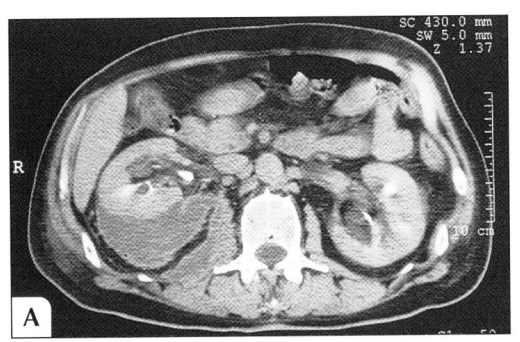

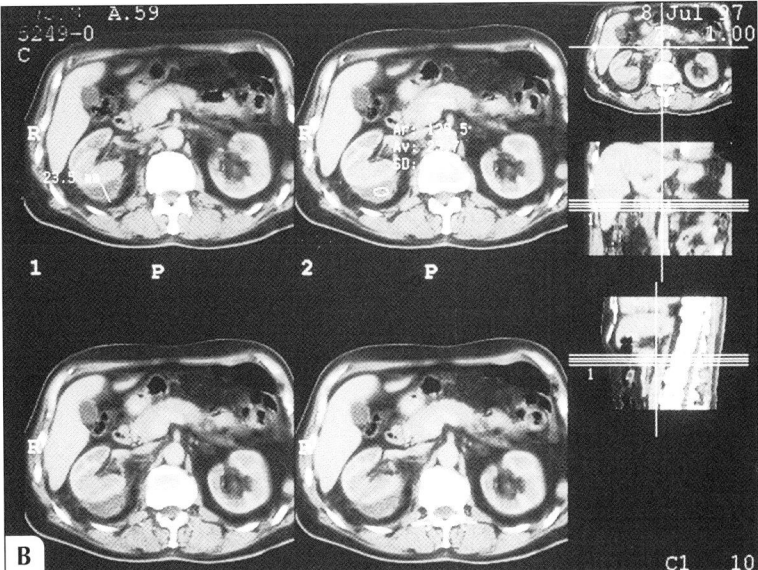

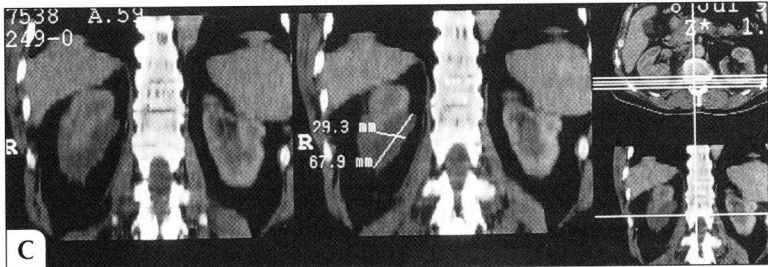

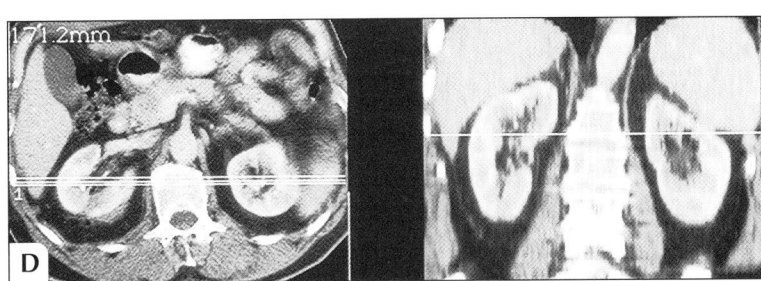

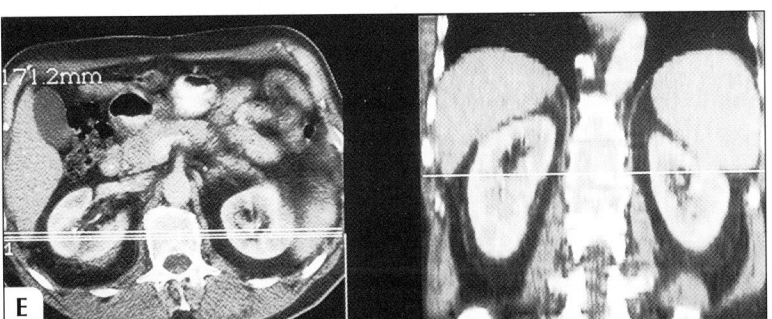

▶ **FIGURE 17-8.** Conservative treatment of posttraumatic hematoma. In hemodynamically stable patients, grade 1, 2, or 3 lesions should be treated conservatively. Early surgery could result in an unnecessary nephrectomy. Conversely, closed hematomas almost always undergo complete reabsorption without complications. This figure shows a large hematoma after a conservatively treated grade 3 renal trauma. **A,** The CT scan from the emergency department. **B** and **C,** CT spiral imaging one month later. **D** and **E,** CT spiral imaging 6 months later. Panel **E,** An excellent CT representation of the normal perirenal space.

REFERENCES

1. Meyers MA: *Dynamic Radiology of the Abdomen: Normal and Pathologic Anatomy*, edn 4. New York: Springer-Verlag; 1994.

2. Korobkin M, Silverman PM, Quint LE, Francis IR: CT of the extraperitoneal space: normal anatomy and fluid collections. *AJR Am J Roentgenol* 1992, 159:933–941.

3. Molmenti EP, Balfe DM, Kanterman RY, Bennett HF: Anatomy of the retroperitoneum: observations of the distribution of pathologic fluid collections. *Radiology* 1996, 200:95–103.

4. Healy ME, Teng SS, Moss AA: Uriniferous pseudocyst: computed tomographic findings. *Radiology* 1984, 153:757–762.

5. Meyers MA: Uriniferous perirenal pseudocyst: new observations. *Radiology* 1975, 117:539–545.

6. Tien R, Shirkhoda A, David R: Circumferential perirenal urinoma mimicking nephromegaly on urography. *Urol Radiol* 1989, 11:92–96.

7. Bosniak MA: Spontaneous subcapsular and perirenal hematomas [editorial]. *Radiology* 1989, 172:601–602.

8. Zagoria RJ, Dyer RB, Assimos DG, *et al.*: Spontaneous perinephric hemorrhage: imaging and management. *J Urol* 1991, 165:468–471.

9. Baron RL, Stark DD, McClennan BL, *et al.*: Intrathoracic extension of retroperitoneal urine collections. *AJR Am J Roentgenol* 1981, 137:37–41.

10. Gerzof SG, Robbins AH, Birkett DM, *et al.*: Percutaneous catheter drainage of abdominal abscesses guided by ultrasound and computed tomography. *AJR Am J Roentgenol* 1979, 133:1–5.

11. Gerzof SG, Robbins AH, Johnson WC, *et al.*: Percutaneous catheter drainage of abdominal abscesses: a five-year experience. *N Engl J Med* 1981, 305:353–357.

12. Hoddick W, Jeffrey RB, Goldberg HI, *et al.*: CT and sonography of severe renal and perirenal infections. *AJR Am J Roentgenol* 1983, 140:517–522.

13. Mendez G, Isoroff MB, Morillo G: The role of computer tomography in the diagnosis of renal and perirenal abscesses. *J Urol* 1979, 122:582–587.

14. van Waes PFGH, Feldberg MA, Mali WP, *et al.*: Management of loculated abscesses that are difficult to drain: a new approach. *Radiology* 1983, 147:57–60.

15. Ball WS, Towbin R, Strife JL, *et al.*: Interventional genitourinary radiology in children: a review of 61 procedures. *AJR Am J Roentgenol* 1986, 147:791–795.

16. Hulbert JC, Hunter D, Young AT, *et al.*: Percutaneous intrarenal marsupialization of a perirenal cystic collection: endocystolysis. *J Urol* 1988, 139:1039–1040.

17. Morano JU, Burkhalter JL: Percutaneous catheter drainage of post-traumatic urinoma. *J Urol* 1985, 134:319–320.

18. Brolin RE, Nosher JL, Leiman S, *et al.*: Percutaneous catheter versus open surgical drainage in the treatment of abdominal abscesses. *Am Surg* 1984, 50:102–106.

19. Porena M, Valli PP, Petroni P, *et al.*: Echo-guided drainage of pararenal and pelvic fluid accumulations: technique, indications, and results. *Arch Ital Urol Nefrol Androl* 1996, 68:5 (suppl), 19–26.

20. Polkey HJ, Vynalek WJ: Spontaneous non-traumatic perirenal and renal hematomas: experimental and clinical study. *Arch Surg* 1933, 26:196–218.

21. Gentry LR, Gould HR, Alter AJ, *et al.*: Hemorrhagic angiomyolipoma: demonstration by computed tomography. *J Comput Assist Tomogr* 1981, 5:861–865.

22. Belville JS, Morgenthaler A, Loughlin KR, *et al.*: Spontaneous perinephric and subcapsular renal hemorrhage: evaluation with CT, US, and angiography. *Radiology* 1989, 172:733–736.

23. Drago JR, York JP, Dagen JE, *et al.*: Spontaneous retroperitoneal hemorrhage secondary to a renal cause. *J Surg Oncol* 1986, 31:31–33.

24. Leib ES, Restivo C, Paulus HE: Immunosuppressive and corticosteroid therapy of polyarteritis nodosa. *Am J Med* 1979, 67:941–944.

25. Kindell AR, Senay BA, Coll ME: Spontaneous subcapsular renal hematoma: diagnosis and management. *J Urol* 1988, 139:246–249.

26. Milutinovich J, Follette WC, Scribner BH: Spontaneous retroperitoneal bleeding in patients on chronic chemodialysis. *Ann Intern Med* 1977, 86:189–190.

27. Pode D, Caine M: Spontaneous retroperitoneal hemorrhage. *J Urol* 1992, 147:311–313.

28. Moore EE, Cogbill TH, Malangoni MA, *et al.*: Organ injury scaling: spleen, liver, and kidney. *J Trauma* 1989, 29:1664–1677.

29. Wessels H, McAninch JW, Meyer A, Bruce J: Criteria for nonoperative treatment of significant penetrating renal lacerations. *J Urol* 1997, 157:24–27.

30. Rauschkolb EN, Sandler CM, Patel S, *et al.*: Computed tomography of renal inflammatory disease. *J Comput Assist Tomogr* 1982, 6:502–505.

31. Zaonta MR, Pahira JJ, Wolfman M, *et al.*: Acute focal bacterial nephritis: a systematic approach to diagnosis and treatment. *J Urol* 1985, 133:752–756.

32. Gold LP, McClennan BL, Rottenberg RL: CT appearance of acute inflammatory disease of the renal interstitium. *AJR Am J Roentgenol* 1983, 141:343–348.

33. Morehouse HT, Weiner SN, Hoffman JC: Imaging in inflammatory disease of the kidney. *AJR Am J Roentgenol* 1984, 143:135–141.

INDEX

COLOR PLATES

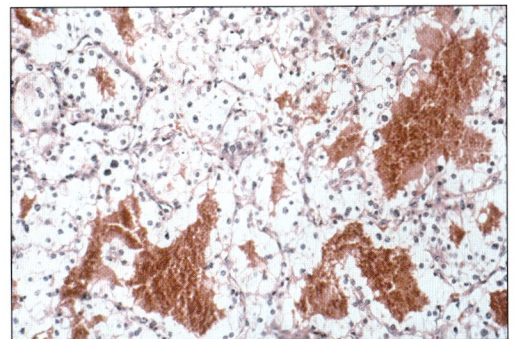

FIGURE 3-19A.

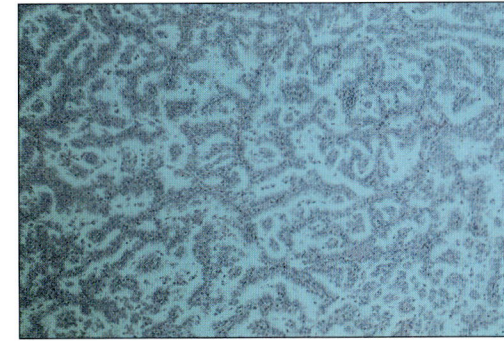

FIGURE 3-19B.

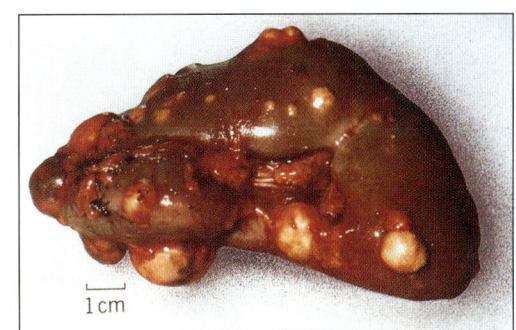

FIGURE 3-26.

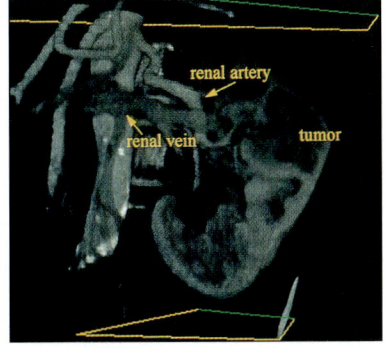

FIGURE 4-3.

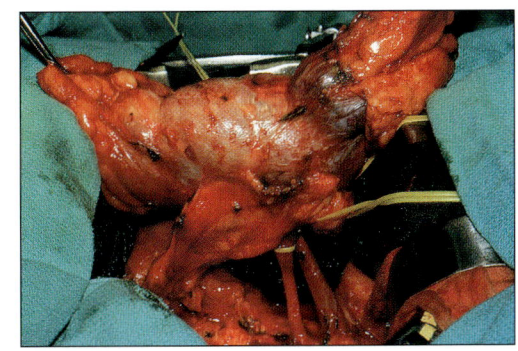

FIGURE 4-7.

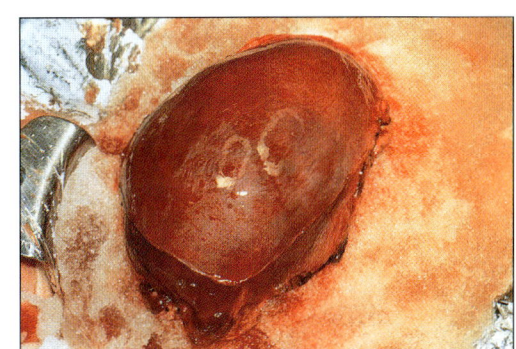

FIGURE 4-10A.

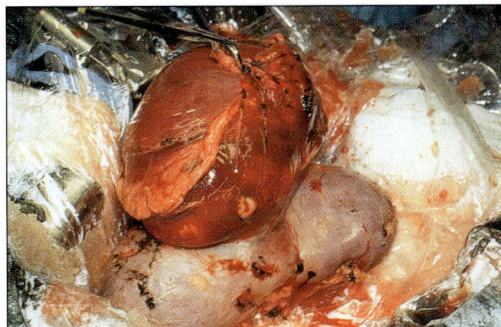

FIGURE 4-10B.

FIGURE 4-12.

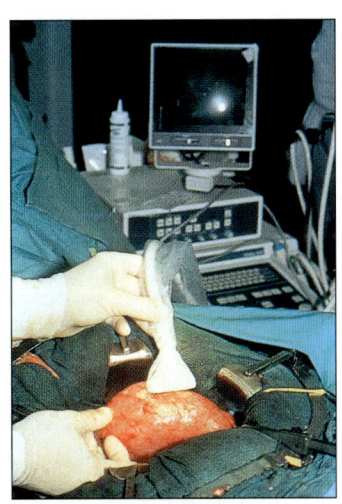
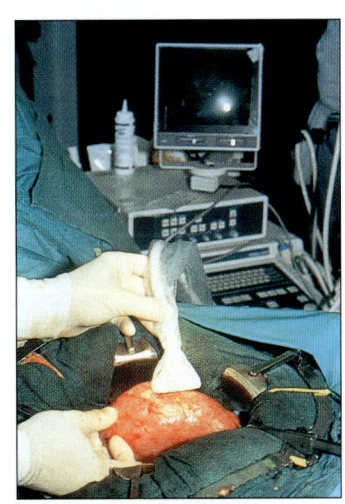

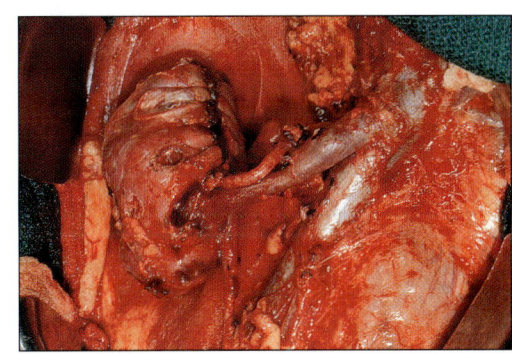

FIGURE 4-19.

FIGURE 5-21.

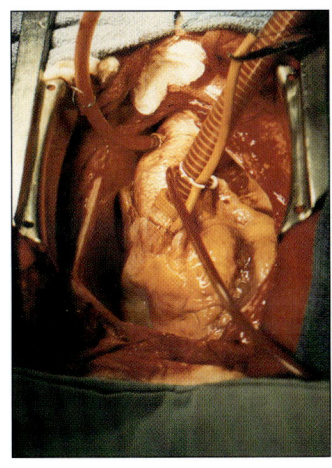

FIGURE 5-24.

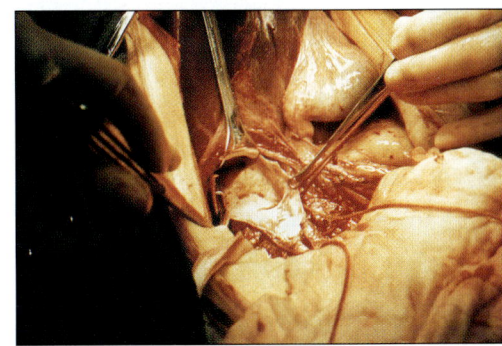

FIGURE 5-23.

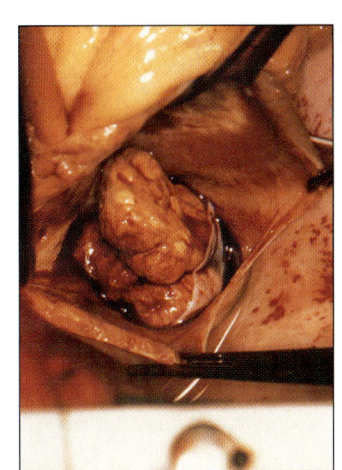

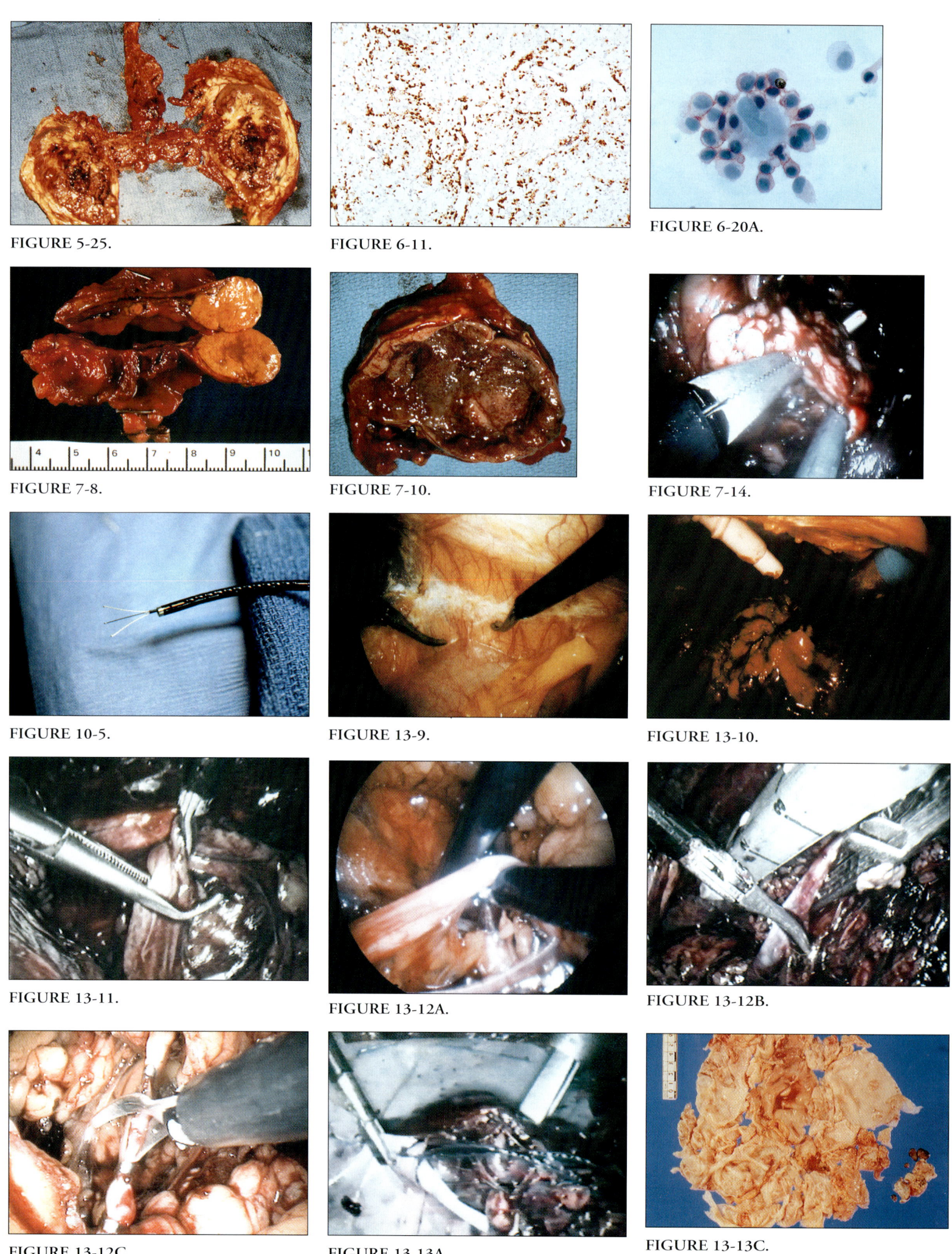

FIGURE 5-25.

FIGURE 6-11.

FIGURE 6-20A.

FIGURE 7-8.

FIGURE 7-10.

FIGURE 7-14.

FIGURE 10-5.

FIGURE 13-9.

FIGURE 13-10.

FIGURE 13-11.

FIGURE 13-12A.

FIGURE 13-12B.

FIGURE 13-12C.

FIGURE 13-13A.

FIGURE 13-13C.

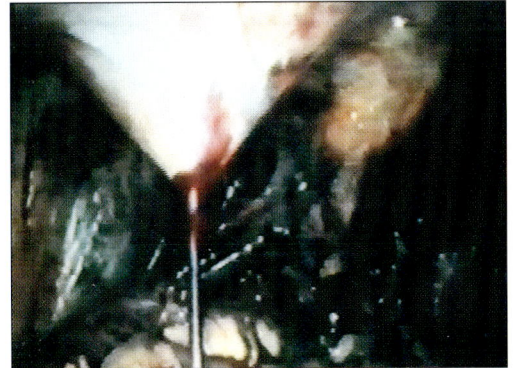

FIGURE 13-14.

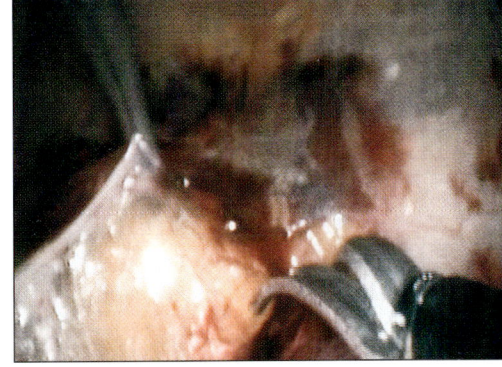

FIGURE 13-19A.

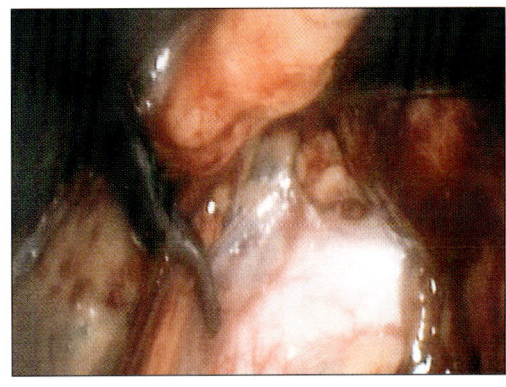

FIGURE 13-19B.

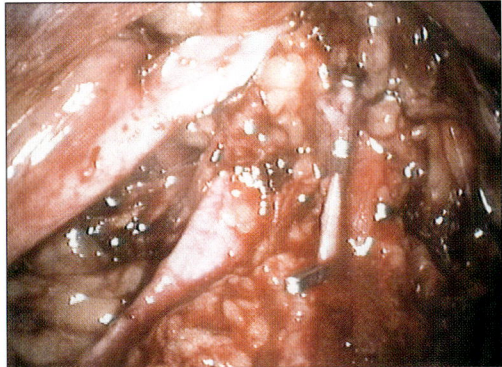

FIGURE 13-19C.

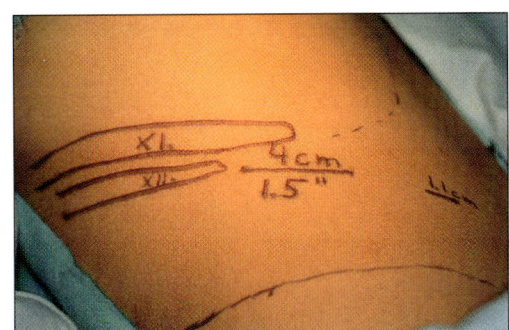

FIGURE 14-6.

FIGURE 14-8.

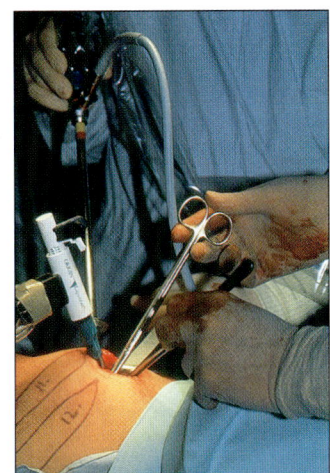

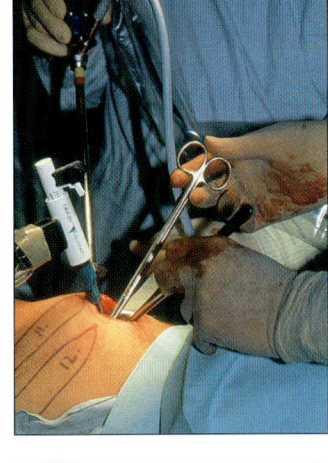

FIGURE 14-9.

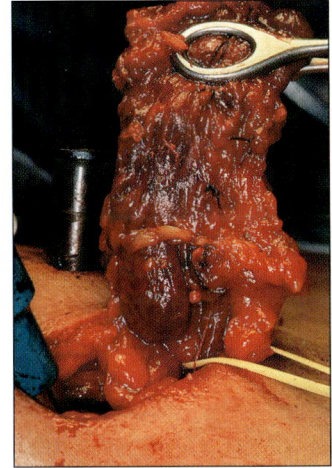

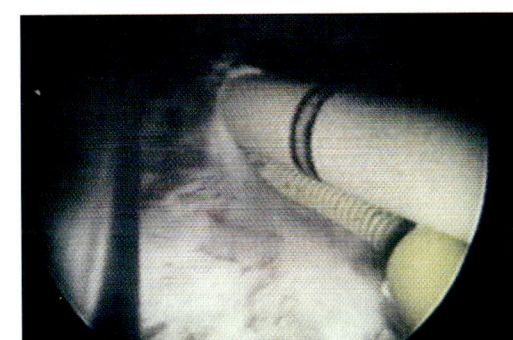

FIGURE 15-2A.

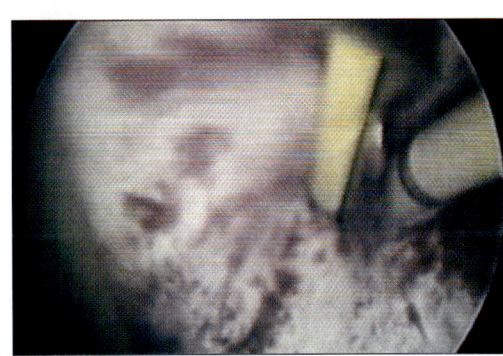

FIGURE 15-2B.

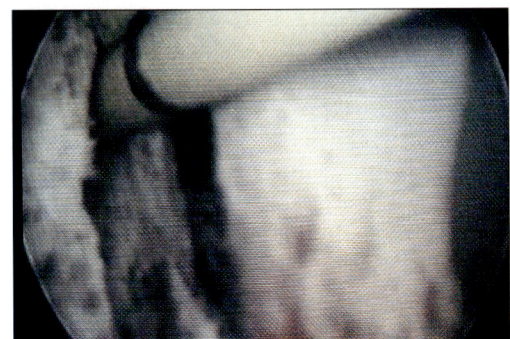

FIGURE 15-2C.

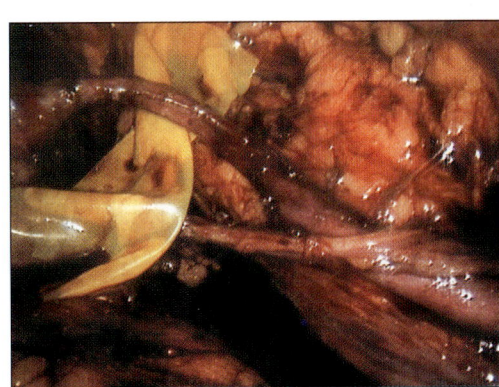

FIGURE 16-1.

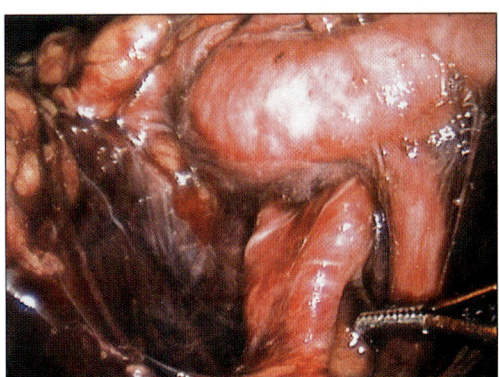

FIGURE 16-2.

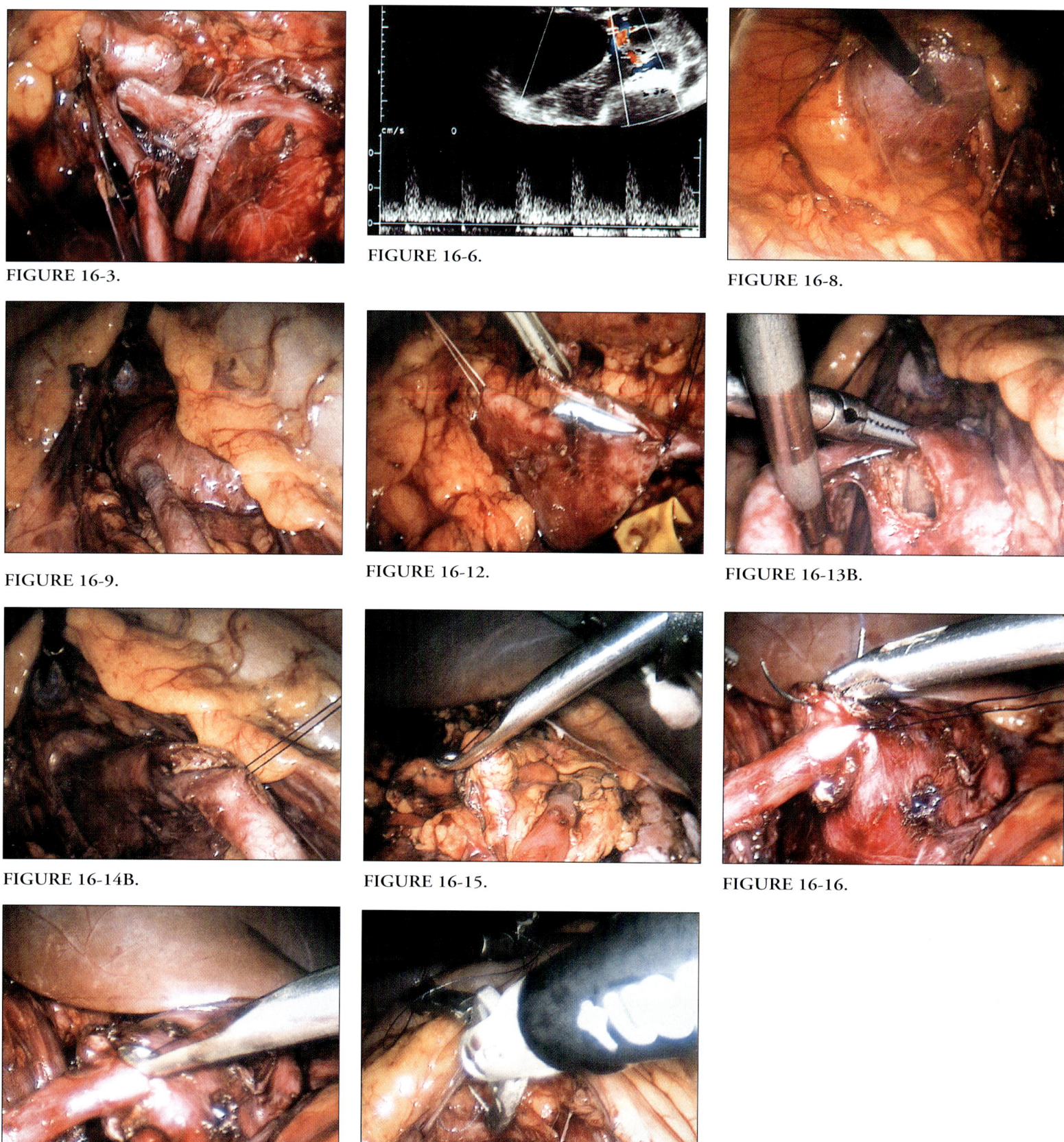

FIGURE 16-3.

FIGURE 16-6.

FIGURE 16-8.

FIGURE 16-9.

FIGURE 16-12.

FIGURE 16-13B.

FIGURE 16-14B.

FIGURE 16-15.

FIGURE 16-16.

FIGURE 16-17.

FIGURE 16-18.